The End of Medicine

Death by Doctor: Why and how doctors are
now paid to kill their patients

Vernon Coleman

Books by Vernon Coleman include:

Medical
The Medicine Men
Paper Doctors
Everything You Want To Know About Ageing
The Home Pharmacy
Aspirin or Ambulance
Face Values
Stress and Your Stomach
A Guide to Child Health
Guilt
The Good Medicine Guide
An A to Z of Women's Problems
Bodypower
Bodysense
Taking Care of Your Skin
Life without Tranquillisers
High Blood Pressure
Diabetes
Arthritis
Eczema and Dermatitis
The Story of Medicine
Natural Pain Control
Mindpower
Addicts and Addictions
Dr Vernon Coleman's Guide to Alternative Medicine
Stress Management Techniques
Overcoming Stress
The Health Scandal
The 20 Minute Health Check
Sex for Everyone
Mind over Body
Eat Green Lose Weight
Why Doctors Do More Harm Than Good
The Drugs Myth

Complete Guide to Sex
How to Conquer Backache
How to Conquer Pain
Betrayal of Trust
Know Your Drugs
Food for Thought
The Traditional Home Doctor
Relief from IBS
The Parent's Handbook
Men in Bras, Panties and Dresses
Power over Cancer
How to Conquer Arthritis
How to Stop Your Doctor Killing You
Superbody
Stomach Problems – Relief at Last
How to Overcome Guilt
How to Live Longer
Coleman's Laws
Millions of Alzheimer Patients Have Been Misdiagnosed
Climbing Trees at 112
Is Your Health Written in the Stars?
The Kick-Ass A–Z for over 60s
Briefs Encounter
The Benzos Story
Dementia Myth
What Doctors Won't Tell You About Chemotherapy
The End of Medicine

Psychology/Sociology
Stress Control
How to Overcome Toxic Stress
Know Yourself (1988)
Stress and Relaxation
People Watching
Spiritpower
Toxic Stress
I Hope Your Penis Shrivels Up
Oral Sex: Bad Taste and Hard To Swallow

Other People's Problems
The 100 Sexiest, Craziest, Most Outrageous Agony Column
Questions (and Answers) Of All Time
How to Relax and Overcome Stress
Too Sexy To Print
Psychiatry
Are You Living With a Psychopath?

Politics and General

England Our England
Rogue Nation
Confronting the Global Bully
Saving England
Why Everything Is Going To Get Worse Before It Gets Better
The Truth They Won't Tell You...About The EU
Living In a Fascist Country
How to Protect & Preserve Your Freedom, Identity & Privacy
Oil Apocalypse
Gordon is a Moron
The OFPIS File
What Happens Next?
Bloodless Revolution
2020
Stuffed
The Shocking History of the EU
Coming Apocalypse
Covid-19: The Greatest Hoax in History
Old Man in a Chair
Endgame
Proof that Masks do more harm than Good
Covid-19: The Fraud Continues
Covid-19: Exposing the Lies
Social Credit: Nightmare on Your Street
NHS: What's wrong and how to put it right
They want your money and your life.
Their Terrifying Plan

Diaries and Autobiographies

Diary of a Disgruntled Man
Just another Bloody Year
Bugger off and Leave Me Alone
Return of the Disgruntled Man
Life on the Edge
The Game's Afoot
Tickety Tonk
Memories 1
Memories 2
Memories 3
My Favourite Books
Truth Teller: The Price

Animals
Why Animal Experiments Must Stop
Fighting For Animals
Alice and Other Friends
Animal Rights – Human Wrongs
Animal Experiments – Simple Truths

General Non Fiction
How to Publish Your Own Book
How to Make Money While Watching TV
Strange but True
Daily Inspirations
Why Is Public Hair Curly
People Push Bottles Up Peaceniks
Secrets of Paris
Moneypower
101 Things I Have Learned
100 Greatest Englishmen and Englishwomen
Cheese Rolling, Shin Kicking and Ugly Tattoos
One Thing after Another
Vernon Coleman's Dictionary of Old English Words and Phrases
Old Man in an Old Car
Vernon Coleman's Commonplace Book

Novels (General)

Mrs Caldicot's Cabbage War
Mrs Caldicot's Knickerbocker Glory
Mrs Caldicot's Oyster Parade
Mrs Caldicot's Turkish Delight
Deadline
Second Chance
Tunnel
Mr Henry Mulligan
The Truth Kills
Revolt
My Secret Years with Elvis
Balancing the Books
Doctor in Paris
Stories with a Twist in the Tale (short stories)
Dr Bullock's Annals
The Awakening of Dr Amelia Leighton
A Needle for a Needle (novella)

The Young Country Doctor Series
Book 1   Bilbury Chronicles
Book 2   Bilbury Grange
Book 3   Bilbury Revels
Book 4   Bilbury Country
Book 5   Bilbury Village
Book 6   Bilbury Pie (short stories)
Book 7   Bilbury Pudding (short stories)
Book 8   Bilbury Tonic
Book 9   Bilbury Relish
Book 10 Bilbury Mixture
Book 11 Bilbury Delights
Book 12 Bilbury Joys
Book 13 Bilbury Tales
Book 14 Bilbury Days
Book 15 Bilbury Memories
Book 16 Bilbury Times

Novels (Sport)
Thomas Winsden's Cricketing Almanack

Diary of a Cricket Lover
The Village Cricket Tour
The Man Who Inherited a Golf Course
Around the Wicket
Too Many Clubs and Not Enough Balls

Cat books
Alice's Diary
Alice's Adventures
We Love Cats
Cats Own Annual
The Secret Lives of Cats
Cat Basket
The Cataholics' Handbook
Cat Fables
Cat Tales
Catoons from Catland

As Edward Vernon
Practice Makes Perfect
Practise What You Preach
Getting Into Practice
Aphrodisiacs – An Owner's Manual
The Complete Guide to Life

Play
Mrs Caldicot's Cabbage War

Written with Donna Antoinette Coleman
How to Conquer Health Problems between Ages 50 & 120
Health Secrets Doctors Share With Their Families
Animal Miscellany
England's Glory
Wisdom of Animals

Dedication

Dedicated, as always, with all my love to Antoinette
Thank you for being you and for everything you do.
Everything you touch you make better
Everyone you meet you make happier
Everywhere you go you make more beautiful

Contents List

Preface

I'm sorry if this is a bit blunt, but there isn't another way to put it.

In *The End of Medicine* I am going to prove to you that doctors have been ordered to murder their patients and whether they realise it or not, that is, I'm afraid, exactly what they are doing.

Now that I have caught your attention, let me put it another way: your doctor has been ordered to kill you or, at the very least, to let you die. Murder or manslaughter, that's the choice. That is what she or he is now being paid to do. And that's exactly what she or he is going to do. Doctors have been turned into killing machines. Doctors are now paid (very well) to kill.

This is the most explosive, terrifying, shocking book you will ever read

Of course, your doctor isn't likely to shoot you, or run you over, or stab you with a carving knife. It's all much more subtle than that. But in the end you'll be dead and your doctor will be richer.

Vernon Coleman

P.S. You can, incidentally, check out everything in this book by going online, reading my previous books or studying the books listed in the short bibliography at the back of this book.

P.P.S. At the end of my book *Truth Teller: The Price* I said that I did not intend to write any more books on medical topics. But everything changed when the medical establishment decided that tackling the alleged threat created by global warming should take priority over the care of patients. When I realised just how far they were prepared to take their devotion to this new cult, I knew I had to write *The End of Medicine*. The title is no exaggeration. The willingness of the medical establishment to abandon the care of patients in order to protect the planet from a non-existent, deliberately manufactured threat had to be exposed. And at the same time I felt that I needed to show how new developments in nanotechnology are being used by the medical establishment to threaten our very humanity and the very core of our existence as humans.

P.P.P.S. You will see the word 'debate' a good many times in this book. No apologies. The key to the success of the conspirators has been their ability to turn news organisations into propaganda machines and to refuse to debate any of the issues which most threaten us. If we fail in our battle against the conspirators it will be because we have failed to force them to engage us in open debate.

Chapter One

As I described in my books *Endgame* and *Their Terrifying Plan*, the mythical threat of global warming was invented by a group of insane megalomaniacs who wrongly believed that the world was overpopulated. The megalomaniacs (henceforth known as 'the conspirators' or 'the cultists') decided that the best way to force people to accept the raft of totalitarian laws which they knew they required in order to push through a depopulation programme designed to reduce the world's population by nine tenths, was to convince everyone that something terrible was about to happen. They knew that it didn't matter what the threat was – a dreadful pandemic or a proposed Martian invasion would both do quite nicely – as long as it could be made to sound convincing and very scary.

The people creating the myth knew that most people will trust whatever they are told by people representing authority whether that authority be a government department or a major State approved broadcaster such as the globally known British Broadcasting Corporation.

Surprisingly, most people are still frighteningly naïve and trusting even though almost every politician in the world has proved themselves to be unworthy of our trust. (Try to think of a political leader you'd trust to sell you a car and you'll see what I mean.) We really should not have any faith in the system because the people running it (whether as politicians, aides or bureaucrats) are irredeemably corrupt and greedy. Today, the mass of people are blind to what is happening, as unseeing as the complacent aristocrats in St Petersburg just before the Russian revolution. They have no idea what is happening, partly because the truth has been well hidden from them and partly because they don't want to know the truth. They know the world isn't the place it used to be and they want someone else to sort it out.

And so the false science of global warming was born as a weapon to terrorise and to bludgeon the public into submission.

Choosing a weather based scare was a cold-blooded decision

because it was easier to 'sell' to the gullible than a Martian invasion, and a better way to lead us into global genocide. And global warming was and is, the biggest fraud in history. It is the excuse of global warming which is leading us into the horrors of Net Zero and the Great Reset.

And global warming is now being used as an excuse to turn health care into a killing machine.

(It's important to understand that when it became patently clear that the world really wasn't getting any warmer and that the fake science created by the conspirators couldn't support the weight of such a transparently fake threat , the name of the threat was changed from 'global warming' to `climate change'. It was a crafty though belated correction for the relaunched weather-based scare enabled the conspirators and their servants to blame every storm, every sunny day and every breeze on 'climate change'. They also needed to rename their scare 'climate change' when it became clear that far from becoming hotter, the world was actually getting colder)

The conspirators do not say things in the way normal people do. Instead of reporting news or releasing press releases they (or, more accurately, their spokespersons) make proclamations, decrees, pronouncements, dictates, edicts, declarations and rulings. And, of course, they use words like sustainable and diversity every few moments. If today's weather is different to yesterday's weather then the explanation must be 'climate change'. If a house catches fire then it was due to 'climate change'. If your fence blows over that was 'climate change'. If a tree falls down it was 'climate change'. If your hat blows off you must blame 'climate change'.

Everyone with functioning brain tissue knows that global warming is a scam. The only people who are still promoting the lie are the small group of scientists and journalists who have been bought, and who are paid to keep promoting the lie, and a variety of specialist companies which give themselves impressive sounding names and earn huge fees by promoting and succouring the myth.

Let's be clear about this: the science shows that global warming doesn't exist. There is no man made weather change. The science shows that we are, if anything, in a long ice age. But the crooks and charlatans promoting the weather myth are using global warming (or climate change) as an excuse to destroy the global economy, to create mass depression, to ensure that countless thousands of innocents die of cold or hunger, to destroy farming, to put an end to travel (except to the regular global warming bean-feasts, usually held in exotic places at taxpayers' expense) and to re-wild the countryside so that we are forced into the horrors of their twenty minute cities.

And it is clear that the evil conspirators and their equally evil servants have, for some time now, been steadily, sneakily, slyly, craftily, deliberately, destroying medical care.

They say it's because of the weather. Most doctors and nurses believe it. But the ones in the medical establishment who have IQs as high as double figures know that the global warming garbage is exactly that – garbage. They aren't destroying health care to conquer global warming. They are ruthlessly, cold-bloodedly and unforgivably destroying medical care to help the depopulation plan.

What better way is there to kill millions than by withdrawing medical care? And what easier and more convincing way than to blame global warming for everything they say they have to do? The sick sycophants who make up the global medical establishment are actually preening and cooing as they boast about how they are destroying medicine, killing people and pushing the trusting into their new devilment – euthanasia. The medical establishment is pushing us, relentlessly and remorselessly, into the sort of society available in China: a technocracy, a world controlled by scientists and technicians; a system built on social credit. And, in case you didn't know, the Chinese system was designed by Klaus Schwab, one of the scariest men in the world, the living embodiment of the truth that you can be a fascist and a communist at the same time, and the founder of the World Economic Forum. Schwab has said that China is a role model for other countries.

Medicine has, I'm afraid, long been run by crooked and ruthless people who are easily manipulated by the prospect of profit. As a result, medicine has retreated, gone backwards, decreased in relevance and failed.

There once was a time when patients had greater regard for a doctor who kept up with advances in theory and practice. But today the opposite is true. Patients are safer if they are treated by a doctor who hasn't taken notice of any judgements or opinions offered by the medical establishment for at least a decade and probably two.

The men and women who end up in the medical establishment are, almost by definition, the dregs of the profession; the least committed to the art and science of healing and the most easily corruptible. They have, on the whole, abandoned clinical practice and the consulting room for the easier and far more profitable corridors of power, and the cosy, tucked away committee rooms and bars where deals are done and decisions made. They mix not with the sick, the fearful and the trusting but with the wheelers and dealers, the movers and shakers, who long ago sold the medical profession to the pharmaceutical industry. They sell their evil in old-fashioned ways. They create problems and then provide us with solutions. They lie brazenly and tell us that they want to help people. They tell us that we're in danger and that they, and only they, can rescue us.

And so now we have the greatest betrayal of all: the destruction of the legacy of Aesculapius and Hippocrates.

Naturally, they are beginning by killing the disabled, the elderly, the frail, the mentally ill and the poor.

But, however fit you are and however young you are, they're after you too.

This book will shock you, appal you and horrify you. It will probably frighten you, too, though I make no apology for that.

And it's all true. You can check out anything I've written on the internet or by using the bibliography at the back of this book.

What is happening is worse, far worse, than anything that has ever happened in history. This is cold-blooded global genocide which will, if we do not stop it, make Genghis Khan's activities look positively unambitious and rather parochial. Indeed, the Rockefeller and Rothschild dynasties, the string pullers behind the scenes, the families which make politicians and mere billionaires jump when they are told to jump, and as high as they are told, make Genghis look comfortably avuncular and relatively harmless.

There is no excuse to say 'I don't know why all this is happening'.

The answers are here in this book.

Now is about to become the most frightening time in history. Never before has man been in such jeopardy.

Finally, consider this: the World Health Organisation's advice to doctors and other health care workers is simply this: 'Don't debate the science'.

As with covid and the covid vaccine, debate is forbidden because any debate would reveal the truth.

The WHO knows that if doctors once start debating the science of global warming (or climate change) they will lose every debate. They know that global warming is a myth. And they know that all the changes which are taking place, and which are predicated on the global warming myth cannot be justified.

Chapter Two

In 1992, the conspirators who attended the Rio Earth Summit officially gave their loyalty to promoting something called sustainable development (though none of them really knew what it meant, though it had a nice ring to it) and called for a reduction in the earth's population by two thirds within 30 to 50 years. (This bizarre and unscientific demand was the origin of the startling Deagel figures, which were produced with the help of the Central Intelligence Agency and the Rockefeller Foundation, and which showed dramatic falls in population numbers for specific countries.)

In 1992, the United Nations' Commission on Global Governance first met and in 1996 the group published a book called 'Our Global Neighbourhood' which described how a global taxation scheme would give the United Nations more power, and enable it to establish an economic security council and a standing army. Excited by this plan, the United Nations created Agenda 21 (later renamed Agenda 30 when Agenda 21 fell by the wayside), a Biodiversity Treaty and its Wildlands Project. These were the forerunners of Net Zero and were an integral part of reducing the world's population.

The Wildlands Project (aka The Wildlands Scheme) called for the conversion of at least 50% of the land area of North America into wilderness, which would be off limits to human beings, with the reduced human population resettled on the remaining 25% of land and living in 'sustainable communities'.

The 50% figure was later increased to 75% and the plan was made global. The aim was a global government and a massive depopulation programme. Global warming was just a manufactured excuse for everything else that was being planned.

The UN's Commission on Global Governance had 28 members and funding from various governments and various private foundations. The members of the Commission included a former American President of the World Bank and US Congressman called Barber Conable; the rather infamous former President of the European Commission, Jacques Delors who was a French politician most well-known for the tabloid headline 'Up Yours Delors'; Frank Judd, a fairly undistinguished member of Britain's House of Commons and then House of Lords; someone called Brian Urquhart who had been a British army officer who became the Under Secretary General for Special Political Affairs at the United Nations and the ubiquitous Maurice Strong, a Canadian who worked for the United Nations and had been an oil man. None of these were household names, people of great achievement or charismatic individuals of great distinction. It seems clear to me that someone hiding behind the curtain was pulling their strings.

The aim always was depopulation.

'Depopulation should be the highest priority of foreign policy towards the Third World,' said Henry Kissinger, rather bluntly and imperiously.

Once they'd succeeded in tricking the world into believing that the earth was really getting hotter, as a result of man's own activities, the conspirators introduced a series of harsh measures ostensibly designed to protect the world from the planet's warming caused by naughty humans. Well-paid advisors produced fake and manipulated evidence proving that the world was heating up so fast that within a very short time the seas would be boiling and the Eiffel Tower, Big Ben and the Empire State Building would all be deep under water.

And for years now the forecasts have been coming thick and fast. Manufactured and entirely spurious climate scares have been common for decades. Scare stories always attract readers, viewers and listeners and the gullible will always believe what they read, see and hear. The people believing what they are told do not seem aware that floods and droughts have always been part of life – as have forest fires. For the cultists, this widespread ignorance of our past is one of the benefits of the deliberate failure of education to deal with history and culture.

Predictions and forecasts made by climate change 'scientists' have been woefully inaccurate – consistently.

Back in 2007, the World Wildlife Fund told us that we had five years to save the world. The global warming hysterics told us that the English county of Cornwall would be a desert by 2010. In 2011, the International Energy Agency said we had five years to avoid

Armageddon. In 2017, the United Nations said we had three years left and in that same year the International Energy Agency also said we had three years left. Some of these merry doomsters were relatively cautious and merely claimed that our planet will be unliveable within a generation. Others were far more specific. In 2020, Greta Thunberg announced that we had eight years left to save the planet. I don't think she explained why it was eight and not seven or nine years before the Four Horsemen would ride into view in their electric cars. (It always seemed to me quite bizarre that a relatively uneducated girl with no scientific background felt able to be so dogmatic. And even more bizarre that anyone listened to her. Was it at all possible that someone was feeding her opinions?) In 2013, a Cambridge professor called Peter Wadhams warned that we might just have until 2015 before all the Arctic ice disappears. He is still making predictions. Mind you, he was optimistic compared to Gordon Brown who, in 2009, taking a tea-break from buggering up the British economy, told us that we had just 50 days to save the planet. And in 2004, the readers of The Observer were warned that by 2020, Britons would be living in a Siberian climate, though I'm not sure how they fitted that into the 'global warming' theory. In 2009, Prince Charles said that we had eight years left to save the planet, so you might imagine that as king he would now be hiding in a cupboard feeling rather embarrassed. However, Charles is made of sterner stuff than most of us and he is continuing with his scaremongering without allowing his past predictions to interfere with his latest proselytizing and enthusiasm for the Great Reset. (Incidentally, if you search the internet you will find a photograph of a Rothschild poking Charles in the chest. The photograph shows clearly who is in charge. And it's definitely not Charles.)

Newspapers, magazines, radio stations, TV stations, celebrities and assorted royalty are constantly telling us that we have a year, a month or half a day before the end of the world. They all have one thing in common. They're always completely wrong. But it is impossible to argue with the cultists because they merely state their belief as though it were a fact beyond dispute and as though it would be an insult to ask for evidence. There is never any debate. It is now generally forgotten but in 2009 emails were leaked from the University of East Anglia's Climatic Research Unit. More emails were released in 2011 and 2013. Known as 'Climategate' these emails revealed group thinking, bullying and the manipulation of evidence. The released emails should have spelt the end for the global warming scam. But they didn't. The hoax continues, supported by endless streams of propaganda from the mainstream media. In 2019, *The Guardian* upped the ante by announcing that instead of referring to 'global warming', the paper would refer to 'global heating' and instead of writing about climate change the paper would prefer to refer to 'climate emergency, crisis or breakdown'. This was presumably done in an attempt to scare people even more, and to promote the lies with more apparent justification.

And now cultists are advised by the World Health Organisation not to debate the science but simply to blast ahead with the warnings. They would, it seems, rather encourage hysteria and terror than use facts to win debates. Using the created threat of global warming the conspirators and the naïve are planning to take us through the horrors of Net Zero and into the Great Reset. They plan, as they have for years, to lock up 75% of the world's land (and natural resources) by a cruel and absurd process called re-wilding. They claim they are giving priority to nature but the people behind this evil fraud don't really give a damn about nature. And there are constant warnings of the horrors and hard times to come. Something called the Financial Stability Board (which is a group of central bankers, ministers and regulators) has warned that the 'financial damage of climate shocks such as floods, droughts, fires or storms could cause a broader pullback in lending and a downturn in investor confidence. Banks could reduce lending, including for recovery to already vulnerable households and corporations.' Well, I suppose it could. But so could an invasion of little green men popping down from Uranus to cause global mayhem. This is unjustified and unjustifiable scaremongering at its tabloid worst.

All this wild, scary stuff merely proves that the whole global warming/climate change thing is a hoax, an international scam of Brobdingnagian proportions. Despite the evidence that global warming is a manufactured myth, the mythmakers will doubtless keep going with their predictions. And, of course, making a prediction about the end of the world is a great way to get publicity and pick up more social media. The trick, it seems, is to pick a date a few years ahead and then hope that by the time we get there, everyone will have forgotten what you said. Discussions are usually one sided because those who question global warming are likely to be thrown off social media sites.

If you are a climate scientist then global warming is the new AIDS. Just as frauds who labelled themselves AIDS specialists did so with such success, you can carve out for yourself a nice quiet corner of the global warming world, produce lots of fake figures, make some scary television programmes and videos, write subsidised books, attend lots of conferences in lovely resorts and become rich and famous. Climate scientists and meteorologists who had previously been stuck in a miserable backwater where they earned rotten salaries and were inspired only by the hope of a professorship or the chance to write a dull tome on weather patterns (or possibly a spicy book on 'Hurricanes I have Known') suddenly became global superstars, charging huge fees for their manufactured threats and receiving so many invitations to appear on television or speak at huge conferences that they doubtless needed agents and lawyers and high powered tax accountants. The lies they tell are endless and self-serving. There isn't a shred of real evidence linking 'extreme weather' and 'global warming' to man's activities but lazy journalists, looking for a pat on the back and a nice bonus are quick to provide the link. 'Global warming' is the most over-promoted minority cult ever seen. The fact is that the heat-wave seen in the 1930s was much more extreme than anything seen today. Extreme weather in the 1940s and the 1960s was much more dramatic than anything seen in the 21st century. There has been no increase in hurricanes or droughts or forest fires.

The cultists attempt to frighten investors away from oil companies by saying that the oil will have to be left in the ground. They use the phrase 'stranded assets'. Company bosses were pressured into signing up to bizarre ESG policies to please the media, even if doing so meant destroying their companies, their employees' prospects and their shareholders' income. The ESG enthusiasts thought they could become members of the elite but they were suckered into destroying shareholder value and their own credibility. They could only become servants of the conspiracy.

And then, in the US, the *Washington Post* published details of a study published in the journal 'Science' which dealt with the earth's climate over the last 485 million years. The study shows the massive variations in weather and temperature which have occurred, and concludes that the earth's temperature is the lowest it has been for 485 million years and has been falling for years. The earth has previously been much warmer than it is now, and the global mean surface temperature has fallen from nearly 100 degrees Fahrenheit at the start of the modern human era to a little over 50 degrees Fahrenheit now. You don't need a degree in weather watching to realise that's a fall in temperature, not a rise. Much nonsense is talked about earth tremors and disappearing islands but the evidence shows these events are nothing unusual. Seismographers confirm that for centuries islands in different parts of the world have disappeared as a result of tidal waves, volcanic disturbances or earth tremors.

The arguments in favour of the existence of global warming are nothing more than snippets of laughable pseudoscience but those promoting it manage to appear deadly serious and most of the mainstream media journalists are so besotted by the idea of an over-heating planet, and frightened of facts that will make them look stupid, that they refuse to debate the issue (just as they refuse to debate or discuss the pros and cons of covid or vaccination.) Anyone who questions global warming will be dismissed as a conspiracy theorist. There's irony for you. Question the lies of the conspirators and you will be a conspiracy theorist. (Remember, as I have pointed out, the World Health Organisation actually advises those promoting the global warming myth not to engage in debate about the science. There could not be better proof that global warming is a scam.)

Doctors, dentists and pharmacists have all worked hard to exceed one another as they sign up to the fraud and produce statements full of their commitment to sustainability and diversity, of course. (In Wales, pharmacists were told they were expected to undergo training in climate change and carbon literary under the Welsh Government's Net Zero requirements.)

There is no little irony in the way that global warming cultists talk about diversity but suppress all debate about their myth. The cultists are doing their best to suppress and destroy diversity of thought because it terrifies them. Through a mixture of stupidity and gullibility they've all chosen to drink the Kool Aid. And now they want us to drink it too.

The conspirators' plan was always a simple one. The theory was that once enough gullible humans had been convinced of the threat of global warming, those gullible humans would be delighted to help destroy the world and turn themselves into slaves of the conspiracy. The most seriously afflicted by the fraud would enrol in the cult and join in the hysteria. They'd glue themselves to roads to delay ambulances and fire engines and they'd interrupt sporting events and they'd throw mixed vegetable soup at works of art to draw attention to themselves. (Throwing soup at paintings is their idea of debate.) They'd spread death and misery and they'd do it sanctimoniously in the name of their imaginary cause. Or at least they thought they were helping their cause. Sadly, the reality was that the extremists annoyed the unconverted so much that the conspirators had to try to shut them up and put a few of them in prison to keep them out of the way. This, of course, was useful to the cultists because a martyred pensioner serving time in jail is a much better advertisement for the cause than a scruffy old bat daring the driver of the Number 11 bus to run her over. (The conspirators realised in the end that 99.8% of the population were cheering on the bus driver and very happy to bring in a verdict of 'not guilty' if they ended up on a jury with him or her in the dock.)

It was, of course, the old trick. You create a horrifying threat and create genuine fear and then you offer a solution which may be unpleasant (nasty medicine) but which will save us people, children and polar bears from extinction.

A short way into what was without doubt the biggest long con in history, the conspirators realised that they'd got their plot slightly wrong.

The world isn't getting hotter after all.

Still, when you've got a long con going you have to be adaptable and so the conspirators merely changed the threat of 'global warming' to the threat of 'climate change'. The suckers who had fallen for the 'global warming' myth didn't blink an eye, they moved seamlessly into accepting the 'climate change' scenario. This was a bit like a con man promising to sell a mark the Eiffel Tower and then half way through the deal suddenly telling the mark that he wouldn't be buying the Eiffel Tower after all but he would be buying Tower Bridge. Or, maybe, a small bridge over a canal in Lincolnshire.

The fact is that the conspirators were lying all along, of course. The weather has nothing to do with anything man has done. Moreover, any change that is taking place is going in the opposite direction: the world is very slowly getting colder not hotter. Oddly enough, on 24th June 1974, *Time* magazine (that's the silly rag which made Little Greta their person of the year in 2019) announced the coming of another ice age. The *Time* magazine warning was actually more accurate than anything else that has been published about the weather in more recent years. Did the conspirators know this? I feel sure that they did. In which case these people are even more evil than we had assumed for they knew that they were making things worse by dimming the sun with a technique which involves injecting particles into the stratosphere. They started to dim the sun (they are already doing this, hence our constantly grey skies and increasingly rare glimpses of the sun) even though the conspirators should have known that if done globally this could result in hundreds of millions of deaths. The conspirators don't do the wrong thing by mistake – they do the wrong thing on purpose. The myth of global warming is a major part of the depopulation plan.

It is, incidentally, interesting to recall that on 2nd July 2020 I published a video entitled 'They're going to starve us and freeze us to death'. The video was removed from YouTube within minutes and not long afterwards YouTube suddenly removed my channel, banned me for life and, quite bizarrely, banned me from looking at other people's videos on YouTube. The script of this video is available in my book *Covid-19: The Greatest Hoax in History*.

The other aims of the conspirators were to use the myth of global warming as an excuse to bring in a world government, to gain total control of the world's resources for themselves, to set up a totalitarian regime which they would run and which would turn the world's population into slaves. This was nothing if not ambitious but the conspirators had two big advantages. First, they controlled most of the money in the world. And second they control the world's media. It also helps that they are insane and, therefore, free not to have to worry about facts or good sense.

A year or two ago, the paragraphs above would have probably resulted in a visit from men in white coats, equipped with a straight jacket and a large syringe full of a serious sedative, offering to take me away to a nice place in the country for a long rest.

Today, we've gone past that. If I get a visit these days it will be from men in uniform, carrying guns, who will take me to a place where men in white coats won't bother promising to help me get better but will merely jab with a lethal cocktail of a benzodiazepine such as midazolam and a narcotic such as morphine. They have already done everything they can to crush me, wreck my reputation and censor me. They've banned me from all mainstream media, from YouTube, from all social media and from most of the internet. And they've made one serious but unsuccessful attempt to kill me.

The mainstream media, which is controlled by the billionaire conspirators and their billionaire pals, constantly tells us that the greatest threat to our security, comfort and survival comes from the Far Right. This is a nonsense; a lie, a classical example of misdirection. The truth is that the biggest threat comes not from the Far Right but from the other end of the political spectrum – the Far Left. It is the Far Left which has taken control of the media and politicians. In fact the world is run by the Far Left. Politicians, bureaucrats, aides and the media are all so Far Left that they are effectively communists. Institutions and Non-Governmental Organisations (NGOs), although ostensibly run by Liberals are also very Far Left. Many of the powerful organisations which now run the world are far left wing in their outlook. For example, the World Economic Forum (which organises the annual shindig in Davos, where politicians and civil servants can meet billionaires and arrange their future employment) is an unashamedly communist organisation. (Kier Starmer, the UK's Prime Minister, has said that he prefers Davos to Westminster). It is important to remember that there is no practical difference between communism and fascism. Both lie at the extreme of the political spectrum and are identical in purpose and outlook and how they operate.

The one clue to the fact that everything that is happening is part of a plan is the fact that it is all happening worldwide. Health care is being destroyed worldwide. Politicians all around the world seem incompetent or crooked or both (I find it impossible to name one leading politician in the world who is not both of these things). Undemocratic organisations such as the United Nations and its subsidiary the World Health Organisation, the EU Commission, the World Bank, the International Monetary Fund, the World Economic Forum and hundreds of NGOs and quangos, all led by unelected individuals, are taking more and more power. Fear is being used as a tool to create obedience and compliance. New laws are being introduced to limit our freedom (they are, of course, all introduced to protect us in some curious way from some imagined or created threat). The conspirators (who already control the central banks) want to eradicate nationalism and introduce global governance without accountability, though I suspect that most of those blindly following the instructions of the billionaire conspirators are unaware of the extent of the plan. When Donald Trump was appointed President of the United States in 2025, he wasted no time in announcing that he intended to annex Greenland, turn Canada into an American state and take over Gaza. All that was just a step towards a World Government.

The cultists who believe in global warming have acquired an enormous amount of power. The majority of people in the world realise that global warming is a hoax but the conspirators have a disproportional amount of power and money. The International Monetary Fund has called for restrictions on economic activity that far exceed the effect of the covid lockdowns (which were always pointless from a medical point of view but, like absurd recycling schemes, designed only to get people used to restrictions and having less freedom). Their plans will lead to massive energy and food shortages, job losses, the collapse of Western civilisation and (the ultimate aim) a massive population decline. There are calls to limit private vehicle use and to ban fossil fuel companies from drilling. The IMF wants all nations to achieve the Net Zero carbon goal by 2030 – this despite the absence of any evidence connecting human activity to global warming.

In order to help the conspirators, banks are using their financial power to influence every aspect of our society. Local branches are being closed to push the world into a digital currency. The Net Zero Banking Alliance, set up by the United Nations, withdrew lending facilities from petrol stations in New Zealand (the new home of the witless and the woke). Obviously, without petrol stations all fossil fuel motoring will have to stop. (Curiously, the Net Zero Banking Alliance may have done a good deal of public virtue signalling but since it was set up, the Alliance has actually increased its financing of the fossil fuel industry. A quick profit, it seems, trumps virtue signalling. And early in 2025 it was announced that a number of major banks had abandoned the Alliance).

The conspirators and their servants do not seem aware that far from being a dangerous pollutant, carbon dioxide (the substance which they claim is destroying the world) helps to keep the earth alive. The pseudoscience which labels carbon dioxide a poison is absurd and serves solely to advance a corrupt political agenda. In truth, rising carbon dioxide levels help expand forests, increase agricultural yields and enhance biodiversity. The claim that carbon dioxide is causing a rise in the earth's temperature is at best wildly exaggerated and at worst a complete lie.

As I have already pointed out, the conspirators are spraying particles into the stratosphere to dim the sun. (I repeat: now you know why the skies over much of the world have been grey for many months now.) Whistle blowers who tell the truth about what is happening are subject to gag orders or put in prison.

There are serious stories around confirming that fires and earthquakes have been started deliberately in an attempt to prove that global warming is real. The threats and warnings are endless and so are the organisations promoting the nonsense. The words 'diversity' and 'sustainability' are everywhere. (I'm hoping to see the phrase 'sustainable diversity' appearing soon.)

The propaganda in favour of the global warming scam seems endless. Natural variations in temperature and weather patterns are misinterpreted and offered as evidence of global warming. The Bank of England has warned that global warming could devastate the values of hundreds of thousands of UK homes and has given doomsday scenarios of flooding. There is no evidence for this prediction other than the result of the fact that houses are being deliberately built on flood plains, and some waterways are not being kept open and repaired and dredged.

And the global warming cultists constantly talk about poor

harvests. There have always been good harvests and bad harvests but this time they are right because farmers are being paid to stop farming while huge areas of farmland are being covered with solar panels and wind turbines.

The biggest irony in the history of the world is that our climate really is now changing. And it is changing because of man. But it isn't the burning of fossil fuels that is changing the climate. It's the deliberate dimming of the sun that is now about to start doing serious damage. Dimming the sun is going to create storms and cold weather and it's going to exacerbate the effect of the coming ice age. And every new storm, or few hours of bad weather, will be blamed on non-existent global warming and honoured with a name so that we can all have three or four named storms in a week.

Already, we know that every time the wind changes direction it is given a new name. Storm Kier is followed closely by Storm Rachel which comes hard on the heels of Storm Donald, if storms can be said to have heels. And so at the end of every quarter, the doomsters can say: 'See in a normal three months we would have had X storms. But now we have had 5X storms and this proves that global warming is real.' It doesn't mean any such thing, of course. Anyone who believes in the nonsense known as global warming is either seriously deprived of brain tissue or in the pay of the conspirators. These people lie about the past, lie about the present and lie about the future. They do not seem to understand that the future is where we will all spend the rest of our lives.

Just look at some of the truths which the controlled media will not share with you:

1) For years now the authorities have not been dredging rivers. Waterways everywhere have been left alone and have blocked. The result, inevitably, is flooding. And to make things worse, houses have been built on flood plains. The result is that the news programmes are regularly full of stories of towns and housing estates being flooded. The cultists blame global warming and the naïve believe them. In fact, the flooding has been deliberately engineered to help sustain the myth.

2) In 2024, the UK paid £1 billion to turn off the country's wind

turbines either because the wind was too strong for the turbines or because there wasn't enough wind to make them go round. The electricity that should have come from the turbines had to be replaced with electricity from fossil fuels. In order to stop wind turbines from getting stuck, electricity is sometimes used to keep the blades going round. The evidence shows that if you take into account the amount of energy required to build and erect wind turbines, they are energy negative. (In other words they require more energy than they produce.)

3) If global warming were real the world would benefit enormously. Far more people die from the cold than die from the heat.

4) The World Economic Forum and the International Monetary Fund would like a permanent, global lockdown to be introduced because they reckon that the lockdowns introduced in 2020 helped reduce carbon emissions and destroy the world economy. Evidence proves that the lockdowns did absolutely no good and a great deal of harm – especially to the physical and mental health of children.

5) Reduced speed limits are being introduced everywhere because the cultists say that vehicles use less fuel when driving slowly. This isn't true. I've owned three cars which did their best mileage when travelling at or just over 70 mph. The evidence shows that travelling slowly results in more dangerous emissions, more accidents and reduced productivity.

6) Hundreds of millions are starving to death in Africa and Asia. This is not because of imaginary global warming but because of Net Zero and the rules and regulations introduced at the behest of the United Nations, the World Economic Forum and the various cultists who believe in global warming. (Incidentally, it is important to remember that, despite all the propaganda, global warming is a minority cult. Most people realise that it is a myth.)

7) Officially and allegedly, global warming caused six weeks of dangerously hot days in 2024. This laughable claim is offered as yet more evidence of a phenomenon increasingly seen as a myth. Other, more honest, reports shown that the UK had one of the most miserable summers ever experienced. But the big lie must always be protected by little lies.

8) The great majority of independent scientists realise that global warming is a myth. Nearly all scientists who make big money of the

global warming myth say they believe it is real. What a surprise.

9) To help support the myth of global warming, the conspirators are blocking the sun (affecting the weather in numerous, unknown ways), they are allowing rivers to become blocked (causing flooding), they are building on flood plains (resulting in flooded homes), they are almost certainly creating fires, hurricanes and earthquakes. If you really don't believe all his is happening then you are probably naïve enough to believe that global warming is real and that the attack on 9/11 was orchestrated by a man living in a cave in Afghanistan. Incidentally, the global warming cultists claim that the fires which destroyed much of Los Angeles were a result of global warming. That's true but not in the way they imply. The fact is that environmental regulations (created as a result of global warming hysteria) stopped the customary burning of wild vegetation around Los Angeles so when a fire started it spread more easily than it would otherwise have done. So once again the global warming cult caused a major problem.

10) The global warming myth has spread since the people promoting the idea have been clever enough to use ordinary people (including children) to promote the nonsense. The advantage of using children to promote the myth is that anyone who criticises what they say (however silly it might be) is likely to be accused of bullying.

11) Weather forecasters who cannot tell you what the weather will be like tomorrow (or even what it is like today) will happily, and with great confidence, tell you what the weather will be like on April 1st in the year 2075.

12) The evidence for the existence of global warming consists of the words 'because we say it is'. Remember that, on the advice of the World Health Organisation the cult's followers are forbidden to enter into debate about global warming. Debate is forbidden because there is no sustainable science. (Sorry, I couldn't resist using the word 'sustainable'.)

13) Oil was created by God with the help of a process called photosynthesis – which requires sunshine. And so my petrol and diesel powered cars are truly solar powered forms of transport. Moreover, petrol and diesel vehicles have batteries which provides the electrical power for the lights, wipers, indicators and cigar lighter.

14) Even after years of heavy investment, most of the UK's electricity comes from fossil fuels and biomass (pellets of wood from trees which were chopped down on another continent and transported vast distances by ship and lorry). Negligible amounts of electricity are obtained from wind and solar developments. In January 2025, the UK Energy Secretary, Ed Miliband, said he wanted 750 square miles of UK farmland to be turned into solar farms, requiring billions of solar panels. He also wanted another 5,000 wind turbines. Someone should tell him that, sadly, even Australia cannot get solar and wind farms to work well. And maybe should point out that the World Bank has reported that solar power has only a very small potential to produce electricity in the UK. Indeed, the UK is one of the worst places in the world to expect to produce electricity from solar panels. The solar panels do however help cover up vast areas of good farmland – thereby reducing the UK's ability to produce its own food supplies. How convenient.

15) There is only one reason to avoid over-using fossil fuels: they are running out. The online warriors who insist (illogically) that there is plenty of easily obtained oil (and that, therefore, it will never run out) should know that one of BPs biggest ventures is the development of the Kaskida oilfield in the US Gulf of Mexico (not a happy hunting ground for BP) which was discovered in 2006 under a mile of water and six miles of rock. The oil is at such high temperatures and pressures that it has taken nearly 20 years to develop the technology to exploit the oil field. The billionaires who want us to stop using fossil fuels (so that there will be more for their yachts and jets) have invested in allegedly sustainable and definitely profitable alternatives. The idea that there is plenty of oil around is a myth.

16) Our local bank, which is always incredibly busy, with long queues, is being closed. It is being closed because apparently everyone wants to bank online. The people queuing at the counters have presumably been queuing to ask the time or say hello to a friend who works in the bank. The result is that thousands of people who used the bank (the only bank for many miles around) will now have to travel around 30 miles (each way, there and back) to visit the only bank branch available in our part of the country. And then the bank will close that branch and we will be ever closer to a cashless society and digital currencies provided by our central bank. Local

shop keepers are refusing to take cash because there is no bank where they can deposit their takings. The cultists who believe in global warming should be complaining about bank closures because they will clearly lead to more travel. Why don't the bank unions protest? Their members will soon all be gone – unemployed and unemployable. (The mainstream media reported, in its usual pathetic craven way, that the branches were being closed because bank customers preferred to bank online using the bank's app.)

17) Plants absorb 31% more carbon dioxide than the global warming cultists admit. The whole science of global warming is based on a fallacy.

18) Methane levels rose during the lockdowns. And so the global warming cultists are insane in thinking that lockdowns helped their 'cause'.

19) The World Bank has given £41 billion to 'climate causes'. What on earth did they use all that money for? A fraction of that amount would have ended famine for a hundred years.

20) Business travellers will spend $1.5 trillion in 2025 – a new record. So, it is clear that all those company bosses who proselytise about global warming are hypocrites – or simply don't believe the global warming message which they share with such empty sincerity.

And so it goes on. The cultists who believe the hoax (and there are fewer of them than you would imagine) share a dogmatic assumption that their view of the existence of global warming is correct and that their view of the world we must create is also correct. The weather cultists don't believe in democracy. Their dogma is extreme and exclusive.

And now they believe that medical care must be cut back to protect the planet from us. We are the enemy.

The conspirators have decided (without evidence, research or permission) that medical care must be restricted in every way to satisfy their absurd pseudoscience. This is totalitarianism. Their arrogance is so complete that they impose their cultish view upon the public without sharing their plans, without debate, without any democratic oversight and without any attempts to evaluate the effect their plans will have upon the public health. The conspirators and their cult followers are as interested in the health and well-being of you and I as serial killers are interested in the health and well-being of their victims.

In the chapter which follows I will explain how global warming is used as an excuse to destroy health care and to kill people – as part of the depopulation programme. Remember, global warming was invented in order to provide an excuse for carrying out a depopulation programme, and for introducing all the restrictions and laws which now control our lives. I will explain precisely how the conspirators are already ordering doctors, nurses and hospitals to cut back on medical care.

And in the chapter after that I will explain how medical care has already deteriorated to the point where it is now true to say that the medical care we have today is worse than the medical care that was available over half a century ago. That's how bad things are already. And unless we stop them, everything is going to get worse – much worse.

Chapter Three

'**D**on't debate the science' – is advice given from the World Health Organisation to doctors. The WHO does not want doctors to 'debate the science' because there is no science supporting the global warming myth and doctors will look very silly if they try to 'debate the science' and, worse still, they will realise they have been sold a lie.

The truth is that anyone who believes that global warming (aka climate change) is real is ignorant, gullible and possibly already a member of a small, potent and dangerous cult.

The destruction of medicine began some years ago but was understated. Changes went mostly unnoticed and appeared to be nothing more than a gentle decline in the quality and quantity of the care provided. But over the last few years the destruction has become more brazen, and today it is impossible to see that the decline is having a very real impact on our lives.

People first noticed that health care was deteriorating during the illogical and dangerous lockdowns which were introduced in 2020 and which were allegedly but falsely, designed to protect us all from a disease worse than death. In February and March of 2020, I warned the readers of my website that the claims that were being made for that year's new flu were wildly exaggerated. I explained in detail how I had come to this conclusion. I pointed out that the UK Government's advisers had agreed that the coronavirus which was being promoted as the new plague was not a dangerous disease – and no more hazardous than the flu. But the Government ignored their own advisers and accepted the bizarre predictions made by someone called Neil Ferguson, a discredited computer scientist. It was clear from then that the fake pandemic was the harbinger of something much more. In April 2020, I published a book *Coming Apocalypse* in which I explained why the covid-19 scare was a hoax. In order to publish the book I had to avoid using words like 'covid' and 'vaccination'. This was another sign of things to come.

The naïve and the gullible, trained to be compliant by the

recycling scam, thought that the lockdowns had been introduced to protect them.

But they hadn't, of course.

The lockdowns were deliberately introduced to create fear, to kill the elderly and the frail and the sick, to train the public to be obedient, to help sustain the absurd notion that it would make sense to make an untested and toxic vaccine compulsory and to initiate a process of destroying health care.

Since the United Nations was founded, back in the 1940s, human beings have been the enemy, and the aim of the self-appointed saviours of the world has been the formation of a world government and the transfer of all power and money to a tiny elite of malignant self-described philanthropists.

It was during the lockdowns which began in 2020 that both general practitioners and hospitals cut back their services very considerably. General practitioners, showing a lack of courage that should have embarrassed them, dressed from head to toe in utterly pointless but expensive PPE apparel and hid under their desks to avoid the flu. Moreover, they took advantage of the fake pandemic to stop seeing patients face to face. Instead, for the first time, many of them insisted on providing consultations exclusively by telephone and by computer. The evidence shows unequivocally that attempting to diagnose and treat patients by telephone, or over an internet connection, is so dangerous as to be worse than useless. (It is worse than useless because it means that real disease is over-looked and the patient is given bad advice – often worse than no advice at all.)

But the lockdowns, and the imagined threat from the well-marketed flu, gave lazy doctors an opportunity to abandon medical care and to introduce a new system of medical care that would help the conspirators with their long-standing depopulation programme.

Any doubt in my mind that the lockdowns were designed and introduced with a malignant purpose disappeared when, early on, I made a video suggesting that because of their reduced exposure to sunshine, most people would benefit if they took vitamin D supplements. The suggestion that vitamin D supplements be taken had another advantage too. Vitamin D helps strengthen the immune system and provide protection from infection. I put the video on YouTube in the hope that it would help those who saw it. All the video contained was advice about vitamin D. And what happened?

YouTube, which was promoting bad advice and suppressing good advice, took down the video and immediately banned it.

Now things have got a good deal worse. The destruction of health care has become official policy and the medical establishment, loyal to a fault to the conspirators, whose overriding aim is to see a smaller world population, (and loyal to the imagined and carefully constructed global warming threat which they do not realise is fake and has an ulterior purpose) are tearing medical care apart and enriching themselves while damaging and killing their parents, apparently without a care. How are doctors enriching themselves? Well, in the UK the average GP earns around £150,000 a year for a 23 hour week and is making a bonus of £50,000 a year or so merely by telling his State employed staff to vaccinate patients. And GPs who are given a prescribing budget can make another bonus by prescribing very few drugs. The money left over at the end of the financial year is theirs to spend on another Mercedes.

None of the things that are happening have anything to do with global warming. I know this for certain because I know for certain that there is no global warming. Everything the cultists say about climate change is a lie, designed to trick you into believing the propaganda – and designed to make you feel guilty and ashamed if you don't go along with their self-serving pseudoscientific nonsense.

So-called weather scientists, arrogant and impervious to the truth, fiddle their results with impunity and the sort of imagination usually seen with confidence tricksters. They say that the weather is hotter and colder than ever before and dismiss evidence proving them wrong by claiming (with remarkable arrogance) that their predecessors made a lot of mistakes when measuring temperatures.

GP's surgeries/clinics are now introducing CCTV cameras. The only explanation I can think of is that the doctors are planning to introduce car park charges – in just the same way that hospital car parks charge hefty fees when patients or visitors park their vehicles. This is, I suspect, another attempt to keep patients (particularly the poorer ones) from attending their doctor's office. Doctors now much prefer patients to consult them over the telephone or the internet. (They claim, naturally, that this is to prevent the mythical global warming. However, it is more likely to be a way to reduce their working hours still further, since it is possible to deal with patients more speedily and at lower cost if patients are forced to accept telephone consultations.) And if you think GPs couldn't possibly be this greedy, just remember that a few years ago quite a number of GPs introduced premium rate phone numbers for patients ringing the surgery to make an appointment or request a repeat prescription of their medication.

If doctors in the medical establishment had been honest they would have said 'We have been told that global warming is real, though the evidence does not support that notion, and so we are refusing the suggestion that we put health care second to attempts to deal with the hypothesis that global warming is real. Meanwhile we will urge the authorities to prove that their claim is real. And we will urge governments to do proper trials to see how medical care can safely be changed if global warming turns out to be a real problem.'

But the medical establishment chose, instead, to accept that global warming as real and to change the way medicine is practised accordingly.

Everything that happens is scarcely believable.

'I can't believe I'm saying this,' said Antoinette, as she reported yet another horror story from the medical establishment's plan to turn health care into a killing machine.

'I can't believe I believe you,' I answered sadly.

The two giveaways that everything that is happening is fraudulent are, first, the fact that the changes are all global and second that the people who support the global warming hoax will not debate it. The mainstream media will not even admit that there is any opposition. And, as I have said earlier, the World Health Organisation has told those who believe in this bizarre and dangerous cult not to debate the science of global warming with anyone.

We should make it clear to everyone that debate is banned, just as it was with the covid-19 hoax. With global warming, as with the covid-19 hoax (and, indeed, as with vaccines and vaccination) the authorities, the cultists and the conspirators know that if they debate these issues they will always lose because all the facts are on our side. Only lies and pseudo-science are on their side.

We have to attack the cultists and demand, repeatedly, that they debate. Unless we do this we will never win and we will be doomed to a life without independence, without self-responsibility and without freedom.

In the rest of this chapter I will list some of the ways in which the global warming hoax is now being used as an excuse to reduce the quality and quantity of health care which is available.

In 2024, medical journals around the world suddenly started to print articles arguing that health care was a major cause of global warming. The hysteria was almost palpable and it became clear that the left wing cultists (more properly known as the born again communists desperate to rule the world for their masters the Rothschilds and the Rockefellers) had recruited the global medical establishment as another weapon against mankind and were using the mythical and unscientific nonsense known as global warming as an excuse to destroy medical care.

I should, perhaps, admit that I find that everything produced by the hysterically woke health care cultists to be terrifying. Almost everything seems designed to delight the conspirators, the United Nations, the World Economic Forum and various assorted maniacs (the sort of people whose idea of an afternoon well spent is an afternoon spent glued to the nearest motorway, holding up a queue of ambulances and fire engines).

Nothing new, it seems, has been done with thought for the safety or health of patients. The assumption is that global warming is real and that dealing with global warming must take precedence over patient care and good clinical practice. The real reason for everything that is happening is very simple: a massive depopulation programme which will reduce the world's population to 500 million. And that means that a lot of people have to die.

Destroying health care is one way the conspirators are going to achieve that aim – though the people who are doing the destroying have no idea what is going on, or how they are being used by a few hundred ruthless, power and money hungry megalomaniacs who lie and deceive and cheat and kill in the same way that most of us breathe, eat and sleep.

In the UK the initial warning shot fired in the direction of patients was a publication produced by the NHS in October 2020. The publication, called 'Delivering a Net Zero National Health Service' 'set ambitions on reaching Net Zero for emissions controlled directly by the NHS by 2040 and for emissions influenced by the NHS by 2045'. I believe that the document is probably one of the most insane but depressing productions I've come across in a lifetime's encounters with insane publications. It seems to me to be based solidly on a mixture of pseudo-science, assumptions, prejudice without any interest in facts or the interests of patients. The publication has what it calls a '10 point green plan for practices'. The first of these is to 'declare a practice climate and nature crisis', though naturally there doesn't seem to be any evidence for the existence of either a practice climate crisis or a practice nature crisis. The next few items include advice to 'optimise inhalers', 'calculate the practice's carbon footprint', 'monitor and reduce your practice's energy usage' and 'consider switching your business banking provider to a green bank'. (A green bank is apparently one which is a 'mission driven institution that uses innovative financing to fight climate change'. Since there is no such thing as climate change, this seems a particularly pointless exercise.) The sixth item on the list concerns 'environmental prescribing and treatment' and the first suggestion here is that doctors 'consider non-pharmaceutical interventions such as 'green social prescribing' or an increase in physical activity. I had to look up 'green social prescribing' and I found that it is 'the practice of supporting people to engage in nature-based interventions and activities to improve their mental and physical health.' Apparently the NHS now employs 'social prescribing link workers' who will connect people to community groups and agencies for practical and emotional support.' Digging a little further I found that this means 'local walking schemes, community gardening projects, conservation volunteering, open water swimming or arts and cultural activities which take place outdoors.' Wonderful. 'You have pneumonia, Mrs Reeves. I'm sending you down to the river to do a little open water swimming in the sewage.' 'You have a vaccine damaged heart, Mr Starmer, so I've prescribed a week's cultural activities for you.' There is also a recommendation to begin 'de-prescribing in frailty' and returning inhalers to pharmacies for safe disposal. I had absolutely no idea what 'de-prescribing in frailty' means so I looked it up on the internet and it seems to mean not giving too many medicines to patients – particularly old and frail ones. This is something I've been writing about since the 1970s but I never thought to describe it as 'de-prescribing in frailty'. It would make a snappy book title. Returning inhalers to the pharmacy for safe disposal seems a good idea though hardly world changing. And there is a suggestion that prescription durations should be appropriate for the course of medication required. This comes under the same heading as telling old people to drink plenty when the weather is hot and to put on a scarf and hat when it's cold. Next we come to a suggestion that doctors 'continue remote consultations where appropriate'. And this was the point in the report where I exploded and threw my reading glasses across the room because remote consultations, although now extremely popular with lazy GPs (who prefer to avoid actually doing what they are paid for) are almost never appropriate. Any doctor providing remote consultations (whether by telephone or computer) should be boiled in oil, hung drawn and quartered, tarred and feathered and then have their licence surgically removed with a spoon. The telephone's place in medicine is to be used as a tool for patients to ask the doctor to come and visit them at home. But that doesn't happen now because doctors, taking full advantage of the global warming myth, don't get out of bed much any more.

The rest of the report was just rubbish. Number 7 on the list was 'Engage, educate and empower patients to take individual action on the climate crisis for the benefit of their health.' Since there is absolutely no evidence that there is a climate crisis, this suggestion was clearly superfluous. And if there were a crisis I'm not quite sure what individual patients are supposed to do about it other than worry. Number 8 on the list is 'promote active transport for both staff and patients'. I had to look this up as well and although I originally thought it might mean walking or bicycling it doesn't. 'Active transport' is defined as the movement of molecules or ions across a cell membrane from a region of lower concentration to a region of higher concentration – against the concentration gradient.' I hope you are confused by this because I certainly am. Number 9 on the list suggested, among other things, 'using scrap paper and paper clips instead of post it notes' and 'opting for naturally wrapped treats such as satsumas or snacks with compostable or recyclable packaging'. I was startled by this. I had never previously thought of the satsuma as having such a significant role to play in medicine and I still can't work out why the satsuma is considered superior to the banana or the orange or the bunch of grapes. There is also a suggestion called 'Revolution Zero' which is defined as using reusable masks. I don't know why they didn't just call it 'using reusable masks' but people who get excited about satsumas probably also get excited by phrases like 'Revolution Zero'. Number 10 on the list is 'Use the green impact for health toolkit' which is, I suspect, the title of the whole thing, including the stuff about active transport, doing something with satsumas and GPs doing their morning surgeries on the telephone without wasting energy by getting out of bed. You will see from all this that the NHS still hadn't quite got its head round the idea of Net Zero in health care. But this was just the beginning and I doubt if anyone involved really thought that the mass consumption of satsumas was going to lead the NHS into Net Zero. The really dramatic stuff was presumably yet to come though those determined to update medical practice did not seem to have worked out that motion, movement and change are not directly or necessarily linked to progress and better care for people or polar bears.

In America, the first formal interest in using global warming to destroy health care came with the realisation that in the US the health care sector was responsible for 8.5 per cent of the country's greenhouse gas emissions. (This figure is much higher than that quoted in other countries by the way.)

The suggestion (which I found in a report from the Ways and Means Committee Democrats and a publication called 'Explainer' and which contained a story under the headline 'How the US Health Care System Contributes to Climate Change' dated April 19th 2022) was that 'Health systems must learn to adapt to a changing climate, but they also can take steps to mitigate the level of carbon emissions they produce.'

The report warned us that 'Greenhouse gases trap heat and make the planet warmer' and that 'human activities are responsible for nearly all the increase in greenhouse gases – primarily carbon dioxide in the atmosphere over the last 150 years.' There is of course not one shred of evidence to support this bizarre and entirely worthless claim. In fact, as independent scientists agree, carbon dioxide is making the planet healthier and helping to produce more natural foodstuffs.

There was then the usual gibberish about 'severe weather, ocean warming and acidification, extended periods of drought and extreme temperatures'. As usual not a shred of evidence was offered for any of these claims.

Readers were told that 'climate change is already devastating the planet' (I think the writers got their ideas from the Greta Thunberg playbook) and that the 'negative health effects of climate induced crises disproportionately impact groups that are already at risk, including people of colour, people with low income, people with pre-existing health conditions, older adults and children'. They didn't explain why people of colour are more likely to be impacted by the 'devastation' they say is already affecting the planet but they did say that 'climate change disrupts the health systems ability to deliver safe, effective care.' Again, no evidence was offered for this bizarre claim.

In March 2022, the Committee on Ways and Means Chair sent out a request for information to hospitals and health systems to find out how climate events had impacted them. The conclusion from the respondents was summed up as 'The climate crisis knows no bounds' which sounds like a bad line from a very bad disaster film.

A majority of respondents told the Committee that they had experienced at least one extreme weather event in the last five years. There was no definition of an extreme weather event but I assume the respondents meant they had experienced a very windy day, a very hot day or a very cold day. I think that an analysis of people in any century would report much the same.

This utter gibberish helped prepare the ground for the destruction of medicine. And with the ground prepared, the next move was to start laying the foundation stones for the takeover of medicine and the deliberate, cold-blooded destruction of health care.

In October 2022, in a paper entitled 'How clinicians can lead climate action to protect patients and the planet', it was argued that clinicians must 'embrace their roles in creating an environmentally sustainable health care system to protect patients and the planet' and that the 'US health care system must be more proactive in mitigating climate change, and clinicians have a big role to play'.

Once again the assumption was made that global warming is real. That's really not how science is supposed to work. You can't just say 'the best way to treat pneumonia is to give patients a bowl of custard' or 'the best cure for gout is rhubarb pie'. You need evidence before making a claim. And there isn't evidence proving that global warming is real. If there was any evidence they'd use it in debates. But the bottom line is that the supporters of the global warming cult don't produce any evidence because there isn't any, and they won't debate global warming because they'll lose and that will be the end of the myth.

The paper published in October 2022 says that there are several reasons why all clinicians should get involved in reducing health care's contribution to climate change.

First, they claim that climate change leads to public health damage (though they offer no evidence) and reducing this damage is a moral, professional and public health imperative for clinicians. And that's rubbish too. Clinicians have one responsibility only: to do the best to diagnose, treat and care for their patients. That's it.

Second, they allege that clinicians are among the most respected professionals in society and can influence patient care, policy and advocacy. They say that 'their leadership role can serve as an example for other sectors that intersect with health, including food, agriculture, transportation, plastics, waste and fossil fuels.' I'm afraid I doubt that clinicians are still respected. The covid vaccine fiasco pretty well destroyed that. And I don't think that even if they are still respected, doctors have any responsibility to promote the dangerous pseudoscience that is leading us directly into Net Zero – something that is causing illness and death on a global scale.

Third, they claim that 'impact from climate change causes preventable harm to patients, the public and the planet'. Once again there isn't any evidence because there isn't any evidence. There's a lot of hot air but hot air isn't scientific evidence. The paper also states that 'Climate change impact could create harm similar in magnitude to that caused by medical errors'. I agree that medical errors cause massive harm (there is strong evidence that one in six people in hospital is there because they've been made ill by a doctor, and no one now disputes the fact that every year millions of patients are killed by doctors) but before making changes to adapt to a non-existent problem, wouldn't it be wise to deal with an acknowledged real problem (the growing incidence of iatrogenesis)?

So, what does all this mean in practice?

Well, it apparently means using environmentally friendly inhalers and yoga, and there's a lot of the usual sort of chatter about 'organisational sustainability efforts'. (I believe it is now illegal to discuss global warming without using the word 'sustainability' on a regular basis.) And there is talk of environmentally friendly products and services and the need to build awareness and enable change. The whole thing sounds like a leaflet published and distributed at a nutty conference for sandal wearing alternative health fanatics. Disappointingly there was no mention of the role of satsumas in the American recommendations.

By 2023, the medical profession was becoming more hysterical. In papers and debates it was repeatedly claimed (without bothering to produce any evidence of course) that 'climate change is the leading threat to global health'. In the UK, the solutions offered included 'moving care out of hospitals' and 'avoiding unnecessary interventions'. It was officially claimed that dealing with global warming had the support of both the public and NHS staff. Once again no evidence for this was offered, probably because none exists.

It was argued that 'one seasonal influenza vaccination has an estimated carbon footprint over 14 times smaller than the treatment of one case of influenza'.

However, this self-serving statement (guaranteed to delight the drug industry) was not accompanied by any evidence that the two are linked. How many patients who are vaccinated avoid developing influenza? (Sorry, we don't have that figure available.) How many patients are killed or seriously injured by flu vaccines? (Sorry, we can't tell you that because it's secret.) This bizarre and unscientific nonsense about the flu jab is a clue to the future they have planned for us. Our designated future will be dominated by vaccines (especially the toxic, unproven, untested mRNA vaccines) and being jabbed with yet more untested, probably toxic vaccines will be compulsory. We will be told that because of global warming we have to rely on preventative vaccination programmes.

It is stated that by discharging hospital patients earlier, huge amounts of money and carbon dioxide can be saved. There is, of course, no evidence that patients who are discharged earlier are more (or less) likely to live. And no one seems to have bothered to find out whether patients who are discharged earlier need to go back into hospital.

It is stated that 'delivering hospital care in a home setting can also bring carbon savings'. And financial savings. But there doesn't seem to be any evidence that hospital patients who are treated at home do as well as patients who are treated in hospital. Isn't this something that should be tested in properly conducted experiments rather than plucked out of the air as something that seems like a 'good idea'?

It was also stated that 'lower carbon alternatives can be sought' in hospitals. And so it was suggested that alternatives to the anaesthetic gas desflurane should be used. Sadly, I haven't found any evidence of experiments proving that the alternatives are as safe and as effective. They may be cheaper and they may have a lower carbon footprint. But do they work as efficiently and as safely? That, it seems, is the sort of question that shouldn't be asked. The policy seems to be to find ways to please the global warming cultists without bothering to make sure that the alternatives are as safe and as effective.

There is a recommendation that 'sustainable alternatives to conventional diagnostic endoscopy should be considered'. Maybe the alternatives will be better. Maybe they won't. Shouldn't alternatives be selected according to whether or not they are safer and more effective?

Newcastle Hospitals NHS Foundation Trust has apparently employed junior doctors in the specialities of paediatrics, oncology and anaesthetics and told them to devote half or more of their time to 'quality improvement related to environmental sustainability'.

Other hospitals are involved in resourcing clinical staff to work on sustainability. Sustainability officers are breeding like rats. And 'environmental sustainability' has been introduced into medical education.

Doctors' representatives claim that one of the reasons for long waiting lists is the fact that hospitals are desperately short of doctors. So, who decided that valuable doctors should spend their time worrying about imaginary global warming instead of actually treating patients?

One group of hospitals has apparently saved over 13 million miles of patient travel and 1,300 tonnes of carbon dioxide during one year by 'delivering 485,000 outpatient appointments (40% of all appointments) virtually'.

What, exactly, is a virtual hospital appointment?

At first glance it sounds as if patients at home are linked up electronically to the hospital so that they can be examined and tested and interviewed in the comfort of their own home. That's what it sounds like: an appointment without an uncomfortable chair, a five hour wait and a lending library of germs.

Actually, since no one else will tell you, I'll tell you what a virtual appointment consists of.

It's a phone call from someone in the hospital – a doctor, a nurse, a clinical assistant or quite possibly the bloke who has popped in to read the meter. A virtual appointment is a bloody telephone call. If you need to go into hospital for an operation they'll do your pre-op examination on the telephone. A telephone call is what they now call a virtual appointment. You can't check a blood pressure or listen to a heart on the telephone. But in a virtual appointment that's all you get. And when they throw you out of hospital and send you home, your post-operative check-up will consist of …guess what? You're right, a phone call again.

'Are you OK?' they'll say.

And because you're polite you'll say that you're OK even if you're not.

And that's it. Your virtual appointments may last no more than a minute. It could take up less time than a wrong number.

That's what the bastards mean by a virtual appointment.

And has anyone done any research to see whether those patients who were treated virtually were as well looked after as the patients who were actually seen in a hospital?

Don't be silly. That would probably be bad for the environment.

The Care Quality Commission in the UK now considers environmental sustainability part of its single assessment framework of health and care providers.

And it is claimed that 'those responsible for building workforce capability at the national, regional and local levels should ensure that environmental sustainability is embedded into training, professional development and guidance for all health care workers.'

What that means, in practice, is that the cult is brainwashing and indoctrinating, students and young doctors and young nurses before they set eyes on a patient. The indoctrination starts at medical school (building on the garbage students have been taught at school). Students are told it's better not to see patients in the flesh because for that to happen someone has to travel. They're told that medicine practised that way is the 'new' way.

Nowhere, nowhere, have I found evidence that patient care takes precedence over this insane devotion to the global warming cult. Nowhere have I found evidence that anyone is testing these crazy procedures to see if they save more patients or are better received by patients.

Quiet, certain, frighteningly self-satisfied, ruthless and largely uneducated and inexperienced individuals, drenched in arrogance and as uncaring as psychopaths, make decisions based on a simple lie – the lie that is global warming. Ask any of these global warming cultists to show you evidence for their belief and they will run a hundred miles at breakneck speed. They are terrified of confrontation – and that is why global warming cultists will never debate the lies upon which their actions are based.

And here's something else. They are going to cut down on using disposable gloves in hospitals. They want everyone to wear masks (which have been proven to do far more harm than good, to cost a fortune and to be bad for the environment and for wildlife) but they want to cut down on staff wearing gloves. Has anyone done trials to see if this is a good idea? Or did a 12-year-old global warming expert think this one up?

A few years ago I discovered a new disease which I called

'Maskitis'. This is the incomprehensibly stupid yearning to continue wearing a mask even though doing so is damaging both to the wearer and to those around them. Maskitis is an obvious and increasingly prevalent version of virtue signalling. The dangers of mask wearing are significant, and Maskitis sufferers are selfish and grotesquely anti-social. The damage mask wearers do to infants and children is well documented.

Medicine used to pretend to be a science. It often failed, but it used to pretend. Decisions were based on clinical observation and assessments of carefully recorded evidence. Much of the evidence was fiddled, it is true, and drug companies have always suppressed inconvenient evidence, but there was a veneer of honesty. That's all gone. All pretence at following the scientific method has been abandoned. Today, all that matters is following the dictates of those promoting the global warming myth.

The aim of health care has become cutting carbon dioxide emissions and saving money. Could these new aims be among the reasons why waiting lists have grown to a point where many patients will die before they are seen? Of course they could.

Virtual appointments have been such a huge success in saving money and cutting down travel (and, I suspect, in killing people) that virtual wards are now being introduced.

We are assured that virtual wards will enable hospital staff to monitor patients 'through physical devices and integrated software'.

Are virtual wards safe? Are they good for patients?

Well, I couldn't find any research about that but I can tell you that a great deal of information has been published about costings and costing models. The estimated cost saving per patient was £742.44. Another study found savings of over 1,100 bed days, which apparently meant a financial net saving o £529,719.

Brilliant, eh?

The global warming freaks are happy and money is saved as well.

And there's a bonus: staff who would not normally be permitted to work because they have a cough or a cold or a broken funny bone can perform light duties from the comfort and safety of their own home where they can do patient monitoring via tablet devices or laptops. How great is that? It means that huge numbers of hospital staff can work from home? They needn't travel to work at all. The patient can stay at home and the medical staff can stay at home. The two groups need never meet at all. No more bedpans, no more dirty bed sheets.

What else can I tell you about virtual wards?

Well they will be led by a GP or consultant physician. So we can be pretty certain that the patient at home in a virtual ward won't ever be seen by a doctor. GPs, remember, are too lazy to visit patients at home these days. And not visiting patients at home helps cut down everyone's carbon footprint.

And the virtual ward will operate from 8 am to 8 pm. So patients will be monitored between those hours. They won't fall ill outside those hours. Or they won't be allowed to fall ill outside those hours. No more annoying night time emergencies. People who disobey the rules and fall ill at night are allowed to die. And that's it.

And one other thing about virtual wards: patients will be involved in decision making. Actually, from what I've seen, they may well be making all the decisions.

And what about virtual surgery, I hear you ask.

Will patients be given a knife and told to remove their own appendix?

Well, we might well come to that but I can tell you that doctors have already carried out a long operation that was completely carbon neutral.

How did they do this?

Well, the surgeons involved cycled and ran to work, thereby offsetting the emissions that would have been released if they had driven to work as usual.

Great eh?

But was that enough to make the operation carbon neutral?

Well, not quite. They also planted some trees in the hospital grounds to offset their carbon footprint.

They did. They planted trees in the hospital grounds to help offset the carbon footprint involved with one operation. Three trees to be precise.

I don't know what to say. I really, really don't. I thought it was a joke and laughed out loud when I read about this. But it wasn't a joke, though I thank them for the merriment it caused.

There was other stuff too.

The surgeons seem excited about the fact that they wore reusable scrubs. Actually, we did that in hospital well over 50 years ago when I was a medical student and a young house surgeon so that was hardly innovative. And we used reusable glass syringes which were sterilised after use. I bet they haven't thought of that yet so I offer the notion as my contribution to the global warming farce.

Another popular new innovation is injecting a liquid anaesthetic into the patient's vein instead of using a conventional anaesthetic through a mask.

Surgeons have used intravenous Valium as an anaesthetic for at least fifty years so this isn't terribly new. We are told that the problem with anaesthetic gases is that they contribute to greenhouse gases. And so it is best for the planet and the United Nations obsession with sustainability if patients can be given a drug intravenously.

But is this always as safe and effective as using a gas? Can you use an intravenous anaesthetic for a patient having major surgery? Isn't it true that intravenous Valium can be dangerous? Will it be suitable for an eight, ten or twelve hour operation?

Please don't ask difficult, irrelevant and annoying questions.

Surgeons are also cutting emissions by turning off the air conditioning and the lights at night.

Really they are.

At night, when no one is working in the operating theatre, they intend to eliminate emissions by turning off the lights and the air conditioning.

Didn't they always do that?

Well, no actually, apparently they just left them on. They weren't paying the electricity bill so why bother to turn off the lights. So turning off the lights at night is a great innovation and a good way to improve sustainability. And save money I'd have thought.

And here's another thing I read.

'One year of kidney dialysis is equivalent to seven return flights between London and New York.'

So?

So what does that mean?

The only possible thing I can think of is just turning off the kidney dialysis machines. That would save more electricity; and dead people, although neither sustainable nor diverse, are very energy efficient and use up very little in the way of fossil fuel unless they are cremated or transported to the graveside in a vehicle of some kind.

Or maybe it could mean that seven global warming nutters shouldn't go to the next global warming conference.

No, probably not.

They're going to turn off the dialysis machine.

They've found another use for virtual wards.

The virtual wards which are getting everyone in health care so excited are apparently going to be great for 'older people with frailty' who can be 'monitored' at home. (Old people who are a bit wobbly are now called 'older people with frailty'.)

There are going to be Health and Social Care Coordinators who will help ensure that people who are ill (especially old people and especially, especially old people with frailty) stay at home instead of going into hospital.

If necessary, a paramedic will be able to go out to see the patient who is at home. A paramedic you note, not a doctor. I can only assume that when paramedics drive round to see a patient, they use up less fuel than a doctor would.

Actually, when I was a GP back in the 1970s and in the 1980s my partners and I, and all the doctors I knew, visited our patients in their own homes at any time of day or night. We were legally responsible for our patient for 24 hours a day and 365 days a year (366 days in Leap Years). We visited them at 4.00 am, we visited them on Sunday mornings and we visited them on Christmas Day. We routinely kept patients at home when they were ill because patients liked being at home and they often got better quicker at home because hospitals can be dangerous places and we were doctors and looking after our patients was what we did. We could be in our patients' homes within minutes of being called. (On one occasion I did get fined £5 for speeding to a patient with a suspected heart attack but we'll gloss over that if you don't mind. A senior traffic policeman gave chase and couldn't catch me but managed to get my car number.) We supervised our patients' nursing care. We sent in a district nurse to attend to dressings and to bathe patients who couldn't bathe themselves. The Meals on Wheels people took in meals which were a damned sight better than anything served up in hospital. And if a patient suddenly became too ill to stay at home, we rang the house surgeon or house physician on call in the local hospital and we arranged for the patient to be admitted to hospital. We rang an ambulance to take them there. Hospitals had an almoner who helped patients if they needed to go into hospital in a rush and needed someone to stop the milk or feed Kitty, and then helped them when they went home.

The simple truth, the bottom line, is that the modern virtual ward is about one thousandth as good as having GPs who do home visits. But GPs don't like doing home visits because doing home visits means getting out of bed and getting dressed every morning and sometimes in the middle of the night. And governments let doctors get away with being lazy and doing a quarter of a job because they want more people to die. Since global warming is a myth, there is no other explanation.

The savage truth about the future of medicine was apparent when in July 2024 the Royal College of General Practitioners in the UK finally succumbed to the lunacy and published a publication entitled 'Green physician toolkit' though it would, perhaps, have been more accurately described as 'How to kill patients, do less work and still feel good about yourself'.

The booklet began by claiming that 'climate change is one of the biggest threats to human health' (no evidence was offered for what seems to me to be an outrageous piece of scare-mongering) and is 'projected to cause an excess of 250,000 deaths per year by 2050' (no evidence whatsoever was offered for this rather bizarre and exotic proposal). Readers were warned that the UK would not be immune from the effects of extreme heat, flooding or the inevitable arrival of climate refugees. (Well it probably won't be immune to arrivals from Mars either.)

The authors of the public claim that 2022 was the hottest year on record causing 3,000 excess deaths. (Naturally, no evidence was offered for this claim which, having lived through much hotter years I do not believe for a second, and there was no mention of the fact that if the weather does become warmer then the number of people dying from cold will presumably fall from the current level of between 60,000 and 100,000. Global warming would reduce deaths not increase them.)

The UK Health Security Agency was quoted as saying that heat related deaths could increase by10,899 per year) between now and the 2050s. Naturally, no evidence was offered for this remarkably specific estimate which would, it should be noted still produce far fewer deaths than the usual cold of a British winter. It is interesting to note that the specific figures quoted are rather reminiscent of the very specific figures quoted for deaths from covid-19 at the beginning of the pandemic hoax.

It is worth remembering that in the 1980s, pretty well the entire medical and nursing establishment was forecasting medical Armageddon. It was said that every family would be touched by AIDS by the year 2000 and that deaths would be uncountable. They got that wrong, didn't they? That wild scaremongering was the forerunner of the fake covid pandemic of 2020.

You will doubtless be relieved to know that the RCGP has produced an impressive list of ways in which doctors are encouraged to deal with the alleged global warming scare. They suggest that doctors 'ensure both initiation of medication and ongoing use is decided in collaboration with patients by using shared decision making guidance'. ('Do you think I should give you an antibiotic for your pneumonia, Mrs Reeves?' 'How best do you think I should treat your cardiac failure, Mr Starmer?'). They want doctors to switch from intravenous to oral antibiotics (though this is surely a clinical decision). And there is the usual heavy duty bureaucracy so popular with global warming cultists. Doctors are encouraged 'to identify your sustainability lead clinical and the sustainability lead on the board' and to 'incorporate climate change and sustainable health care as a standing item in all clinical governance meetings'. Doctors are told to 'make sure to use the right bin' and to 'think twice before making a request (for blood testing)'. And doctors are told to reduce unnecessary prescriptions. I'd have thought that cutting out all unnecessary prescriptions should have been part of every doctor's professional life since they first slung a stethoscope around their neck in earnest.

And there is the killer (literally) advice to offer remote consultations and remote monitoring where clinically appropriate. Lazy doctors have leapt upon this advice as an excuse to stop seeing patients but actually remote consultations are never, ever appropriate.

Doctors are told that they should 'where appropriate look for opportunities to communicate digitally, thus reducing road transportation-related pollution'.

And this, of course, is why doctors no longer visit patients at home and subsequently why there is no effective health care in Britain. (Without GPs doing home visits neither the ambulance service nor Accident and Emergency Departments can cope).

There is advice to switch patients with asthma to inhalers containing a steroid (though I have not seen any research evidence offered to show that this is safe or effective). Doctors are simply told that 'Most people are open to moving to a new Maintenance and Reliever Therapy inhaler and regime when recommended by their asthma healthcare professional.' Of course they are. Most people would stand on their head in a bucket of custard if told by their 'asthma healthcare professional' that it would cure their asthma. (The phrase 'asthma healthcare professional' is used because in many medical practices it is now nurses who initiate prescribing regimes, though this can sometimes have even more disastrous outcomes than when prescribing is initiated by a doctor.)

And there is also a list of some tips from the World Health Organisation. Doctors are told to tell their patients about how global warming is a threat to their health. (Apparently four people have died in Italy due to extreme heat.) But by far my favourite tip is number ten on the list: 'Don't debate the science'.

I know I've mentioned this before in this book. But this is such a significant recommendation that it deserves to appear in neon lights.

That advice says everything doesn't it?

Don't debate the science because if you do then your patient will make you look like a fool and you'll lose all credibility.

Naturally, just about every organisation has produced its own advice. Anaesthetists have been told that inhaled anaesthetics such as nitrous oxide are potent greenhouse gases and nitrous oxide contributes to the depletion of the ozone layer. And so anaesthetists are told to avoid inhaled anaesthetics and to use intravenous and regional anaesthesia 'when clinically appropriate'.

It seems to me to be reasonable to assume that inhaled anaesthetics have been in use for over a century because they were the safest way to put patients to sleep. But, no, suddenly they must be abandoned to satisfy the nutters who have bowed the knee to the myth of global warming.

One report I saw carried the headline: 'What do doctors think of the new guidelines?'

And underneath was this answer: 'The changing climate is directly impacting our minds, brains and bodies. It's not just around us but within us, as doctors our role is to support patients to learn and understand how this will impact their individual health and our collective public health.'

And who were the doctors who said this?

Well actually it was an anonymous 'Health for Extinction Rebellion' campaigner.

Another report I saw suggested that doctors tell their patients that 'when cars burn petrol they emit toxic air pollutants that can be bad for your health. Remember to carry an inhaler, avoid busy roads where possible and consider wearing a mask outside.'

I'm not sure what this has to do with global warming but telling people to wear masks is stupid since the evidence shows that they do more harm than good. And why no warning about electric cars – the 'silent killers' on our roads?

And doctors are advised to 'be alert to the mental health impacts of climate change, including eco-distress and depression/anxiety/PTSD related to flooding'.

(Actually, of course, the mental health impacts of climate change are all the result of absurd, pseudo-scientific propaganda from global warming cultists.)

There is tons more of this but I'm afraid that even in the interests of research I can't bear to read any more of it.

Antoinette found and printed out a huge wad of waffle from medical organisations (and pseudo medical organisations) but I'm afraid I can't look at any more of it. It is meaningless drivel, written (if that is the right word) by people who have been indoctrinated and are part of a dangerous cult which seems devoted to the destruction of health care and the killing of most of the world's population.

Changes are ordered and insane proposals are made without any attempt to see if they are the right thing to do. There is no science involved. No one says 'Let's try getting rid of anaesthetic gases and see if more people die when we use intravenous anaesthetics.' No one says 'Is it safe to give steroids to every asthma patient?' There is no art, no science and no common sense in medicine any more. (And there was little enough of it in the past.)

I can't bear to look at any more of it and I'm going to take it out into the garden and have a bloody great bonfire with flames and lots of lovely black and grey smoke. (Note: to the officious: that is probably what used to be called a 'joke', a 'tease' – back in the days when such things were allowed.)

When I get back from my bonfire we will together study the way the global warming myth has already done massive damage to health care and the way that insane and indoctrinated doctors have abandoned art, science, knowledge and tradition and have instead adopted dangerous and untried policies which are, I believe, intended to kill people, and which are doing that very effectively.

Chapter Four

This chapter is a sad compendium of deceits, frauds, criminal indifference, laziness, neglect, bad practice, contempt for patients, and a planned behavioural patter which proves that the aim of the medical profession today is not to heal but to kill. In this chapter I will describe the seemingly endless number of ways in which the quantity and quality of health care have been deliberately and steadily destroyed. I will show how doctors and nurses have been lied to and deceived by a corrupt medical establishment. Everything bad that has happened has been done in the false name of global warming (as the WHO effectively admits in its advice to doctors, there is no scientific evidence for the existence of global warming) to force us through Net Zero and into the Great Reset.

Destroying health care is a vital part of a long established depopulation plan. The conspirators want to reduce the global population to 500 million. The result is that the quality of medical care is in steep decline and is now worse than it was 70 years ago.

When I was a medical student I was taught to try to find a single disease to explain all of each patient's symptoms. It didn't always work, of course. Multiple pathology is fairly common among the elderly and it is not infrequently impossible to tie up all the signs and symptoms into one neat diagnosis. But it's a good general rule, and it often does help lead to a diagnosis.

Moreover this notion can be applied to medicine in general.

It is patently clear that everything in medicine is failing: GPs no longer do night calls or see patients at home; hospital A&E departments cannot cope; waiting lists are so long that many patients will die before they are even seen by a specialist, let alone examined, diagnosed or treated. Health care today is full of examples of callousness and uncaring. A sense of vocation seems to be as rare as tenderness, sympathy or good medical practice. I sometimes get the feeling that medical and nursing training has been taken over by the ghost of Josef Mengele.

All of these problems are connected because there is a single cause. You're stuffed. I'm stuffed. But the conspirators are doing just fine, thank you.

None of these things is happening by accident. There are no coincidences.

Health care is being deliberately destroyed. And I have absolutely no doubt that this is an essential part of a global conspiracy.

Drug companies and the medical establishment have been hand in hand for years but they have now become far more lethal. Killing people is the name of the game for the medical establishment (now obsessed with the myth of global warming) and the pharmaceutical industry which is and always has been obsessed with money.

It is vital to remember that the drug industry has never been interested in curing people. There is no profit to be made out of making people better. The big profits come from making people ill, and keeping them ill for as long as possible. And so drug companies and the medical establishment (which is controlled by the drug companies) always suppress anything which might cure serious health issues. (It has since the 1970s been claimed that the drug ivermectin might cure cancer. But no solid research has been done and so this product is not recommended or, rather, allowed. I don't know what it can or cannot do and nor does anyone else. Doctors who prescribe ivermectin for cancer are likely to lose their licences. Meanwhile, pharmacological crap such as statins, hormone replacement therapy and anti-depressants, which all do great harm and no good, are recommended and prescribed with reckless enthusiasm.)

The conspirators know exactly what they are doing. Their aim is simple: they want to kill as many people as possible, as quickly as possible. The medical establishment in countries around the world traditionally consists of ignorant, lazy, greedy and people whose loyalty is easily bought and who have kowtowed to the conspirators – undoubtedly promised that they will be rewarded with great honours and much wealth and a place in the New World Order. They, in turn, have told the rank and file, the GPs and the hospital doctors, that they must reduce the number of patients they see, spend no time travelling to visit patients, stop doing out of hours visits and, to protect the planet, stay at home and treat patients via telephone calls and the internet. As a reward for having to do their morning surgery while lying in bed and their evening surgery while lolling in front of the television, and not having to work so hard, and for abandoning all their professional responsibilities, the rank and file doctors have been rewarded with vast salaries and huge fees. In Britain, for example, the average GP now works a 23 hour work and is paid £150,000 a year plus huge additional fees, including £50,000 a year for authorising vaccinations. Doctors who are able to read knew that the covid-19 vaccine was dangerous and didn't work but to their eternal disgrace they were bribed by the huge fees they were paid. (Despite this largesse, GPs in the UK have been complaining about their huge workload and the stressful nature of their lives. They also want a huge pay rise. As far as I can tell, these protests and demands have been made without any sense of irony.)

Medicine has always been an art as much as a science but in recent years the 'art' got pushed aside by the science. And now medicine isn't a science either. Medicine has become a fake science, a fraud run by bureaucrats, crooked businessmen and mad technocrats.

(It is alarming to note that in his first six months as Britain's Prime Minister, Kier Starmer set up 25 new Quangos and has ordered 67 'reviews'. I suspect that a lot of the people hired were simply chums and colleagues. No one is elected democratically to serve on these powerful and very well paid units.)

Everything is happening cold-bloodedly and quite deliberately. And there is one simple explanation for everything. As I have explained the medical establishment has (either through naivety, stupidity or corruption) been convinced that global warming threatens mankind's future. The official answer is 'depopulation'. And so medical care is being carefully and systematically destroyed.

The authorities let doctors do less work, they encourage them to kill their patients and then they say it is done to save the world from global warming. All of this is being done without any public consultation or authorisation from elected bodies. The policy to kill people, or to allow them to die, is being made by extreme left wing pressure groups. There has been no debate about the changes being made. And instead of asking doctors to measure the effects of the changes, the pressure groups have simply told doctors that they must inform patients of their responsibilities to save the planet from global warming. ('I'm not going to treat you Mrs Rayner. You have to die. But it's for the good of the planet.')

The process of destroying medical care has been going on for around 50 years – since the myth of global warming was created and adopted as a way to scare everyone and introduce the concept of Net Zero. I'm not kidding when I say that medical care has never been as good as it was 50-70 years ago.

The medical profession has always been corrupt and has often advocated and promoted treatment methods which do infinitely more harm than good. It isn't all that long ago that doctors were promoting cigarettes as a healthy way to improve respiration and fight chest diseases. But things are worse today than they have ever been. Today, it is possible to hire doctors to promote any product the drug companies put on the market. Indeed, you can hire a doctor to promote just about anything you like – and to do so knowing that he or she will do so with quiet and convincing sincerity.

The doctors who promoted the toxic covid-19 vaccine were largely paid by governments and drug companies. Most still insist that the covid-19 vaccine is safe and effective when the facts show that it is neither. The USA's own database for vaccine injuries and deaths (VAERS) showed that more people have already been injured or killed by covid-19 jabs than by all other FDA approved vaccines combined for the previous thirty years. And the USA has paid out billions of dollars in damages for vaccine damage and deaths. Frighteningly, despite this evidence, software billionaire Bill Gates, who masquerades as a philanthropist and a vaccine scientist when he is in truth merely an investor in vaccines, is now pushing for more mRNA vaccines to be used. He doesn't seem worried by the fact that the first attempt to use mRNA vaccines has been a total disaster. And that is being generous. Within days of being appointed President of the United States, Donald Trump announced that he was giving $500 billion of American taxpayers' money to a new Stargate initiative designed to build AI infrastructure and develop mRNA solutions. I assume that Trump knows that covid-19 mRNA vaccines produced more adverse effects (including deaths) than any other vaccines (though the truth about the vaccine injuries has been suppressed by the mainstream media). Any attempt to create, promote and give mRNA vaccines must surely be assumed to be a plan to murder more citizens. The medical establishment has been protecting the tawdry reputation of vaccines and vaccination programmes for many decades. Any doctor who has even dared to question the value of vaccination has been excoriated by the medical establishment (which consists of a nicely corrupted covey of self-appointed but solipsistic defenders of the universal conspiracy) and few now dare to stick their heads above the parapet. Vaccines have been protected because they are, and have always been, the almost secret weapon in the armoury of the conspirators.

Back in 2020, I warned that doctors who prescribed the then new and experimental covid-19 vaccine would likely be sued (and also imprisoned) if it turned out, as I expected, that the vaccine caused harm to those who were injected. I warned that doctors' insurers would not be able to cope and that thousands of doctors would go bankrupt.

It seems that my warning was accurate.

According to a ruling by the European Court of Justice in early 2025, all health care professionals who urged individuals to be vaccinated, or who carried out vaccinations, are both civilly and criminally liable.

It was ruled that doctors could have chosen whether or not to administer the vaccines, and could have advised against them, so they can be considered liable for their actions.

(This ruling could result in those doctors who were subject to disciplinary proceedings because they opposed vaccinations, or because they criticised the vaccines, being exonerated.)

The ECJ ruled that since doctors were not obliged to prescribe or administer the vaccines they must take responsibility for their actions.

The Court confirmed that doctors have the right to choose the safest and most appropriate treatment for their patients and doctors have a responsibility to assess in individual cases whether or not to administer the covid-19 vaccine. It seems that any national rules which conflicted with this principle were illegitimate.

It is difficult to estimate what damages might have to be paid out if patients claim that their health was severely and permanently damaged by the vaccines. It seems likely, however, that the sum per patient could run into millions of pounds/dollars/euros. I doubt if doctors' insurance companies would have enough money to satisfy millions of claims (with each patient demanding millions of pounds) and so the vast majority of doctors in the UK, the US, Canada, Australia, the EU, etc., etc., would go bankrupt. In the UK, doctors who go bankrupt because of professional misconduct may lose their licences to practice and this is probably true in other countries. The end result could well be that human doctors would have to be replaced by robots and computers. (It is important to remember that the conspirators' style is to create a problem and then offer a solution. In this instance the problem will be an absence of doctors and the solution will be their replacement with cheaper, more efficient robots and Apps on smart phones and computers.)

And if GPs are sued, it seems likely that bodies which suppressed the truth about covid might also be sued. The BBC boasted that it did not interview anyone who criticised vaccines and vaccination. And YouTube removed all my videos and closed my channel because I told the truth about the vaccine. Social media outlets banned me for the same reason. And so the BBC, YouTube, etc., etc., might all be sued for hiding the truth and suppressing vital information. Similarly, medical licensing bodies (such as the General Medical Council in the UK) might be sued and go bankrupt.

In the EU, the Committee for Medicinal Products for Human Use has recommended marketing authorisation for a self-replicating mRNA injection. It has been claimed that during the clinical trials, five deaths were reported and it is alleged that 90% of those who were injected suffered adverse events. This amount of damage again suggests that the aim of drugs, drug control agencies and doctors is now not to keep patients healthy but to kill them.

The vast majority of doctors know absolutely nothing about vaccines. They promote them, give them and defend them because they are well paid to do so. Any doctor who authorises multiple vaccinations on infants or children or who authorises the giving of the covid-19 vaccine is consumed by greed and so irresponsible that she or he should be arrested and charged with manslaughter. Sadly, this will not happen because the drug industry owned medical establishment, working for the conspirators, will always defend vaccination programmes however much evidence there is to show that they are ineffective and dangerous.

The medical establishment promotes almost anything made by the drug industry. If a big drug company made a product entirely out of pig shit, called it Pigshitium and said it was great for producing weight loss I can guarantee that doctors would queue up to say wonderful things about it.

The truth, of course, is that the medical establishment is almost always wrong.

The medical establishment always gives the impression that it is right about everything. And journalists always assume that the medical establishment is always right because it is, well, the medical establishment.

But, I repeat, the evidence proves quite firmly that the medical establishment is nearly always wrong – until it is forced by circumstances or by campaigners to change its view.

Thanks to the egregious errors made by the medical establishment (some of which I will list in a moment) doctors now kill or injure more people than cancer or heart disease or infections. Thanks to the medical establishment, one in six hospital beds are occupied by patients who have been made ill by doctors. And four out of every ten patients who receive a prescription drug suffer serious and sometimes lethal side effects.

Those who prefer to look at scientific evidence, rather than merely accepting decisions handed down by the pharmaceutical industry and passed on by the medical establishment, are dismissed as renegades and abused as discredited by people who arrogantly assume that they know everything and are always right because they're who they are.

The medical establishment makes a lot of big errors and is, indeed, wrong more often than it is right.

The medical establishment (and its enthusiastic and uncritical supporters in the mainstream media) recklessly promoted and defended the experimental covid-19 vaccines, even after the vaccines had been proved not to work but to be responsible for numerous serious side effects and many deaths. The number of deaths alleged to have been caused by covid-19 (the rebranded flu) was at least ten times larger than the real count. (National mortality statistics show this to be true everywhere.) Government statistics show that the number who died from covid-19 was almost exactly the same as the number who would usually be expected to die of the annual flu. It is telling that during the covid-19 fake pandemic, flu almost completely disappeared.

The doctors and journalists who believe that the medical establishment is always right stood firm in their arrogant certainty (a certainty based on ignorance, greed and prejudice) even as the evidence accumulated showing that they were wrong and that the covid-19 vaccines were doing a great deal of harm and no good at all.

The willingness to support and defend the pharmaceutical industry's reckless claims is bizarre since a little research would prove that the medical establishment is wrong more often than it is right. Moreover, it can easily be shown that the medical establishment is particularly likely to be wrong when it promotes a new remedy or a new diagnosis or a new treatment with uncritical and exceptional enthusiasm, while criticising anyone who dares to murmur any criticism. In addition, the members of the medical establishment will remain fixed in their collective ignorance and will never, ever debate or discuss their views with those who dare to question their certainty.

Here then are just some of the many instances when the medical establishment got it wrong in the past:

For centuries the medical establishment built all its knowledge and assumptions upon Galen's work. The problem was that Galen based all his conclusions on the anatomy of the pig rather than the anatomy of the human body.

Doctors used to believe that blood-letting was a universal panacea. They used leeches and scarifying to remove blood from weak patients and invariably hastened their deaths.

For centuries doctors used purgatives as another universal remedy. Sadly, the purgatives they used with such enthusiasm did no good and a great deal of damage.

Doctors used to treat cancer by giving patients grey lizards to swallow.

Cyanide, mercury and arsenic were all routinely used as medicaments – often with fatal results.

The medical establishment refused to accept that scurvy was caused by a lack of vitamin C until they were forced to accept the link by James Lind.

The medical establishment used to argue that smoking was healthy – and was particularly useful in the treatment of chest troubles.

The medical establishment's approach to nursing and hospital management resulted in a 42% mortality rate in the hospital at Scutari. After Florence Nightingale arrived, and shocked the establishment with her methods, the death rate fell to 2%.

Until nitrous oxide was used as an anaesthetic, doctors used to give their patients alcohol before performing operations.

The medical establishment promoted barbiturates as safe and effective – until doctors were forced to accept that barbiturates were dangerously addictive. (Before the barbiturates they claimed that bromide was safe – and were wrong about that. After the barbiturates they claimed that benzodiazepines were safe – and were wrong about that too.)

Doctors routinely prescribe anti-depressants despite the existence of a mass of evidence showing that they don't work.

The medical establishment approved of electric shock therapy. And then it was found that electric shock therapy was useless and dangerous.

The medical establishment used to promote the removal of yards of intestine. And then they found it was dangerous. Today, surgeons remove healthy sections of intestinal tract to 'help' slimmers, and remove perfectly healthy breasts to prevent breast cancer.

The medical establishment supports psychiatry and psychotherapy, despite the evidence showing that talking to a hairdresser or barman is more likely to be useful than talking to a psychiatrist or a psychotherapist. Similarly, behaviour therapy used to be popular. Until it wasn't.

Heart surgery (particularly bypass surgery) used to be considered essential for patients with heart disease. It has now been shown that most of the time it does more harm than good.

The medical establishment used to promote brain destructive

surgery (such as frontal lobotomies) until it was shown that these did massive harm.

The medical establishment favoured the use of Intensive Care Units and Coronary Care Units but these were shown to cause massive stress in vulnerable patients. The result was that some patients were better off being ill at home.

Doctors used to prescribe amphetamines for weight loss until the amphetamines were shown to be dangerous.

Thalidomide was approved and promoted by the medical establishment.

Doctors ignored hygiene in the operating ward and the delivery room until they were forced to change their working methods by doctors such as Wendell Holmes, Semmelweis and Lister.

Doctors enthusiastically prescribed massive quantities of drugs such as Opren, Distalgesic, phenylbutazone and practolol until they were shown to cause serious side effects.

Doctors used to give patients convulsions and treat them with modified insulin therapy until the medical establishment finally accepted that therapies were dangerous.

The medical establishment used to approve doctors who gave hallucinogenics such as LSD to patients.

The medical establishment used to treat the mentally ill by punishing them until it was shown that this did no good at all and was, indeed, counterproductive.

Steroids were routinely and excessively prescribed for children with mild asthma – until the serious side effects became clear. (Doctors are now once again using steroids to treat asthma – because they are said to cause less global warming than the drugs which have been used for the last few decades.)

The medical establishment used to recommend routine tonsillectomies, circumcision, back operations and hysterectomies – until it was found that the operations often did more harm than good. Similarly, operations for hernias were performed unnecessarily until they too were found to cause too many problems. And D&C was a routine operation for women until it was discredited.

Radiation was thought by the medical establishment to be harmless until it was shown not to be harmless and to need to be treated with great care – both in X-ray form and as radiotherapy.

And so on and on and on.

I could provide hundreds if not thousands of similar examples proving without doubt that the medical establishment is dangerously corrupt and is nearly always wrong until it is forced to change its collective, dishonest mind. The establishment is more concerned with the financial wellbeing of the drug industry than with the health of the patients it is paid to protect.

Today, of course, the medical establishment (and the mainstream media) promotes the covid-19 vaccine – despite the fact that it is useless and dangerous and its introduction and dissemination is undoubtedly part of a conspiracy to terrify and to kill billions of people.

The bottom line is that the medical establishment is always wrong until it is forced to change its mind. In a few years' time the establishment will (in the remote chance that they are allowed to do so by the conspirators who now control our world) accept that the covid-19 vaccines are toxic and dangerous. 'How could we have possibly known?' they will ask, pitifully. I hope someone points to the videos I made in 2020 in which I warned, in precise and accurate detail, of the problems the vaccines would cause. Sadly, by then it will be too late for the people who were killed or injured by the vaccine.

People don't know all these things because the conspirators, who control the drug industry and the medical establishment, own the mainstream media. All battles about the truth are propaganda battles. The conspirators demonise and lie about free thinking truth tellers. TV and radio stations and newspapers have become propaganda vehicles.

Life is full of puzzles.

Some mysteries cannot be solved.

For example, why do supermarkets always stock the same number of custard filled doughnuts as they have of jam filled doughnuts when they must know that the jammy ones always disappear first – leaving a pile of the custard filled variety.

Store keepers must know that most people want the jam ones so why do they order equal quantities of both?

That's a mystery to which I doubt if I will ever find a solution.

But some mysteries are more easily solved.

For example, it isn't difficult to see what the coronavirus hoax was all about.

The lockdowns, the masks, the social distancing, the closure of hospital departments, the closure of schools, the closure of businesses and the absurd restrictions on our free movement had absolutely nothing to do with a virus known to be no more deadly than the flu.

Anyone who says this in public is, of course, immediately demonised as a conspiracy theorist and bullied and libelled everywhere.

But it is clearly the truth – and it's a truth which the establishment, those promoting the myth that covid-19 was a serious, deadly global pandemic did not want spreading.

Actually, the truth is a rare commodity these days.

The chaos that was caused around the world is unnerving – and the greatest threat to humanity since the Black Death. The difference is that the Black Death was a natural disaster. The covid-19 hoax was contrived, artificial and deliberately exaggerated. As always these days the hoax was global – affecting citizens in the US, Germany, France, Italy, Australia, New Zealand, Canada, Brazil, the Middle East, UK – and so on.

The disaster in Africa went almost unnoticed and yet it was truly a disaster of unimaginable proportions killing millions. This man-made disaster was always going to be worse than any natural disaster; worse than any tsunami, any plague or any volcanic eruption.

African countries introduced lockdowns and did all the stupid things they were told to do.

And inevitably things went terribly wrong.

Cases of malaria and tuberculosis went undiagnosed and untreated and both are now spreading and killing millions. Maternal mortality soared and so, did infant mortality. Around 10% of Africa's population will descend into extreme poverty. The number of deaths from starvation has soared. Was that really by accident? Of course not! It was part of the depopulation plan. In 1980, three billion people went to bed hungry. Today, despite or because of the efforts of the United Nations and its various bodies, the figure is higher.

Proof that the chaos was avoidable comes from Malawi. The wise government there did not impose strict lockdown rules even though the prediction was 50,000 deaths. The result was that out of a population of 19 million, there were just 176 covid deaths. And that is yet more proof, to add to Sweden and Japan, showing that the lockdown measures were a total disaster. Curiously, at one point even the World Health Organization announced itself to be opposed to lockdowns.

So, apart from killing people, and thereby helping to reduce the size of the world's population, what was the point behind the covid-19 arranged hysteria and carefully orchestrated panic?

The answer, of course, is simple.

The plan was to disrupt our lives and redesign the world to suit the Agenda 21 lunatics, and to please the billionaires who are still greedy and want to be trillionaires. I believe that people like the Clintons and Obama in the US and Blair in Europe have been behind much of what's been going on – though these are just the handmaidens of the elite conspirators (the Rockefellers and the Rothschilds).

The plan was to alter the social fabric of every country in the world, to ruin the financial security of everyone not already a billionaire, to abolish private property, to destroy health care, to eliminate privacy and to terrorise the world into accepting a new world order. (It is worth noting that the UK Government excluded hedge fund managers and city deal makers from the quarantine rules.)

The elite want to reinvent teaching and to put an end to education. Schools are going to be turned into prisons and will eventually disappear entirely. In the future, education is going to be controlled through the internet. Closing schools was part of that plan. Teachers who voted to keep schools closed were doing precisely what the billionaire conspirators wanted them to do.

The aim was, and is, to force populations everywhere to accept mandatory vaccines – preferably an endless series of mRNA vaccines. The idea was to push us into a position where the majority would queue up and bare their arms to risk their lives for a hope of some normality. In future, medicine is going to consist of regular, mass vaccinations and very little else. Vaccinations will become compulsory. Those who do not have up-to-date vaccine passports will be locked out of the digital world which the conspirators have planned.

They will use vaccination programmes to control all movement and stop us travelling. They want to put an end to private cars – though they may let a few valued individuals to operate electric cars. They will control electricity supplies through smart meters. Trains, aeroplanes and buses are doomed. They want to store us in high rise towers in twenty minute cities. They want to close the countryside to us and keep rural areas empty.

Our food will be made in factories, not grown on farms for they want us to stop eating food grown the old-fashioned way.

I haven't eaten meat for over 30 years and I have campaigned for decades to stop animals being farmed for meat but I am desperately concerned about the changes being made to our diet. How safe will all this new food really be?

I have real doubts about the safety of genetically modified food but unless we grow our own food that's what we will be forced to eat.

They want to change the way we work – with millions of jobs being handed over to robots. Those training as doctors, lawyers and teachers have a decade's work ahead of them at best. They will all be replaced by computers and the internet.

They want us all to be dependent upon the state. With everyone receiving a fixed weekly wage – just enough to live on.

They want us to live in tiny, poorly built apartments. They want to remove ambition and hope from our minds. They want us to learn to blame ourselves for everything that goes wrong. People who feel ashamed are easier to control.

And, more than anything perhaps, they want to reduce the world population by 90% or so. Billions are going to have to die though I have a suspicion that there aren't going to be many politicians or billionaires lined up in the world's morgues.

They want to introduce a global social credit programme (such as has already been introduced in China) so that we are penalised if we misbehave and rewarded if we do as we are told. We will be penalised for what we eat, how much we spend or even who our friends are. Everything we do will be watched and assessed. The World Economic Forum planned the social credit programme used in China and we will be next.

They want to crush and destroy all opposition. They want to

eradicate the elderly and the sick. They want to eradicate national sovereignty. And in Europe they have been using the European Union to do that.

They want to increase the role of the State in raising children.

Much of this has already started.

Hospitals have for some time now been putting 'Do Not Resuscitate' notices on patients over the age of 65 – or in some places over the age of 45.

I know that there have been plans for a one world government for centuries. I know how far back the evil can be traced. But Agenda 21 (updated to Agenda 30 for Sustainable Development when the first deadline passed), and the immediate threat to our humanity and our survival, is more recent.

It really got going with the formation of the United Nations at the end of World War II.

Then there was the formation of the Club of Rome in 1968 and the World Economic Forum which was originally founded in 1971 and which changed into its present form in 1987.

In 1976, the United Nations quietly announced its plan to control the world's land and to manage the world's population.

The World Commission on Environment and Development first announced its commitment to sustainable development in 1987.

And then in 1991, the Club of Rome announced that since humans are very often best motivated by an enemy of some kind they would need a global enemy – something the citizens of every country could share.

And they chose global warming – to which they allied food shortages and water shortages.

The beauty of this was that they could blame us for everything that happened. We were our own worst enemy.

We could be targeted as the authors of our own downfall.

And then in June 1992, at a conference in Rio de Janeiro, a total of 178 countries signed up to a plan to target global warming. The plan was put forward by an oil and mining billionaire.

Bang.

That was it.

I know all about the evil people who have been trying to control the world for centuries. And I know about the current links to the Luciferians. It seems that even the United Nations has a bizarre

Luciferian link.

But the problem we face at the moment really came to the fore in the last half a century. The bad people have been working on it since then. Global warming has been the key they have used to open up the new normal – the global reset – the new world order.

Many have been distracted by a number of problems which were built up to take our attention.

But we're awake now.

We know what the plans are.

They want to take us through the destructive horror of Net Zero and into a Global Reset.

They want to kill most of us and change the lives of the remainder to fit their purposes.

The medical profession is being used to do much of the killing.

Food shortages are already a huge problem in the UK. Indeed, for many, basic foodstuffs are becoming a luxury and the cost of a weekly food shopping bill has soared. The problem is mainly the weather. Constant wet weather and grey skies mean that most of Britain's food has to be imported – at huge expense. The wet weather is simply yet more proof that global warming is a myth. The grey skies have been caused deliberately by the geo-engineers spraying powder in the sky to block out the sun. The end result will be that we all have to eat the factory produced food being prepared by the billionaires. For farmers the end is nigh. Soon farmers won't have to worry about the U.K. Government's new inheritance tax because there will be nothing to inherit.

The global warming cult was invented because a small group of toxic conspirators believed that the world is overpopulated and cannot produce enough food. There is ample evidence to prove this is nonsense. If it were true, why have farmers throughout Europe been paid NOT to produce food but to set aside valuable farm land? For many years farmers have been paid to do nothing on vast acreages of their land. And why do global warming cultists now want 75% of all land to be abandoned to 'nature' and allowed to be overgrown with weeds?

The enthusiasm for vaccination is probably the most unscientific aspect of health care. It is more akin to witch doctor medicine than anything relating to science. Vaccines are not properly tested before being used and no tests are done to see if vaccines are compatible with one another or with other prescription drugs. No long-term tests are done to see how much the immune system is affected. And, perhaps most bizarrely of all, the same dose of a vaccine is given to everyone – children and adults, men and women, young and old. No attempt is ever made to alter the size of a vaccine dose according to the size of a patient. It is well known with other drugs that size and age are significant factors but doctors make no account of these differences. (Actually, of course, no attempt is made to titrate dosage against weight or age with most drugs. So, for example, the same, standardised dose of antibiotic will be given to an 18-year-old weighing 7 stone as will be given to a 45-year-old man weighing 28 stone or a 90-year-old woman weighing 6 stone. You don't have to understand much about medicine or science or the human body to realise that this is unscientific.)

But here is the killer.

No one has ever tested to see if all the different vaccines are safe when given together.

No one has tested to see if vaccines are safe when given with commonly prescribed drugs.

No one teaches vaccinators to pull back the syringe to check that they are not injecting straight into blood vessel. (I warned about this before the mass vaccinations with the covid-19 vaccine began. I believe it was this mistake which led to the deaths of patients within minutes of being vaccinated.)

No one checks to see if diseases such as cancer are commoner among the vaccinated than the non-vaccinated.

The assumption is that vaccines are good and anyone who asks questions will be branded an anti vaxxer – which the conspirators want regarded as a form of terrorism

In 2025, a British television company seemed proud of itself for 'exposing' a scandal relating to the drug diethylstilboestrol. This isn't a new scandal, of course. It was many decades ago, back in the last century, that I first exposed the scandal of a drug called diethylstilboestrol which was given to women in the 1960s and 1970s. It wasn't until much later that it was found that the drug caused breast cancer in the women who took it. Even more worrying was the discovery that the drug caused adenocarcinoma, a type of vaginal cancer, in the daughters of women who took the drug. My worry today is that doctors are using new drugs (such as the mRNA vaccines) without any idea of the short, medium or long term consequences. Will the mRNA vaccines cause problems for the children of the people who were vaccinated with it? I don't know and nor does anyone else. I am sure that the covid-19 vaccine is causing rapidly growing cancers among the generation who took the drug. But what about the next generation?

If vaccines really worked the authorities would not be promoting them. After all, the politicians and the medical establishment (controlled by the conspirators) want us dead. Why would they want to inject us with something which might protect us from ill health? Vaccines are given because they injure and kill.

It should be remembered that most of the health professionals who gave the covid-19 vaccine to the naïve, the gullible and the fearful did not have the jab themselves. They knew that covid-19 was merely the annual flu. And they knew that flu vaccines are worthless at best and often do more harm than good.

There is good reason to believe that all cases of poliomyelitis being diagnosed in the world today, and for the last 40 to 50 years, were caused by the polio vaccine. If medicine were a science this would be debated. But medicine isn't a science and so it won't be mentioned or discussed.

In the 1660s, the richest doctor in England was a man called Thomas Willis. His most popular prescription was a drink made of the dung of horses, pigeons, cocks and oxen. Patients with jaundice were given a tonic made of sheep and goose dung. He recommended rat droppings as a cure for constipation. Special patients, the ones who could afford the treatment, had dog shit smeared on their chests.

If there had been any medical journals around at the time they would have doubtless published enthusiastic accounts of these remedies. And if drug companies had been invented they'd have bottled rat droppings and sheep and goose dung tonics on the market before you could say 'thank you doctor'.

Willis wasn't the only doctor around with exotic prescriptions to offer. A Dr Cotton believed in putting dead pigeons on the heads of his patients. In 1689 he put a dead pigeon on the head of a woman with convulsions. The pigeon remained in situ for five days, quietly rotting.

Nothing much changes, does it?

Today, thanks to science, (most) doctors no longer tell their patients to drink medicines made from horse shit. Instead they inject their patients with scores of different products which are just as daft, and potentially far more dangerous, as the dead pigeon treatment. The products they inject with such enthusiasm have never been shown to work or to be safe – especially when given, in vast quantities, to babies and small children.

These 21st century dog shit remedies are called vaccines, and doctors are so enthusiastic about them that dissent is not allowed. Indeed, any orthodox trained medical doctor who questions their efficacy or safety is likely to lose his or her licence to practise.

(The funny thing is, however, that in the UK only 27% of health care workers allow themselves to be given the flu jab. The other 73% say 'no thanks, I'm not having that toxic rubbish injected into me'. The authorities complain about this but they shouldn't be surprised. After all health care workers see what happens to the gullible who allow themselves to be jabbed.)

However, it is clear to anyone with functioning brain tissue that to claim that vaccines in general are not linked to autism, brain damage and immune system problems is like arguing that vehicles are not linked to road traffic accidents.

So, for example, the scientific and statistical evidence shows that to claim that the covid-19 vaccine has saved many lives and done more good than harm is an absurd and indefensible lie. (However, the UK's Covid Inquiry still refuses to allow me to give evidence – evidence which would prove that the whole inquiry is a sham.)

Doctors who insist on vaccinating their patients are ignorant, crooked or easily bought.

I would heartily recommend that if your doctor wants to vaccinate you then you should tell her that you'd rather have a pigeon put on your head, if it's all right with her. A pigeon on your head might not cure you but it'll be a damned sight less likely to kill you than a vaccination. And, just for the record there is as little evidence assessing the value of the pigeon-on-the-head-regime as has been done to assess the value of mass vaccination.

When will any network TV or radio station have the courage to set up a live debate (with me on one side and the entire medical establishment on the other) to assess the value of vaccination? The debate must be live to be fair and national to be significant.

The title of the debate could simply be: 'Does vaccination do more harm than good?'

And let the public vote at the end of the debate.

At the end of the debate one side or the other will be permanently discredited.

If I lose I'll look a fool.

If the pro-vaccination supporters lose then governments, drug companies and doctors will have to apologise and pay out trillions of dollars in compensation. They'll also have to close down a multi-billion dollar industry.

And so I'm afraid that my challenge will never be accepted.

Governments, drug companies and the medical establishment don't have the courage to debate because they know they will lose.

And the very absence of any debate proves that vaccination is dangerous and useless.

If parents don't do with their child what the State orders them to do (have them vaccinated at the right time, for example) then representatives of the State (with guns if necessary) will take the child away and arrest the parents if they dare to complain. This is happening all around the world.

In several States in the USA, hospitals can now do what they like with patients, and relatives (however close) have no rights. Hospitals have been putting DNR notices on patients without anyone's permission and so patients are effectively kidnapped, poisoned and murdered. No one is allowed to protest or stand as an advocate for an infirm or mentally ill patient. Protests merely bring in security officers and lawyers. Hospital staff see the disabled, the mentally ill and the elderly as helpless and without rights. This is medical murder on an industrial scale. And it's being done partly to save money but mostly to speed up the depopulation programme which is justified by the mythical risk of global warming.

Long, long ago doctors didn't always tell patients if they had a serious disease such as cancer. They made a judgement about whether or not the patient could cope with the news and then used euphemisms to soften the blow. These days, doctors seem to take great delight in telling patients the worst news in a very blunt way. (Though there will always be a nurse on hand with a box of tissues ready). Doctors don't sugar coat their diagnoses and they offer little in the way of hope. It is a sin not to offer all patients some hope. When I was a GP I had two patients with terminal illnesses who lived for many years after they had been abandoned by hospital doctors. There is good anecdotal evidence that many patients lived much longer when they didn't know what was really wrong with them. Susan Hill, the writer, tells how her mother was told she had 'ulcers'. She had a kidney, a large section of bowel and bladder and her uterus removed. The surgeon told Ms Hill's mother that she would get well and she did – enjoying three years of excellent health. And then a friend referred to the illness by name. Susan Hill said that her mother was horrified and 'shrivelled and died in eight weeks'. A doctor who works a good deal with cancer patients said this: 'Tell the patient the truth, but only as much as they can bear and never, ever, remove hope.'

When I was a young hospital doctor I sometimes prescribed alcohol for patients who could not sleep. I actually used the hospital's prescription sheets to write out a prescription for a glass of sherry or a glass of Guinness. Patients received one glassful and no more. You might find this surprising or even shocking. But today, in nursing homes, care homes and hospitals, the staff are allowed to give addictive benzodiazepine tranquillisers to patients who cannot sleep – and to give these powerful drugs without a prescription from a doctor without telling the patient or asking their permission. 'Just take this,' insists the staff member (who may or may not have any qualifications). And the patient accepts and swallows. At least when I prescribed sherry or Guinness the patient knew what they were getting.

In the UK, civil servants have used the term 'digital native' when recruiting new members of staff. The term 'digital native' implies that an applicant has grown up with the internet. This policy has meant that citizens in their 50s and older are not represented in or by the civil service and their interests are not represented when decisions are being made. This blatant ageism is responsible for much wider concerns relating to ageism and the way that older citizens are mistreated.

My book on vaccines (*If anyone tells you vaccines are safe and effective they are lying: here's the proof*) so worries the authorities that it has been widely attacked and suppressed ever since it was first published. It has for years been the world's best-selling book on vaccines but it has never been reviewed, discussed or even mentioned in any mainstream publication. Joe Biden's White House tried to have the book banned. No one has ever successfully disputed any of the facts the book contains. Indeed, it is probably because the book is accurate that they want it banned. (Quite a number of my books have been banned. The books usually come up as 'unavailable' which is apparently the euphemism of choice. The Chinese Government banned all my books. I would rather my books were burnt. At least then they have a moment of existence and one or two may escape the flames. Modern, ruthless bans mean that books tend to disappear completely. I used to be a bestselling author in China and I wrote a column for a massive selling newspaper. I wrote an article on vaccines. The Chinese Government duly banned all my books and banned all publishers from publishing any of my books. And, of course, my column disappeared. I used to have publishers and agents in 26 countries. The words 'used to' are significant. They've all gone.)

Doctors are frighteningly ignorant about the side effects associated with drugs. This can only be because doctors are effectively taught and controlled by the pharmaceutical industry. I have been retired from medical practice for some years but whenever I talk to doctors I am astonished at their ignorance and inability to understand basic medical issues. Most doctors do not, for example, understand how infections are spread. (This is why infections run through hospitals quickly and regularly.) Most doctors didn't understand that the covid-19 test was useless and dangerous. And most didn't realise that during the so-called pandemic there were no more deaths than there are in a normal year. Most didn't realise that the majority of deaths blamed on covid-19 were actually caused by something else. (Patients who were diagnosed as having covid-19 were said to have died of covid-19 even if they had been run over by a bus. The test for covid-19 was, of course, entirely useless and misleading.) And doctors' ignorance about side effects is, to be honest, scary and bordering on terrifying. I once discussed a particular drug's side effects with a consultant oncologist who looked at me as if I were insane before dismissing the side effects as impossible, saying: 'The drug isn't intended to do those things.'

Medical schools are designed to protect and perpetuate myths. Any student who asks difficult questions or who questions the status quo will be in danger of failing her or his exams. Big questions, which might threaten the status quo in some way, are not welcome. Teaching programmes are narrow and designed to avoid upsetting the pharmaceutical industry. Any student who shows signs of caring or being passionate about medicine will be thrown out. If this were not the case the current batch of junior hospital doctors would not have gone on strike (for more money) with such apparent enthusiasm. Today's young doctors have more in common with train drivers than with healers.

The medical establishment has raised several generations of health care professionals who have been trained not to care much about anything except themselves and money and who are devoted to doing as little work as possible, paying as little tax as possible, taking no responsibility for anything (except themselves) and never, ever questioning authority except when they think that by doing so they may be paid more money for less work.

There seems to me no doubt whatsoever that the change in the way students are trained was planned to fit in with the newly developed plan to cut back health care and to turn medicine into a killing profession.

Allowing GPs to stop doing home visits, to stop night time or weekend calls and to remain shut on bank holidays mean that GPs now work the sort of hours that part-time librarians work. Their consulting rooms are shut on all weekends and holidays and are not infrequently closed to patients for up to four days at a time. It is clear now that GPs were allowed to change the level of their availability to patients as part of the plan to destroy health services.

The medical establishment is, of course, aware that it is the closure of GP services which is responsible for the flood of patients seeking help from overcrowded Accident and Emergency departments. It is the same problem which is putting great pressure on the ambulance service. It is absurd to claim (as is now claimed belatedly) that allowing GPs to stop doing home visits has anything to do with alleviating global warming.

Patients who need medical help (and who could be visited at home by a GP) now need to visit the surgery or, if their doctor is one of the many now refusing to see patients at all, to visit their local hospital. The closure of small, local hospitals (in England sometimes quaintly known as cottage hospitals) means that most patients live much further away from their local hospital and, therefore, the number of miles travelled has increased not fallen. But then the cultists promoting the nonsense known as global warming have never been known for their intelligence. (And global warming is a 'cult' not a science.) The closure of local hospitals, by the way, was a deliberate though early part of the destruction of health care. At the same time as small, local hospitals were closed, local nursing services (whereby district nurses were regularly available for the home treatment of patients) were also cut back or relegated to history.

The number of beds available in British hospitals has been falling in roughly the same proportion as the immigrants pouring into the country has increased the population. At the same time as the number of beds has fallen, the number of nurses has also fallen and the number of highly paid administrators has increased dramatically. This is no accident but yet another part of the plan to reduce the quality and quantity of professional health care.

You're not going to believe this but I promise you it is true. There are plans afoot to create virtual accident and emergency departments. Patients who are sick or injured (and who have been betrayed and ignored by their 23 hour a week general practitioners and who must therefore seek help from their local hospital) will not need to go to the hospital at all. (Or, rather, they will not be allowed to go to the hospital). There is talk of community response teams being set up in the hope that they will reach people's homes within two hours. (As a GP I always reckoned to be in someone's home within 15 to 20 minutes if I was called out. If the caller said it was an emergency I could usually get there more speedily.) Where the response team is not considered necessary, patients will be given advice on the telephone. ('Do you have sticking plasters and aspirin in the house?' 'Can you sew?')

The trouble with doctors today is that they have no dignity and they have no respect. They have no self-respect and they have no respect for their patients. They have no sense of vocation. They have no sense of what is right and what is not right. It has always seemed to me that the primary guiding principle for any doctor is that he should provide his or her patients with the type of care that she would hope would be provided for herself or her loved ones if she or they were sick. I cannot believe that today's doctors behave that way.

The Department of Health and Human Services in the USA has reported that about 6% of the 130 million people admitted to Accident and Emergency hospitals in America each year are misdiagnosed. And around 2.6 million of those are harmed as a result. Please read that sentence again. Read it aloud to anyone standing or sitting within hearing range. You will not be surprised that a recent Boston study has found that Chatbots are now better at diagnosing patients than both doctors and Chatbot-assisted doctors. AI can deal more effectively with all sorts of patients. Through their incompetence and their lack of care, doctors have opened the door for AI controlled medicine. The snag, of course, is that using AI to replace doctors would probably require more electricity than America has available. The current AI system, popular with students having their homework done for them, already uses up 16% of all America's electricity.

Today, well over twice as many people are killed in hospitals by infections as are killed on the roads.

It isn't difficult to understand why.

Filthy wards, unhygienic practices, scandalously poor cleaning (I've seen ward cleaners merely sweep dust and dirt under the hospital beds), grubby operating theatres and staff who never wash their hands is the reason there are more serious infections in British hospitals than anywhere else in the world.

If you live in Britain and have to go to hospital for any operation or procedure, you now have a 50% chance of getting a worse disease from being in the hospital. That's official. And if you do survive the experience and get to go home there is a 20% chance that you will leave malnourished. I find that quite astonishing. One in five National Health Service (NHS) patients leaves hospital officially malnourished. Some patients don't eat because the food is inedible and looks unappetising. For others the taste and quality of the food is irrelevant; they stay hungry because no one helps them eat it. Staff dump food on a patient's table and then collect it, untouched, half an hour later. The patient, starving hungry, hasn't eaten because he or she was too weak to reach the food. Staff even put food in front of semi-conscious patients and then walk away. And so, in the 21st century NHS, patients slowly starve to death. One NHS patient who was blind couldn't see the food put before her. No one bothered to tell her that the food was there or to feed her. NHS hospitals are now so badly run, so filthy and so unprofessionally managed that they are likely to do more harm than good.

Nurses will no longer feed patients in hospital because they claim that feeding patients is beneath them and unfitting for their new professional status. Staff members who are not nurses are not allowed to touch patients – they are only allowed to sweep the floor around the beds and, occasionally, if they're lucky, help themselves to a biscuit or a chocolate from the boxes which are always available at the nurses' station. (Ward offices are considered old fashioned)

The nurses who won't feed patients won't help them drink either. It is, therefore, commonplace for someone to deliver a tray full of food to a bed bound patient, place it on the bed tray and then remove it, untouched, half an hour later with the words 'Weren't you hungry, love?' The patient, hungry and thirsty can only murmur a gentle protest. If a patient is in hospital and seriously ill they will probably die of starvation unless relatives or friends go in to feed them. When my mother was ill in hospital with normal pressure hydrocephalus (which nine neurologists failed to diagnose until it was too late – even though the diagnosis was given to them) my eighty odd year old father had to drive to the hospital three times a day, every day, to feed her.

It sounds unbelievable but the evidence has shown for years that many patients who have heart attacks are better off staying at home than going into hospital. As hospitals become increasingly overcrowded and badly run this is truer now than ever before.

It is, of course, the failure of GPs to provide a 24 hour service which is one of the reasons why hospitals cannot cope. Accident and Emergency departments are full with patients who could have been dealt with in five minutes with a visit from their GP.

None of this is happening by accident. The plan to depopulate the world by killing the old, the weak, the disabled and the frail has been going on for some years. The apparent failure of health services has been managed deliberately and cold bloodedly.

The astonishing thing is, of course, that those who are destroying health care, suppressing essential truths, promoting lethal lies and providing services designed to kill rather than cure (and who are recommending or giving dangerous vaccines which they must know will do more harm than good), will also suffer from the consequences of their actions. And their loved ones will suffer too. Maybe those involved, the servants and handmaidens of the elite, believe that they will be invited to share the world being reserved for the billionaire conspirators. I'm afraid they are wrong.

There is now a well advanced plan to get rid of anaesthetics as you and I know it. The safety of surgical procedures, and even childbirth, will be dramatically reduced. A 'gas and air' mixture known as Entonox was commonly used for pregnant mothers giving birth. It had very few side effects and was widely used. Specialist obstetric anaesthetists recommended it but it is now being abandoned because of fictitious global warming.

Safe anaesthesia for general surgery is being abandoned. You'll be lucky if you get a stick put between your teeth to bite on. New techniques are being used to replace the old ones but please don't expect anyone to have done research to compare the new ways of putting patients to sleep with the old, well-tried techniques.

I've known for some time that climate change cultists are wicked and insane. Despite wild claims which are made by the medical establishment there is no evidence that global warming endangers mankind. Like the fake covid pandemic and the pseudo-vaccine, it's a confidence trick. But the cultists will do anything for their cause.

The medical establishment is planning to stop using well tried, safe, anaesthetic gases and replace them with anaesthetics which aren't as safe or as well tried – or with nothing.

Spokespersons for the medical establishment claim that traditional anaesthetics such as gas and air are bad for the environment. A few wicked, dangerous global warming cultists want more sustainable anaesthetics to be used in operating theatres, dental surgeries and delivery wards – even though patients are going to suffer and thousands of people are almost certainly going to die as a result.

The cultists want to replace traditional anaesthetics with what they call 'sustainable anaesthetics' and the favourite seems to be sevoflurane – because it is allegedly a bit kinder to the weather than the traditional, safe for humans stuff.

Now let me tell you about sevoflurane.

It can't be given to patients who have heart disease, heart arrhythmias, kidney disease, lung disease or liver disease or a pile of other problems. And it's not safe for use in patients taking any one of nearly 200 well-known prescription drugs – though of course how many doctors will check before giving the damned stuff? None is my guess.

So you've got to be really fit and healthy and not taking any pills for it to be safe.

What other alternatives are they offering?

Well you can have a local anaesthetic. The sort you have if you need stitches in your finger – though this will probably not be much fun if you're having an open heart operation or your compound fracture sorted out.

Or you can have an intravenous injection of a drug such as ketamine or midazolam or some other benzodiazepines such as Valium. Midazolam is, of course, part of the infamous kill shot already used to murder countless thousands of older folk. And the problem with intravenous benzodiazepines is that they can be very tricky to use and do have a tendency to kill people.

In addition to claiming that anaesthetic gases cause global warming, the cultists claim that gases might harm nurses and doctors although there is no evidence that that has ever happened. This bit of scaremongering has, I suspect, been designed merely to encourage doctors and nurses to abandon well tried and tested techniques and to introduce new forms of anaesthesia or to revive old methods such as the bottle of whisky and the stick between the teeth.

I didn't mind the climate change cultists so much when they were just flying off to conferences or gluing themselves to policemen. They're stupid people who have been brainwashed and wound up by the conspirators like toy soldiers marching to oblivion. They've been suckered by the pseudo-science and by the bought and paid for mainstream media.

But what is happening with anaesthesia is seriously insane. The cultists who believe in this horrendously dangerous pseudo-science won't debate it. As with the toxic pseudo jab – the covid-19 vaccine – the mainstream media has been paid to promote the fraud. Everything is being forced through at breakneck speed. The conspirators, the globalists are pushing this through as part of the Great Reset. Health care must be destroyed – unless you're a billionaire or one of the chosen few. The climate change cultists want to drag medicine back several centuries and at their behest we're heading back to the Middle Ages. And so if you really need an operation (and you're not too old) well, maybe they'll bang you on the head or give you a slug of whisky or laudanum.

The medical establishment has stated categorically, and without bothering to produce a shred of evidence, that global warming is the most serious medical emergency in the world today. They've said that to protect us all from global warming, doctors must do fewer diagnostic procedures and treat fewer patients. If you thought the long waiting lists and delays were accidental, think again.

Doctors who sell out, lie and do not bother to think for themselves (and their patients) are well rewarded – both financially and reputationally. Those who do their own research, think for themselves and are honest are punished and eventually destroyed.

General practice in the UK was reorganised a few years ago. The result is that the vast majority of patients end up seeing a different doctor every time they need medical help.

It has been shown that (as all patients and all doctors over the age of 50 already knew) it is much better for patients if they see the same doctor every time they visit a surgery (or, more likely, enjoy the delight of an internet zoom consultation or a diagnostic chat on the telephone).

A review by Exeter Medical School found that patients were more likely to be candid about their symptoms, live healthily between consultations and complete courses of treatment if they saw the same doctor every time they sought help. The Exeter study analysed the results of 22 different studies carried out in nine countries. The conclusion was that seeing the same doctor meant significantly fewer deaths.

And so we should not, I suppose, be surprised that exactly the opposite is now happening. A patient who seeks medical help will just see the doctor they're given. Or, since the average family doctor now works a derisory 23 hours a week, they will see the nurse or practice assistant to whom they are allocated. (Assistants may or may not have any medical training.)

The system is not designed to heal people. It is designed to kill people. And it's doing that very well.

The quality of health care in Britain has deteriorated to such a point that it is probably fair to warn visitors that Britain no longer offers health care. The mentally ill are dumped on the streets without any treatment other than large doses of benzodiazepine tranquilisers or antidepressants (neither of which work). And the physically ill must take pot luck.

And the consequences are often fatal.

A 28-year-old student nurse who fell ill died after waiting 12 hours to be seen in an Accident and Emergency unit. She arrived at 10.14 pm but did not receive an X-ray until 7.30 am the following day. She died of bronchopneumonia and septicaemia. She was, let me remind you, just 28-years-old. A 43-year-old mother of four died after her planned surgery was cancelled three times at the last minute. She died of an obstructed bowel, and the coroner said that she would have survived if she'd been treated earlier. Actually, maybe she'd have survived if she'd been treated at all. In the UK, the Royal College of Emergency Medicine has predicted that at least 14,000 unnecessary deaths (a year) are due to delays in Accident and Emergency departments. The Labour Government has, entirely for political reasons, de-prioritised emergency care in order to reduce waiting lists for non-urgent treatment.

Britain's health service hospitals are the new killing fields of Europe.

In the UK in 2024 it was revealed that failed asylum seekers, undocumented migrants and asylum seekers were being given priority in NHS hospitals. They were allowed to skip waiting lists for treatment and be seen within fifteen minutes in Accident and Emergency departments. All these immigrants were given full health assessments, treatments and referral to consultants without any delays. Illegal immigrants were also being given immediate access to GPs and dentists. It is difficult to avoid the feeling that this plan was devised to create racism and discontent among tax payers who had paid huge sums for the failed health service in the UK and who were often forced to wait months to see a GP, years to see a consultant, years to be diagnosed and years to start treatment. Anyone who questions this practice, or who dares to question any aspect of immigration, will be dismissed as being Far Right, will be condemned as racist and, if they share their views too widely, may well end up in prison.

After the UK Government stopped giving the annual heating

allowance to pensioners, the Health Secretary advised impoverished pensioners to turn on their heating and wrap up warm in the cold weather. On another occasion a second MP, the Labour Party's Health Minister, told a pensioner who didn't vote for his party that he hoped she would die before the next election.

Hospital accident and emergency departments routinely put elderly patients at the back of the queue to be seen. Anyone over 70 has to wait until younger patients have been seen. The result is that older patients (however frail they might be and however serious their problems might be) often have to wait days to be assessed (let alone treated). And so an increasing number of elderly patients (with broken hips, chest infections, heart attacks and strokes) die before they are seen – even though their problems may be easily remedied. Ambulance services are just as bad. A 95-year-old woman was left on a cold pavement on Christmas Eve in 2024 despite having a broken hip. She waited, lying on the pavement, for more than five hours. An 84-year-old man lay on his driveway with a broken hip for three hours before an ambulance arrived. It seems that broken hips (particularly in the elderly) are no longer considered a priority. Heart attacks and strokes aren't considered priority illnesses either which rather begs the question about what precisely is considered a 'priority' illness worthy of a ride in an ambulance. (Though if an illegal immigrant fell and had a broken finger nail they would receive immediate priority treatment so maybe the answer for those who need an ambulance is to struggle to speak English and to say they've just arrived in England after a long and perilous boat journey across the Channel.)

Pensioners with progressive diseases are losing health care funding for vital care. The elderly come first in the queue when cuts are being made. No one has said what constitutes an elderly patient. In some hospitals 50 is considered elderly. This is, of course, a breach of one of the basic principles of medical care which is that patients should be seen according to the seriousness of their illnesses or injuries. This is what triage is all about. When I was a student in the 1960s, I attended a meeting at which an American doctor had described how appalled he was to discover that hospital doctors had treated riot policemen before demonstrators when there had been injuries after a demonstration. It was generally agreed that this was a serious breach of one of the basic tenets of medical practice. And yet this is how hospitals now operate. And no one seems to care.

At the end of 2024, undertakers admitted that they were busier than ever. They said a big thank you to the doctors still prescribing the covid-19 vaccine – unofficially the world's most toxic and useless pharmaceutical product.

There is much bewilderment among intelligent doctors and scientists as to why so many doctors kept quiet about the lies being told when the covid-19 hoax and the fake pandemic unfolded.

So, why did so many doctors kept quiet about the covid-19 vaccine and continued to prescribe a product which has been accurately described as the most dangerous and damaging single pharmaceutical product ever marketed? The covid-19 jab did not do what the establishment promised it would do but, at the same time, it caused countless thousands of deaths and serious injuries among the patients who were injected.

There are two explanations for the fact that so many doctors ignored the evidence and did what they were told to do by dishonest advisors within the medical establishment and bought and paid for journalists and celebrities.

The first explanation is that all over the world doctors were extraordinarily well paid to give the covid-19 jabs. Hospitals were given bribes (labelled as bonuses) which were dependent upon the number of patients they injected. Doctors were bought off, and dissuaded from asking too many questions, by being paid well over the normal fees for giving vaccinations. Those doctors will, in due course, appear in court where they will be unable to mount any sort of defence. To say that they behaved unprofessionally and greedily is a massive understatement.

The second explanation is that doctors were too terrified to speak out against the medical establishment because they saw what had happened to colleagues who dared to share their views with their colleagues and the general public and who had had their licences removed by the official licensing authorities and, in addition, been vilified by the media.

The truth, so well hidden during the last three years, is that the medical establishment was, as it has been for decades, controlled by the pharmaceutical industry and instead of looking at the facts, licensing authorities around the world merely did as they were told to do. Numerous doctors lost their licences, and their livelihoods, because they dared to speak out and tell the truth. The majority of doctors, seeing what had happened to those who spoke out, kept quiet and betrayed their patients, themselves and their profession. Those gutless wimps should be ashamed.

In the United Kingdom doctors are licensed by the General Medical Council, an organisation which is, in theory at least, a charity but which appears to have some of the worst qualities of a quango, a government department and an enforcer for the drug industry. I believe that drug companies control governments, they control the medical establishment and, it appears, they may also control the UK's medical licensing authority – the General Medical Council.

Fifty years ago, the General Medical Council was infamous for providing the Sunday newspapers with a regular diet of scandal and sleaze. The GMC specialised in striking off doctors who had been found abusing drugs or having sex with their patients. Occasionally, they would take aim at doctors who could be accused of advertising.

(I should mention, at this point, that in the 1970s, I attracted the attention of the GMC as a result of my writing a series of novels which I had written under a pen name. Responding to a complaint from a drug company, the GMC wrote to me and I was threatened with the removal of my name from the medical register. Since I was at the time an NHS GP with no private patients and since the novels had been written under a pen name which was a fairly well-kept secret (if not, apparently, from the GMC) the case against me fell apart quite quickly. This did not, however, prevent the GMC from targeting me on other occasions when they received complaints from drug companies which objected to my more academic books (such as 'The Medicine Men' – published in 1975) in which I had exposed the close links between the pharmaceutical industry and the medical establishment. Over the years I have been subjected to a constant stream of unsuccessful complaints and lawsuits from drug companies.)

More recently, the GMC has become infamous for its extraordinarily one-sided defence of the exaggerated covid pandemic and the pointless but enormously dangerous covid vaccine.

When the fake pandemic was first promoted with enthusiasm in February and March 2020, I immediately described the covid scare a hoax. The figures available proved without any question that the danger of what was clearly merely a rebranded annual flu had been massively exaggerated by people who had a bad track record at assessing the relevant figures. In the UK, the Government's own official advisors agreed with me, dismissing the covid-19 infection as being no more dangerous than the annual flu. Their expert advice appears to have been ignored in favour of advice from a mathematician with a terrible track record.

I have been writing about drug companies and medical deceits since the 1960s and I can spot a medical fraud a mile away. Naturally, the conspirators behind the exaggerated risk (and I use the word conspirators deliberately) did not like my description of the covid scare as a hoax (a video I made with this title was seen by many millions within days) and I was quickly demonised and lied about in the media. The GMC couldn't take away my licence because their own administrative rules meant that, as with many doctors, my retirement from active practise meant that I'd had to give up my licence. But younger doctors, those still in practice, were to feel the full wrath of the drug company controlled medical establishment.

So, for example, consider the case of Dr Mohammad Adil who was a respected surgeon working in the NHS. When Dr Adil criticised the Government line on covid, the GMC responded by taking away his licence – meaning that he could no longer practise as a surgeon or, as a doctor in any capacity.

Today, Dr Adil still doesn't have his licence. The cost to him has been extraordinary. And we should not forget the cost to the NHS. If we consider that in that three years he could have performed 1,000 operations a year – not an unlikely number – then his banishment means that thousands of patients have been denied the operations they needed.

Dr Adil is not alone. I know of several other doctors in the UK who have had their licences removed for criticising the absurd and indefensible covid policy. (Later I wrote to the three judges on the

Court of Appeal on Dr Adil's behalf but I did not receive a reply and Dr Adil did not win his appeal.)

Exactly the same thing has been happening around the world where licensing authorities have ignored the scientific evidence and punished doctors who have dared to share the truth with the world – usually on social media. It is this unscientific bullying, and the widespread publicity given to the consequences, which has contributed to the fact that thousands of doctors who share their doubts and fears have kept quiet – frightened that they too would lose their licences and their livelihoods. A doctor without a licence to practice is as useless as a sweep without his brushes or a taxi driver without a cab.

On the other hand, it is extraordinary that the GMC appears to have taken no action whatsoever against doctors who did not care about patients but allowed themselves to be bribed to vaccinate with an unnecessary and dangerous drug. Nor has it punished doctors who went on strike, demanding an inflationary 35% pay rise, and abandoned their patients – thereby breaking every moral, ethical and professional commitment.

The GMC's decision to deny Dr Adil his licence was always unjustifiable.

First, there is the question of free speech. Article 19 of the United Nations Charter states clearly that 'everyone has the right to freedom of opinion and expression'. There is no codicil limiting the rights of doctors. The GMC's decision is in direct opposition to this fundamental human right. It has been argued that doctors have a special responsibility because of their position and training but this strengthens rather than weakens the UN charter. Doctors have a special responsibility to speak out when they believe that something is wrong. And, of course, you can't have a little bit of free speech any more than a woman can be a bit pregnant. You either have free speech or you don't. To say that a doctor cannot criticise the medical establishment is as nonsensical as saying that an opposition party politician cannot criticise the Government. The licensing authorities which have removed doctors' licences for speaking out are undeniably in breach of the UN Charter. How a lawyer or a judge can justify allowing any licensing body to deny an individual's right to protection from the UN Charter is, I confess, a mystery to me. Doctors are entitled to share their views with the public and the public is entitled to decide whom to believe.

It is worth noting, by the way, that right from the start, in early spring of 2020, the doctors supporting the Government and drug companies steadfastly refused to debate in public and the mainstream media took an entirely biased, unbalanced one-sided line in reporting the fake pandemic. The BBC even stated that they would not interview anyone questioning the value of vaccination whether they were 'right or wrong'. I have frequently challenged vaccine supporters to a live, national public debate. None have had the confidence or the courage to accept the challenge.

Second, the GMC has assumed that the Government and the medical establishment must always be correct and beyond criticism. This is dangerous nonsense. One doesn't have to go very far back in history to find numerous examples of times when the Government and the medical establishment have been completely wrong and, as a result, patients have suffered until doctors had the courage to stand up for the truth. When Dr John Snow gave chloroform to Queen Victoria there was an uproar in the medical establishment because it was felt that women should not be given anaesthesia during childbirth. Electroconvulsive therapy, leucotomies and the removal of vast lengths of the intestine were all approved by the medical establishment but later condemned. It was because of the medical establishment that tonsils were removed without good reason. No one knows how many children died as a result. A good deal of unnecessary heart surgery has been performed on patients because of bad medical practices promoted by the medical establishment. It was because of bad medical practices condoned or encouraged by the medical establishment that millions of patients became hooked on barbiturates and then benzodiazepines. And I wonder how many of those who have condemned Dr Adil know that widely used and previously approved vaccination programmes have been condemned as worthless and dangerous.

History shows that the medical establishment has been wrong more often than it has been right, and if the GMC stops doctors criticising the Government and the medical establishment (known to be linked to the pharmaceutical industry) then nothing will ever change for the better.

If we go back a little further in medical history we come across individuals such as Dr Semmelweiss whose work on women lying in labour wards changed medical practice and saved thousands if not millions of lives. Dr Semmelweiss was, of course, viciously attacked by the medical establishment. There are many more examples in my book *Medical Heretics*.

The undeniable truth is that history shows that the medical establishment has always suppressed the truth and promoted profitable lies. Nothing has changed. The medical establishment still promotes medical procedures which don't work, while suppressing essential but inconvenient truths. The GMC's fundamental mistake appears to me to have been to have assumed that its loyalty should be to the pharmaceutical industry and the medical establishment rather than to the welfare of patients.

Third, and more directly perhaps, the evidence now shows quite clearly that the medical establishment's official line on covid-19 was completely false. Everything that the establishment has said and done has been wrong and dangerous. The General Medical Council and all those who supported its decisions seemed to have assumed that the establishment was right.

If they had looked closely at the evidence they would have known that the UK Government's own scientific advisers decided, back in March 2020, that covid-19 was not a major threat. They would have known that Government statistics show that the number of people who died from covid-19 was no greater than the number who die from flu every year (a disease which had mysteriously and conveniently disappeared). Indeed, the number of deaths from what was clearly a rebranded flu was no greater in 2020 and 2021 than it was in some previous years. Moreover, it is now clear that the absurd policies of lockdowns, social distancing and mask wearing were without any scientific foundation, were unnecessary and dangerous and were in part responsible for the entirely predictable increase in deaths which marked 2022 and will continue for some years to come. The PCR test was never intended to be used as it was, and has been proven, beyond any doubt, to be of no more value than a coin toss. It is clear that the closing down of schools and businesses was also entirely unnecessary and has done massive, long-lasting damage.

Worse still, it is now abundantly clear, and generally accepted by intelligent, well-informed doctors and scientists, that the covid-19 vaccine was never properly tested, was never fit for purpose and is the most dangerous and deadly pharmaceutical product ever marketed. Largely because of links with the pharmaceutical companies involved, the Government and the medical establishment misled the public and the health professions.

Finally, there is one other rather shocking reason why the GMC should not have made any rulings about Dr Adil or any other doctors who criticised the official line on covid-19 and the covid-19 vaccine.

Remarkably, it seems to me that the General Medical Council has itself been behaving quite improperly. Its disciplinary actions must surely now come into question.

The General Medical Council (in my view one of two big enemies of patients in the UK – the other is the British Medical Association) has invested nearly £1,000,000 in fast food and drink firms and, worse still, has invested large amounts of money from doctors' fees in drug companies. And one of the companies in which it had shares was one of the companies making a covid-19 vaccine.

How can the GMC judge doctors' behaviour in relation to covid and covid jabs when it has a vested interest in the financial success of vaccine manufacturers such as Astra Zeneca?

It seems to me that it cannot.

I believe that any doctors who have lost their licences for criticising the fake pandemic and the toxic covid jab should be reinstated immediately since the GMC is clearly 'contaminated'.

It could surely be argued that the GMC, which has money invested in vaccine manufacture, has a vested interest in protecting vaccine making and should not, therefore, discipline doctors whose actions might have damaged the earning potential of any companies in which it has invested its own money.

The GMC can be compared to a judge punishing someone for criticising a product in which he himself has a financial interest. Indeed, I would argue that the GMC, and its vast army of overpaid, and, it seems to me, sometimes arrogant, pen pushers has abandoned its role as a guardian of the public and become an enforcer for the pharmaceutical industry.

Those doctors who had the wisdom to see that the Government and the medical establishment were wrong, deserve praise not punishment.

Those who had the courage to speak out should be applauded and it is they, not the promoters of a 'vaccine' that does not do what it was promised to do but which has caused many deaths and much illness, who should be honoured.

In a free and progressive society, criticism of the establishment should never be subject to censorship.

My conclusion can only be that the General Medical Council is unfit for purpose and should be closed down immediately. It is not fit to hand out dog licences, and certainly not equipped to control the licensing of doctors. It has failed to do its job: to protect the public and it appears to me to have acted more in the interests of the pharmaceutical industry than the interests of patients.

I believe that other licensing bodies around the world may, on investigation, be shown to have similarly failed their publics and I hope that they too will be investigated.

Actually, the General Medical Council became a serious threat to patients even before it took upon itself the duty of destroying the careers of the few honest doctors in Britain.

There was a time, not long ago, when British GPs provided the best home doctor service in the world. Patients could telephone their doctor 24 hours a day, seven days a week (including Christmas Day), ask for a home visit and get one. Patients prepared to visit the surgery could expect to see a doctor the day they called.

Those were the good old days.

Today, it is easier to find a plumber than a doctor at nights and weekends. The absence of out of hours GP services means that patients wanting emergency help out of office hours must visit their nearest major hospital and spend hours queuing in the A&E department. In some areas the waiting time is 16 hours. In practice, patients may be forced to lie in an ambulance, parked outside the hospital, for more than a day before room can be found for them in the accident and emergency department. Patients who might otherwise have been saved are dying while waiting for treatment.

It is generally assumed that the sudden deterioration in the quality of general practice is the result of the deal done between the Government and the British Medical Association, the doctors' trade union. The deal allowed doctors to opt out of providing night and weekend cover and, for most of the country, spelt the end of the traditional 24 hour a day cover. Those who looked a little closer assumed that the deal was itself an inevitable result of EU employment laws which regulated the number of hours employees could work.

But although the EU laws are partly responsible for the sudden deterioration in the quality of the NHS they aren't the whole answer; there is another organisation which deserves a good part of the blame: the General Medical Council.

The General Medical Council, the GMC, seems to me to behave as an enforcer for the drug companies and the Great Reset.

The GMC used to consist of a little more than a file clerk, who kept the register of doctors who were qualified to practise medicine, and a committee of rather pompous individuals who sat in judgement when erring doctors were accused of 'having extra marital relations' with their patients on the consulting room couch.

In those simple days, the filing clerk kept a list of doctors and stored the list in a couple of filing cabinets. Every year the GMC published a couple of thick, red books which listed all the doctors on the medical register. The whole thing cost next to nothing to run. As recently as 1973, the GMC's total income was £662,579. I doubt if that would pay the current organisation's phone bill.

Today, in contrast, the GMC is a vast organisation with a huge budget and a seemingly insatiable yearning for power. It employs a host of administrators with ideas well above their station, though most have little or no experience of medicine in practice.

The new GMC does nothing to improve the quality of medical care (it does nothing about dirty hospitals, the over prescribing of antibiotics or the fact that doctors are now officially encouraged to murder elderly patients who have been in hospital for too long) but its staff constantly make statements about how doctors should practise medicine. So, for example, the GMC has decided that it no longer approves of the Hippocratic Oath, which it considers rather old-fashioned, and it has happily overseen the disappearance of the principle of medical confidentiality.

The real problem with the GMC, however, is that it has been given the job of licensing doctors. And as a result, the GMC probably kills more people than influenza. It is no stretch to say that the GMC is such a threat to the nation that it should be classified as a terrorist organisation.

For no obvious reason, but probably in order to satisfy Agenda 21 requirements, it was decreed that some form of regular testing should be introduced so that doctors in practice could be assessed.

The GMC was given the job of finding a new way of assessing medical practitioners and designed an entirely bureaucratic system (called 'revalidation') which was guaranteed to increase its own power and its own income. The inept, the incompetent, the corrupt and the cruel will pass the test easily. Drug company cheerleaders will sail through. The revalidation scheme is perfectly suited to the dishonest, the cheat, the silver tongued and the rogue. Revalidation appears to have been designed to ensure a massive deterioration in the quality of medical care and a dramatic increase in the number of patients dying unnecessarily.

To pass their appraisal, doctors have to fill in reams of forms and find a few dozen patients and colleagues prepared to sign report cards. The scheme is a bureaucrat's dream and a practitioner's nightmare; it seems to have been designed by the sort of people who have six ball point pens in their breast pocket and its rigidity has made life unbearably difficult for thousands of doctors, such as locums, ships doctors and retired practitioners, who do not fit neatly into the system.

Some parts of the revalidation procedure astonished me. So, for example, the GMC asked for details of all my motoring offences – which included details of a 1984 speeding offence and a £5 fine I received in 1977 when an officious policeman spotted me hurrying to a suspected heart attack patient. (My astonishment abated when I discovered that Ms Lindsey Westwood, who was in charge of the GMC's revalidation programme was, just two years prior to these enquiries, working for the Traffic Penalty Tribunal as an appeals manager. I found it staggering that the person the GMC had put in charge of checking the fitness to practice of every doctor in Britain had previously been checking parking tickets for a living.)

The GMC's power and money grab has been enormously successful; they've designed a scheme which has built them an empire. Doctors now have to pay the GMC a huge sum a year to be registered and licensed. There are fees for everything imaginable and the power and money grab has been enormously successful. The GMC has a multi-million pound income. And the income is guaranteed to grow.

The problem is that by distracting doctors from the work they should be doing, the revalidation scheme will, I believe, result in vastly more deaths than before.

The GMC's new method of assessing medical practitioners has made many doctors hate their jobs and it is pushing doctors into early retirement, with a growing number choosing to retire in their 50s. Doctors already had enough forms to fill in. The revalidation scheme has turned doctors into full-time form fillers. A survey of GPs showed that 78% thought that the revalidation programme was a waste of money.

In the 'old' days, a doctor who retired would often work at his former practice as a locum; covering for holidays or sickness. His expertise, local knowledge and intuition would not be lost. In local emergencies, such as a flu epidemic, he could be called upon to help out. But the GMC's new revalidation scheme makes that impossible. Once a doctor has retired he can no longer practice at all. The doctor who retires at 55 must stay retired. As a result locum doctors, many of whom don't speak English properly, have to be imported, at enormous expense, from other countries.

The GMC isn't just killing patients; it's destroying the NHS too.

It is perhaps not surprising that the GMC now provides private medical care for its staff.

According to Seamus Bruner in his book *Controligarchs* (which I thoroughly recommend): 'Most of the thought policing which resulted in suppressing the views of doctors questioning the covid hoax and the covid vaccine, came from Big Tech's social media monopolies – namely, Twitter, Facebook, Instagram, Google, and YouTube. People noticed that videos were taken down, posts were slapped with warning labels or outright deleted, and users were suspended en masse.'

Mr Bruner goes on to add: 'As it turned out, the pharmaceutical companies were coordinating with the tech giants. Big Pharma operatives were specifically concerned about their patents and an activist movement that sought to make the vaccines free to all. They contacted Twitter employees requesting an intervention. Twitter then shielded Big Pharma accounts, including Pfizer's and Moderna's, from negative posts…'.

It wasn't just the drug companies, of course. President Biden openly spent $267 million on censorship and Biden's White House tried to have my book on vaccines banned. I believe that the bottom line today is that if a video creator producing videos with medical content has a channel on YouTube then they are approved by the CIA and the drug companies. Today, my website www.vernoncoleman.com is constantly blocked and hidden. (My other main website www.vernoncoleman.org had to be taken down after a 'bad actor' succeeded in infiltrating the site.) One reader visited my website recently and a notice came up on his screen saying: 'Do you really want to visit this site?' No one has ever found any errors of fact on my website or in my videos.

A writer is his own currency and depends upon his reputation to survive. My reputation was deliberately devalued for the modern crime of sharing the truth.

There is no doubt that the incidence of many cancers is increasing among young people. And many of the cancers which appear are fast growing 'turbo' cancers. Doctors looking for an explanation refuse even to consider that the covid-19 vaccine may be the cause and journalists obediently also ignore the link.

The BBC, which is a government run propaganda machine if ever there was one, does what it is told, reports what it is told to report, suppresses what it is told to suppress and demonises and lies about those it is told to demonise and lie about. The BBC has succeeded in carving for itself a dominant position in British broadcasting because it never has to worry about earning any money. It receives funding from the Government and also collects money from citizens by a protection racket called the licence fee. (Not paying the licence fee is, bizarrely, a criminal offence. Those who do not pay the fee are likely to receive threatening letters and visits from hired thugs and eventually taken to court and possibly imprisoned.)

Independent publishers, website owners and broadcasters are at a huge disadvantage for they must try to collect revenue to sustain their operations. The BBC is even allowed to sell a range of books, magazines and DVDs which it ruthlessly promotes. The aim of the BBC appears to be to control the news and to protect the conspirators.

It has been suggested that the British Government should introduce a 'kitemark' scheme to give approved news content a UK regulatory stamp of approval. Some media executives claim this would be the end of news. But there is no news in the mainstream media – only propaganda.

Many alternative news organisations on the internet are receiving funding from pressure groups and drug companies. Even if writers and editors give their time and work for free it costs at least £1,000 a year in regulatory fees and so on to run a modest website. Major sites admit that only 0.1% of their users will give any money. So if a site has 20,000 regular users only 20 are likely to give money. If they each give £20 the site will receive £400 a year. Even big internet sites which have a million regular visitors do not receive enough money in subscriptions and donations – and so (like fact checkers) many must rely on advertising and sponsorship and on payments from drug companies, foreign governments and others. You can probably spot which websites, podcasts, etc., have sold out by looking to see how professional and well-staffed they seem to be when compared to the number of readers or listeners they have. Most of the sites, platforms, podcasts on the internet are compromised in some way. In my view anyone who discusses medical matters on YouTube must be approved by the drug companies and the security services.

Intimidating or coercing a civilian population is called terrorism in the USA. So those who promoted the covid vaccine with lies are terrorists.

There is no doubt that the incidence of many cancers is increasing among young people. And many of the cancers which appear are fast growing 'turbo' cancers. Doctors looking for an explanation refuse even to consider that the covid-19 vaccine may be the cause, and journalists obediently also ignore the link. The simple fact is that anyone who doesn't even consider the role of the mRNA vaccine in the development of these cancers must be a bought and paid for drug company shill.

One survey showed that 19% of vaccinated children suffer adverse reactions. But doctors still keep giving vaccines and defending them, and the medical establishment bans doctors who try to share the truth. Criticising the medical establishment (and the liberal left) is a career killer.

The Government in the UK constantly tells patients to call 999 if they or anyone in their home shows signs of having had a stroke. The Government says that it is vital to get rapid treatment for strokes. And the Government's advice is wise. Unfortunately, patients now often have to wait days for an ambulance (particularly if they are elderly). Indeed, the official policy in the UK is that patients who have 'merely' had a stroke won't merit an ambulance and will have to make their own way to hospital. And if they do eventually reach a hospital they will have to wait hours or, more likely, days to be seen. The only remaining question is this: should patients who have a stroke drive themselves to hospital or should they ride there on their bicycle? And I suppose it would be nice to know what medical conditions are regarded as serious enough to warrant an ambulance.

Back in 1974 it was decided that there must, in future, be the same number of female doctors as there are male doctors. There is no law ruling that there should be as many male nurses, models or ballet dancers as there are female nurses, models or ballet dancers but there is a rule that there must be as many women doctors as there are men doctors. It was decided that this absurd and extraordinarily sexist law would be enforced by introducing sexual discrimination into medical school selection policies. More female students were accepted than male students. As a result, well over half of all new medical students are now female. The aim is not just to produce as many women doctors as male doctors but to make the total number of women doctors equal to the total number of male doctors. Since there have traditionally been far more male doctors than female doctors, the changes are being made quickly and dramatically by training more women than men. Forcing medical schools to take a greater percentage of girls than boys has been disastrous; there are always fewer girls than boys applying and so medical schools have struggled to match their quotas. Moreover, there are far fewer women who genuinely want to be doctors – and students who aren't driven by a real vocation make terrible doctors. Naturally, no one dares protest about this obscene and dangerous example of sexual discrimination, despite the fact that it is producing very real problems. The decree that medical students should be selected not according to vocation or intellect but according to chromosome resulted in massive changes to the whole philosophy of medical care and, allied to the changes in working hours introduced as a result of legislation introduced by the European Union, destroyed the concept of continuity of care. I have no doubt that the insistence that medical schools give preference to women is one of the fundamental reasons for the deterioration in the quality of medical care. Women doctors want to work part-time; they want to be home when their children come in from school, they want to be there to make tea, they don't want to work at nights or at weekends or on bank holidays. They want to have a year off every time they have a baby. The result is that most female GPs prefer to work only part of the time. And so the average working week of a GP is now 23 hours. And it was largely because female GPs didn't want to do house visits or out of hours calls that GPs stopped providing 24 hour cover for 365 days a year. This change has destroyed health care by putting pressure on hospitals (particularly Accident and Emergency Departments which must now do the work previously done by GPs) and on ambulances. I find it rather difficult to believe that the people who insisted that the number of women doctors should be massively increased did not foresee this problem.

Doctors are preparing the way for AI doctors and robot doctors. It has been shown that computers and robots are better at all forms of treatment than human beings. Robots perform surgery more reliably, more safely and more effectively and prescribe treatments such as drugs with fewer mistakes. And, surprisingly and disappointingly, robots and AI 'doctors' offer more empathy and sympathy than human beings can manage. Students just beginning their medical education are probably wasting their time because there won't be any need for human doctors by the time they qualify. The same thing goes for student nurses for robots can do everything a nurse can do but can do it better. The conspirators and the medical establishment will find it as easy to programme AI 'doctors', 'surgeons' and 'nurses' to kill patients who are regarded as useless or unnecessary as it did with human practitioners.

Euthanasia is being introduced worldwide (and as usual, when this happens, you can tell that the conspirators are behind the development). And, of course, in every country, the same lies are told by those trying to 'sell' euthanasia to the indigenous population. The people promoting euthanasia say it is painless, quick and efficient. They say that euthanasia will not be offered to children or the mentally ill or to people who are simply poor or unemployed. They say that no one will be coerced. All these are lies but, of course, there is never any adequate public debate and so these lies are not exposed. It is worth noting that execution by injection has been reported to be far from painless. Individuals who are injected with the drug used to induce paralysis may still be able to think, for example, and are often in great distress. Giving a drug to cause paralysis has been used as a form of torture.

The conspirators used lockdowns and school closures to create depression among teenagers (and, indeed, younger children). These depressed young people (many of whom are still depressed and anxious) will be perfect candidates for euthanasia programmes. Nothing is happening by accident. Everything is planned.

In some countries euthanasia is offered to patients suffering from manic-depression (aka bipolar disease). When patients are in a down phase they will be more likely to accept euthanasia.

Hospices everywhere are being closed for lack of funding. When hospices close, the patients are invariably offered euthanasia as an alternative. In the UK, hospices were hit by a new tax in the Labour Government's first budget. The new tax meant that even more hospices would have to close. The new tax was designed not to affect government employees in any way. The Government then followed up with new laws guaranteed to ensure that even more hospices closed. And as if all that wasn't enough the Labour Government reduced their funding. The dire straits of hospices everywhere is all deliberate, in an attempt to push the sick into euthanasia.

Millions of elderly people have no access to the digital world and do not even have access to the internet. Such citizens are a hindrance to those who are desperate to create a digital world. This is another reason why cultists want to get rid of them, why they are withdrawing health care from the elderly, why they are encouraging the elderly to enrol in a euthanasia programme and why they are putting Do Not Resuscitate (DNR) notices on their medical records if they are admitted to hospital. (When doctors and nurses try to persuade patients to refuse resuscitation they often claim that resuscitation is painful and can frequently leave the patient with severe injuries. These are lies.)

It should be understood by everyone that euthanasia is being introduced worldwide because it is part of the depopulation plan. That is the only reason for it. Chris Whitty, the Chief Medical Officer in England, said that people must not face a bureaucratic thicket if they chose to die.

Kim Leadbeater, a British MP, who introduced a private members Bill entitled 'Terminally Ill Adults (End of Life) Bill has said that 'someone feeling they are a burden has a legitimate reason to apply for euthanasia'. I like the word 'apply' because it makes the whole thing sound like joining a tennis club. Leadbeater's Bill is worded to limit the number of applicants but Britain's membership of the European Convention of Human Rights means that in practice almost anyone will be entitled to apply. (It is illegal to offer something to one group of people only.) Leadbeater will choose members of a House of Commons committee to discuss her Bill, which will be voted on by MPs who won't, I suspect, have the foggiest idea of the implications of what they are voting for or against – or, indeed, the long-term and global implications of what they are voting for or against.

MPs (most of whom knew very little about the subject) voted for the Bill but probably thought that they were merely allowing the Bill to begin an arduous journey before becoming law.

The next step in turning the Bill into law was for a committee of MPs to look into the issue more closely. The committee has the responsibility of scrutinising the Bill. But Ms Leadbeater, who introduced the Bill, had a considerable amount of power over the committee. In fact she chose who would sit on the committee and most of the MPs she picked, and who have a known view, voted for her bill.

And she picked the witnesses who would give evidence.

The witnesses were picked in secret and I'd bet that a surprising number of the witnesses backed euthanasia.

As I have already explained, doctors have been deliberately killing people for years.

First, there was the Liverpool Care Pathway – a scheme whereby doctors were allowed to kill off the elderly, the frail, the vulnerable and the sick if they were considered to be an unproductive waste of space. The Liverpool Care Pathway was supposed to have been discarded. But it hasn't been. Doctors still use it to kill patients who are regarded as a nuisance.

Second, there were the Do Not Resuscitate notices which were and are used as an excuse to kill anyone who has an illness which needs a lot of medical or nursing care. Patients are supposed to be given the option of whether or not to agree to a DNR notice. 'Sign here and if you feel poorly we'll put you out of your misery'. Note the word 'supposed'. In practice doctors, and especially nurses, slap DNR notices on anyone they decide should be dead.

And then came Leadbeater's 'Kill by Doctor' Bill – in my view, the official approval of genocide; the slaughter of the innocent and the infirm – the very people doctors should protect. I believe it is a Bill which will put an end to the final vestiges of dignity and decency in medical practice. Doctors are supposed to care for patients, not to kill them.

There is, I fear, one point that Leadbeater's committee might not hear.

Nine out of ten people who attempt suicide and fail will not die of suicide. They will change their minds and often live long and successful lives.

Many, many famous and enormously successful people have tried to commit suicide and failed. The world would be a sadder and bleaker place if they had been allowed to take advantage of a legalised euthanasia programme.

Euthanasia is being promoted as offering dignity and control.

But in a growing number of countries all over the world the same lies are told and everything you think you know about euthanasia is almost certainly wrong.

Euthanasia is about saving money, collecting organs for the super-rich, killing disabled children, killing the mentally ill and reducing the money spent on caring for the poor and the disabled and patients in pain. Euthanasia isn't painless and it's all about saving money and harvesting organs for the rich.

I'm not exaggerating.

They killed one man because he was deaf. They've already killed people who were poor. And they've killed people who tried to change their minds. Euthanasia victims have died screaming – struggling to live. They'll kill children who say they want to die – without their parents' permission.

Euthanasia victims are listed in the official statistics according to whatever disease they had last. So, someone with diabetes who is euthanized will have died of diabetes and not of euthanasia. This is the same trick they used to pretend that covid was killing millions. And it is similar to the trick that they used when it was claimed that thousands were dying of AIDS in Africa, when many were really dying of TB. Early in 2020 I pointed out that the rules, and the entirely useless PCR test, had allowed the authorities to label patients as having died of covid even if they had actually been run over by a bus or killed by an axe wielding madman.

As I write, euthanasia is already legal in Belgium, Canada, Luxembourg, Netherlands, New Zealand, Spain, Colombia and parts of Australia as well as Switzerland and some States in America.

A disabled woman in Canada was offered a place on her nation's euthanasia programme because it was easier than adapting her home to her needs. A Canadian man who was facing eviction from social housing was accepted onto the country's euthanasia program. A mother was accused of selfishness when she wouldn't allow them to kill her disabled but life-loving daughter.

Euthanasia is the next stage in the conspirators' plan to use doctors as slaughter house technicians.

This is what the conspirators have been working towards for decades and they're preparing to turn the world into one big Jonestown.

Euthanasia or death by doctor is the most evil, cold-blooded massacre since Genghis Khan made genocide fashionable.

They're planning to kill children without telling their parents. They're planning to kill anyone who can't look after themselves. They're planning to kill anyone classified as disabled. And in case you haven't noticed they've been busy expanding the list of people who are now officially classified as disabled. They're planning to get rid of hospices and to abandon palliative care because it's much quicker and cheaper to kill people than it is to care for them.

Forget the self-serving myth that euthanasia is painless and dignified.

There are no standardised methods for euthanasia and so, as a result, there are frequent cases of prolonged and distressing deaths. Patients being euthanized vomit, wake up from comas and can take up to seven days to die. No one knows what to do if an initial attempt at euthanasia fails. What should be done if a patient is semi-conscious? Should another attempt be made to kill them?

The same drugs which are used for killing prisoners on death row are sometimes used to kill patients who have consented to euthanasia. But if paralysing drugs are used, the patient appears calm, peaceful and quiet – but that doesn't tell us what the patient is experiencing.

Unlike with prisoners, monitors are not used when a patient is being killed. This means that there is no evidence about what is happening.

Experts fear that patients being killed may suffer intolerable, unbearable physical or psychological pain.

The relatives of a woman in her 30s heard screams when she was supposedly being euthanized. The woman was suffocated with a pillow after drugs failed to kill her.

An elderly, demented woman in Belgium was euthanized after her family decided that she should be killed. The doctor laced her coffee with her sedatives – while she was chatting with her family. The doctor gave another sedative by injection. The woman then stood up. Family members held her down while the doctor injected her and killed her. Judges declared that 'the doctor did not need to verify her wish for euthanasia.'

Complications which have been recorded during euthanasia include: vomiting, tachycardia, sweating, gasping. One patient became unconscious 25 minutes after swallowing lethal medication but woke up and regained consciousness 65 hours later.

Lethal injections cause severe pain, a sensation of drowning and quiet, unspoken terror in the overwhelming majority of cases.

And doctors are using euthanasia to rid society of individuals who are regarded as a nuisance. A woman needed a wheelchair ramp in her home. Her caseworker offered her a medical assisted death instead. A student went to hospital for help with her debilitating feelings of depression and hopelessness. The staff member she saw told her that psychiatrists were in short supply. 'Have you considered euthanasia?' she was asked. A 61-year-old woman suffered from depression after a concussion sustained in a car crash. She was offered, and accepted, death by doctor as an alternative to treatment. A 61-year-old Canadian was killed by a lethal injection in 2019. His health problem was hearing loss. No medical personnel contacted his relatives 'out of respect for patient confidentiality'. A man with a degenerative brain disorder was offered euthanasia so often that he began recording hospital staff. In one recording, a hospital ethicist told him that his care was costing the hospital 'north of $1,500 a day' and asked if he had 'an interest in assisted dying'. A woman took her daughter to a hospital emergency room. Unprompted, the doctor informed the woman that her 25-year-old daughter, who has cerebral palsy and spinal bifida, was a good candidate for euthanasia. When she said No, the doctor called the mother selfish. Euthanasia is being offered to the mentally ill. Since there is now a major global epidemic of mental illness and general misery, this is a perfect background for selling euthanasia.

And they're killing children.

Naturally, the world being what it is these days, the authorities will not tell the parents of those children what is being planned. The parents will only know after the event. They'll get an email. 'You may have noticed that your 12-year-old son did not come home from school today. This is because he enrolled in our Suicide for Students programme and we helped him to kill himself this afternoon.'

How many children (and particularly teenagers) do not sometimes wish they were dead? 'My boyfriend has broken up with me. I wish I were dead.' 'I've been bullied on Facebook so much. I wish I were dead.'

No problem, here at the Justin Trudeau Let's Kill the Children centre we can deal with that for you. Like Mr Trudeau himself, it'll just be a little prick. Just put your satchel and your lollypop down, lie down and your problems are over forever. We'll ring your mum and dad later and tell them that you won't be coming home. They can collect your body from the Justin Trudeau Morgue.

The incidence of state sanctioned suicide is soaring – though as I've explained, they fiddle the figures and the real figure is even higher.

Millions of younger people have been encouraged to regard every moment of temporary unhappiness or disappointment as a sign of a serious mental disorder. Doctors in the UK are now writing nearly 500,000 prescriptions for powerful, largely unsuitable antidepressant drugs to be given to children.

Millions of prescriptions are written for children said to be suffering from autism, Asperger's or ADHD.

This is a perfect background for selling euthanasia.

The media has created fear and sadness and a sense of powerlessness and worthlessness. They have created the concept of a life not worth living. Is it really a coincidence that the subject of euthanasia is being promoted heavily by the media and by politicians at the same time as fear levels are at their highest for a very long time?

And physical disabilities now merit euthanasia too.

Back in 2010 the British Government quietly changed the legal definition of disability. Lots of people thought this was kind of them.

You are now automatically classified as disabled (and, therefore, likely to be a suitable candidate for euthanasia) if you have, among other many things:

Any visual impairment
Any physical or mental impairment
Any difficulty in communicating with other people
Any difficulty in filling in forms

Any difficulty in preparing and eating food
Any difficulty in sitting down or standing up
Any difficulty in using a computer
Any difficulty in getting washed and dressed
Any difficulty in following instructions
Long covid – even though it doesn't exist
Menopausal symptoms
And, of course, ADHD, autism, dyslexia

Millions welcomed the change. The disabled can be permanently off work and receive benefits. But, although they may not yet realise this, disabled people are candidates for euthanasia, whether or not they are willing to be killed.

Campaigners speaking on behalf of the disabled have for many decades warned that the legalisation of assisted suicide would lead to society devaluing the lives of people who are disabled or elderly. The usually unspoken fear was that patients would be made to feel guilty if they didn't kill themselves (or allow themselves to be killed).

It's happening.

Death is seen as a viable alternative to costly and inevitably futile medical treatment.

A paper in Canada concluded that Medically Assisted Death could dramatically reduce annual health spending.

Vulnerable people will be killed (or will be expected to do a Captain Oates to save money and resources).

One third of those taking part in Canada's euthanasia programme perceived themselves to be a burden on their family, their friends and on their caregivers. Many worried about the amount of money that was being spent on caring for them.

Unsurprisingly, euthanasia is rapidly becoming one of Canada's fastest growing causes of death.

A woman who was living on disability payments and who had failed to obtain affordable housing ended her life under Canada's assisted-suicide laws. 'The Government sees me as expendable trash,' she said.

Canada's Supreme Court ruled that the previous law which excluded people with disabilities from the death by doctor scheme was unconstitutional.

Amazingly 27% of Canadians believe that euthanasia should be expanded to include people who aren't ill but who are poor. And 28% of Canadians would offer 'death by doctor' to the homeless.

Euthanasia was supposed to be offered only to people who were terminally ill. But who knows what is incurable and what isn't? A cure may be just around the corner. The patient's problem may disappear without treatment. The diagnosis might be wrong. The doctor may not be aware that a cure is available. An available cure may be deemed too expensive. I've known patients diagnosed as having weeks to live who were still alive a decade later.

With mental health problems, the worries are even greater. But there won't be a chance for a better day. The sensitive and the vulnerable will be dead.

The elderly are being killed off first, of course, being made to feel guilty if they don't submit to euthanasia. Conditioning, propaganda and predictive programming are all being used to promote the idea that older citizens have a duty to die when they reach 70 years of age.

Enthusiasts like to claim that doctor assisted suicide is essential because people are living longer and, as a result, the global population of elderly people is growing out of proportion. The only sensible thing to do, the argument goes, is to kill off the excess old people to preserve space and resources for the young.

As I first explained back in the 1970s, that's a myth.

Improved sanitation facilities and better drinking water supplies meant that the number of babies dying – and the number of women dying in childbirth – fell dramatically at the end of the 19th century and the start of the 20th century. That is what has resulted in a bigger population and more old people.

Life expectation for adults has not risen appreciably during the last century.

So why are so many countries legalising death by doctor?

The conspirators claim that it is necessary to reduce the size of the global population. They want to cut the world's population down to 500 million. This is a lie, of course. There is plenty of food to feed billions.

The conspirators have two fundamental policies: 'End global poverty by killing all the poor people' and 'End disease by killing all the sick.'

You have to follow the money if you want to find the truth.

The disabled and the elderly are now widely regarded as of little or no financial value.

And then there are pensions, of course.

Many of those who receive State pensions believe (quite erroneously) that the money they have paid in taxes has been put aside to pay their pensions. But pension programmes are simply huge Ponzi schemes. State pensions are paid out of today's taxes. In twenty years' time, pensions will be paid out of the taxes which are paid by workers in twenty years' time. If the size of the aged population can be cut, the annual savings will be measured in billions of dollars.

After thousands of elderly people were murdered in hospitals and care homes during the lockdowns – I called it murder at the time – politicians boasted with glee that the financial savings, in unpaid pensions, would be huge. The more people they kill, the more money they'll save.

The pro-euthanasia programme is nothing to do with reducing pain or distress: it is all about saving money.

It is a lot cheaper to kill people than it is to provide palliative care.

Take a look at what is happening in Holland.

The advocates of killing-by-doctor in Holland don't like to use the word 'kill', of course. They much prefer anodyne phrases such as 'physician assisted suicide' or 'aid in dying'. You can call it 'medically assisted suicide' or 'death with dignity'. But don't call it killing or murder. They've mastered the art of state approved slaughter.

Doctors will kill people of any age and they will kill people who are demented or depressed or who have long-term, chronic disorders. An 18-year-old with psychiatric problems was killed by doctors.

They will, indeed, kill just about anyone. They'll even kill you if you are just 'tired of life'. A petition, signed by a number of prominent Dutch citizens, has suggested that euthanasia should be available to everyone over the age of 70 who feels a bit worn out.

Plans were announced for a law that would allow 'assisted suicide' if a patient 'felt that they had completed their life' (whatever that means). It was said that the needs of older people should be met if they were struggling with mobility problems, a loss of independence, fatigue or loneliness. It was argued that meeting their needs shouldn't involve walking sticks, wheelchairs, dietary help or companionship but death by doctor.

Today, they'll kill you if you are demented or have an existential problem you can't cope with. They'll kill you if you are lonely or depressed or not much use.

Older patients are deprived of food, water, diagnosis or medication. And then, when they feel pretty damned uncomfortable and miserable, they're offered a death pill.

'You've had a long life, why are you hanging on when your time is up? You're using up valuable resources.'

And they'll kill children as young as 12-years-old.

The enthusiasts promoting 'death by doctor' in Holland now even have a 'Euthanasia Week' where they can share propaganda promoting euthanasia.

Individuals can make a 'Living Will' or 'Advance Directive' in which they sign up for euthanasia at some future time. Don't try to change your mind because living wills are legal documents which cannot be easily rescinded.

One patient fought back while doctors were giving her a kill shot. The relatives held the patient down while the needle went in. The patient was screaming as well as fighting. Courts later cleared the doctors (and presumably the family) of any crime.

And look again at what is happening to hospices and palliative care around the world. Funding for both is disappearing. There's plenty of money for gender displacement clinics but none for hospices or palliative care.

Hospices have to find three quarters of their funding themselves. Just imagine the outcry if, for example, infertility services or cosmetic surgery clinics relied on jumble sales, car boot sales, bucket collections and charity shops to survive?

The aim is clearly to reduce palliative care just as the availability of euthanasia is increased. The same thing is happening all around the world.

What the world desperately needs, of course, is more mobile palliative care services with doctors and nurses available to visit patients who are dying and who are in their own homes.

But the opposite is happening.

Just a few decades ago, doctors in Britain visited their patients at home during the daytime, during the evening, at weekends and on bank holidays. Nowhere in the world was there a better 24 hour a day GP service than in Britain. Today, the average GP earns over £150,000 a year with a £50,000 vaccine bonus and works just 23 hours a week. Accountants and librarians work longer hours than GPs.

Health care in Britain has been deliberately destroyed. Today, there is more untreated illness and more people suffering from chronic illnesses (and suffering unnecessarily) than ever before.

Because there is no 24 hour service from GPs, patients who are ill have little alternative but to call for an ambulance or visit their nearest Accident and Emergency hospital department. Many of these patients have problems which could be dealt with by a GP in five minutes but the vastly increased pressure means that the average waiting time for an ambulance has gone in many areas from minutes to hours or even days, and in Accident and Emergency departments patients wait days to be seen and are then treated on trolleys in the corridor. It is now by no means exceptional for patients to die while waiting to be treated. Each year over 100,000 people over 70 wait more than 24 hours in A and E – just to be seen by someone.

Turn up at a hospital and they'll likely offer you instant death instead of hours of waiting and pain.

The same deterioration has taken place around the world and it has led to a dramatic increase in the number of people agreeing to have Do Not Resuscitate notices placed on their medical records and accepting euthanasia as the only viable option.

And there is one other reason why the establishment is so keen on euthanasia: it will release a good many organs for use. If people are left to die naturally, their organs will deteriorate and begin to rot but if they are selected at the right time, their organs can be harvested in good condition – as they're needed.

Organ donation started out as optional and voluntary but has become the default position, with citizens having to opt out of giving their organs – possibly while they would like to be still using them.

There is no little irony in the fact that patients being encouraged to die might themselves be saved if they were considered important enough to be treated as organ recipients rather than as organ donors.

Doctors have been told to suggest organ donation as, if not an incentive, kind of 'consolation' for the person's own loss of life.

Since organ transplantation is extremely expensive, and health services are cutting costs, it is inevitable that the organs taken from patients who have been murdered by the State will be reserved for politicians, senior civil servants and billionaires.

Oh, and one other thing: organs can only be extracted and used for transplantation if the donor patient is still alive. You can't take organs from a dead person who has died in a car crash. But you can take as many organs as you can carry from a euthanasia victim.

Euthanasia is now global. In America, death by doctor is being pushed by politicians, lobbyists and lawyers. Death by doctor is being sold as freedom, as a choice, as a human right.

The right to die has become the duty to die. In Oregon and Washington, well over half of requests for assisted suicide cited 'feelings of being a burden' as significant reasons for their requests.

Just how enthusiastic would anyone be if doctors simply shot their patients in the head instead of injecting them? Doctors agree that the quickest, simplest, most painless, most dignified and cheapest way to kill people is to shoot them in the head.

Or maybe gas chambers could be introduced. They are cheap and effective and can allegedly be used to kill a number of people at a time.

Here is an Open Letter which I wrote to Kim Leadbeater MP. Ms Leadbeater introduced a Private Members Bill advocating euthanasia, to the House of Commons. At the time I wrote the letter, a House of Commons committee was discussing the Bill. The members of the committee, and the witnesses called to give evidence, were all chosen by Kim Leadbeater.

Open Letter to Kim Leadbeater MP
From Dr Vernon Coleman
February 2025
Dear Kim Leadbeater,
I have a suspicion that you think your Euthanasia Bill is a 'good' thing. I rather hope you do think this and that your motives in sponsoring it are honourable. I know the Bill is really called the 'Terminally Ill Adults (End of Life) Bill' but I'm afraid your title is laughably misleading and quite inaccurate. If your Bill becomes law it will not be long before the service you are promoting will be

available to the anxious, the depressed, the disabled, the unemployed and the poor. It will be available to the young and to the old. And it will be available to those who are far from the end of their lives.

How do I know this? Because I've studied what has happened in other countries where euthanasia has been introduced. The initial idea is always that euthanasia will be available only to patients who are at the very end of a long process of dying. The idea is that patients at the very end of their lives will be liberated from their pain and suffering and will be allowed to die in quiet dignity.

But that's not what happens. It is definitely not what happens.

Look at every other country which has introduced euthanasia. Look at Canada where people are being murdered because they are jobless and poor and without hope. People are being killed for social reasons. Euthanasia will be available for patients with mental illness in 2027. Is that what you have in mind? And Children with autism, Asperger's and ADHD will be quietly euthanized. Killing the long-term sick saves a lot of money. A Canadian Armed Forces Veteran who was injured in Afghanistan has reported how at least six veterans in Canada have been offered euthanasia after asking for help. One asked for care and received a letter saying: 'If it is too difficult for you to continue living, Madam, we can offer you medical assistance in dying'. One veteran called a crisis hotline and was offered 'assisted suicide' as a solution. And this is already happening in the UK too. A 25-year-old veteran was in crisis and asked for help. A doctor (in the UK, remember) suggested assisted suicide. The police have been contacted. Check it out.

And look at how the 'Do Not Resuscitate' instruction has changed in Britain. This too was introduced with good intentions. The idea was patients who were dying and beyond help would not be resuscitated time and time again, simply delaying the inevitable. But today 'Do Not Resuscitate' notices are routinely slapped on the notes of patients who are disabled, awaiting surgery for an entirely curable problem or suffering from mental illness. Check it out. You'll find horror stories everywhere. Even adults and young children are labelled 'Do Not Resuscitate' if a doctor or nurse feels their lives are worthless. There are, I'm afraid, more Dr Shipmans around than you realise. And there are a good many Nurse Shipmans too. The NHS already treats the elderly as subhuman. In Accident and Emergency units the elderly are made to wait for days to be seen. There is no triage. The elderly, however ill, must wait and wait and wait. During the covid lockdowns thousands of old people were murdered. (No, that's not hyperbole. By any definition, they were murdered.)

If you really think that euthanasia is painless and dignified then I'm afraid you need to do a little more research. It's neither. Check out the problems prisons have with execution in America. If you really think that euthanasia (as offered in your Bill) is only going to be offered to Terminally Ill Adults then you are extraordinarily naïve. Read the evidence in Dr Jack King's book 'They want to kill us'. Look at what always happens when euthanasia legislation is introduced.

Your plan to employ a panel of social workers, psychiatrists and retired judges to decide whether or not an applicant is suitable for 'death by doctor' is one of the most frightening ideas I've ever heard. What do social workers, psychiatrists or judges know of this? What do they know of 'terminal' illness? When I was a GP I had two patients who were diagnosed as having terminal cancer. Both lived for more than a decade after they had been abandoned by hospitals. (Both had strong reasons for staying alive.) Older GPs, who, like me, practised in a different time, could tell you similar stories.

Like all doctors who worked in general practice as it was practised in the days when doctors helped look after dying patients in their own homes (before being a GP meant working 23 hours a week sitting at home in front of a laptop) I have a considerable amount of experience of this subject. Doctors don't like to talk about these things because it worries people and, legally, it's a difficult area, but no good GP ever allowed a patient to approach their death in pain. The idea of dying patients in agony is a myth created for the purpose of promoting your Bill (and Bills like it around the world.) No one needs ever be in intractable pain. Pain control is (or should be) available and can free patients and often give them more life than they knew they had, or that your Bill will allow them. Patients are only in unbearable pain if their pain control isn't being managed properly. The fear that painkillers will cause addiction is a nonsense for it has been shown that patients in genuine pain do not become addicted. The real problem today is that a clique of cultists within the medical establishment, who mistakenly believe that prescribing drugs contributes to global warming, have encouraged doctors to cut back on their prescribing. And, of course, your own government is deliberately and cold bloodedly destroying palliative care. Hospices are closing because changes introduced by your colleagues mean that they cannot afford to stay open.

If you continue to push this Bill then your name will forever be associated with the legalised murder of the disabled and the weak. You will be remembered as the Midwife of Death. Your Bill has nothing to do with compassion and whatever you may think there will be no safeguards. Your legacy will be State controlled murder. Is that really what you want? Your bill has nothing whatsoever to do with easing the lives of people in too much pain. Do you really want people to be killed because they consider themselves to be a burden?

Did anyone encourage you to promote this Bill? Does it not occur to you that you are part of the depopulation plan which is so dear to some of the so-called elite? Your Bill is nothing more than practical eugenics with the bonus that it will save money for the State. Remember too that the vast majority of those who try to kill themselves but fail go on to regret their mistake and to have enormously satisfying lives.

As the years go by, your Bill will be extended more and more. You may think that history will look on you kindly. It won't. History will see you as the midwife for legalised murder. Your name will be reviled even more than Shipman's. If your Bill goes through you will be personally responsible for the deaths of thousands who had much to offer. I guarantee that within five years at the very most you will be responsible for children, the disabled, the poor, the jobless and the depressed being murdered. Euthanasia programmes always start with limits. But the limits never last.

Finally, did you know that the Nazis ran a euthanasia programme for a while? After a short period Hitler abandoned it because he considered it morally indefensible.

Yours sincerely,

Dr Vernon Coleman

Suicide by doctor isn't legal yet in the UK but Britain has an excellent substitute. Back in the 1990s something called the Liverpool Care Pathway was introduced. This allowed doctors and nurses to kill anyone over 70 by the simple expedient of not giving them food or water.

Officially, the Liverpool Care Pathway was put out of bounds as being unethical, painful, distressing and wicked. But doctors and nurses still use it. And they speed things up with a kill shot of morphine and midazolam. This was very popular during the covid fraud and was used to free up whole hospital wards so that nurses and doctors could get on with rehearsing their TikTok dance steps.

And then there are the Do Not Resuscitate notices (DNR notices). DNR notices have been put on patients' notes without their permission and even against their wishes.

It is vital that you do not allow doctors or nurses to write DNR on your medical records or on the records of anyone you know. The letters DNR stand for 'Do Not Resuscitate'. DNR notices were introduced decades ago with the idea that patients who were moribund would not be dragged back to life time and time again.

When I was a junior doctor working in hospital we would take a crash cart to every patient who was dying and we would try to bring them back to life. This did not always seem to be good medicine. Patients who were clearly dying would be brought back to life and then kept alive artificially. This was often distressing for the patient (if they were aware of what was happening – which they usually were not) and distressing for relatives and friends. The problem was that medicine had progressed faster than medical ethics or common sense.

And so a system was introduced whereby patients who were not going to recover (because there was too much brain or heart damage or because other organs had failed and were irreparable) would not be brought back to life time and time again but would be allowed to die peacefully. Patients who had metastatic cancer and who were clearly dying would not be given antibiotics if they developed pneumonia.

And so the letters DNR were written on the patient's medical records, usually in red ink. And the records would, of course, be kept confidential in the ward office, where the ward sister and the ward clerk oversaw what was happening.

But then the letters DNR slowly began to appear on the medical records of patients who were ill but not dying. Doctors and nurses began to make 'life and death' decisions. And in the last few years there has been a veritable explosion in the use of DNR notices. Today, DNR notices are put on patients who have routine and curable problems. Many patients having routine surgery are asked if they want to be resuscitated. The doctor or nurse who is asking will usually lie and say that resuscitation is a painful procedure. They talk of the risk of broken ribs and the danger of a broken sternum (even though it is rare for ribs to be broken and almost unheard of for the sternum to be broken).

Patients who go into hospital for what are called 'minor' operations (there is no such thing as 'minor' surgery, but you know what I mean) are asked to agree to a DNR notice being put on their records. Patients over 70, 60 or even 50 years of age are routinely given DNR notices if they need to go into a hospital or care home. And individuals who have health care problems such as diabetes or with mental health issues of any kind are routinely (and often without their knowledge) given DNR notices. The DNR system has travelled a long way and is being used to kill as many patients as possible. If you or a relative goes into hospital or a care home please make sure that you do not accept a DNR notice.

Nothing that is happening in medicine is happening by accident. The destruction of medical care (with the absurd claim that doctors must stop treating patients because of the global warming myth) is accelerating rapidly. Encouraged by the medical establishment, your doctor wants you dead – especially if you are elderly, frail, disabled or mentally ill.

In 2025 it was reported that UK's Labour Party Chancellor of the Exchequer, Rachel Reeves had increased the amount of financial support offered to vaccine manufacturer Astra Zeneca from the initial proposal of £40 million. Astonishingly, Astra Zeneca said the sum was enough and waltzed off in a huff. (At which point Reeves should have told them they would not in future be allowed to sell their damned products to the NHS.) Astra Zeneca is a £180 billion company which has forecast revenue of $80 billion by 2030 and makes such huge profits that it paid boss Pascal Soriot £14.7 million last year. Soriot has been paid nearly £120 million in the last decade. Reeves, happily throwing taxpayers' money at Astra Zeneca, is the woman who cut the winter fuel allowance for OAPs, leaving thousands of impecunious old people to freeze to death. In February 2025 it was revealed that three out of four pensioners in the UK were living in cold homes because they couldn't afford to heat them. Between 60,000 and 100,000 will die of the cold in the winter. (Compare this to the few dozen who might die of heat if global warming were real.)

I have no doubt that euthanasia, supported by the media, will be legalised in the UK very soon.

Who will decide who can or should die? Will it be patients themselves, relatives, nurses, social workers or just any old neighbourly busy body? Suicide has gone from illegal to optional. How soon will euthanasia become compulsory and for whom?

When euthanasia is made legal worldwide then Pandora's Box will be open. And no one will ever be able to close the lid. The laws will enable doctors to kill people who are deaf or diabetic or 16 and feeling fed up with the world.

Who is going to be trained to help with euthanasia?

The problem, of course, is that good, caring doctors and nurses are trained to keep people alive and refuse to kill their patients. Most hospices refuse to have anything to do with euthanasia.

This will leave patients in the hands of people who are not experts in end of life care or of pain management.

Either euthanasia will be provided by a small group of itinerant doctors who will travel around the country killing patients they don't know – the modern equivalent of the professional hangmen who used to travel around with a supply of rope.

Or euthanasia will be provided by technicians who have as little as six hours' online training. I suspect that many of the people who will be attracted to work as hired killers will be psychopaths, murderers and assassins who will enjoy killing people.

Remember that the vast majority of people who attempt to commit suicide and fail, later give thanks that they have failed. With 'death by doctor' that possibility is lost. Remember too that many people think of suicide as a long stop solution to life's sometimes apparently insoluble problems. 'If things really get too bad I can always escape by killing myself.' Most people, of course, never take the ultimate escape option. But when the State and the medical profession make things very easy, and your doctor offers immediate and allegedly painless suicide as an option the uptake will show a dramatic rise.

Can doctors bring up the subject of assisted death without influencing their patients? Or frightening them unnecessarily? Is it really a doctor's job to offer to kill their patient?

Discussing euthanasia would make a great TV or radio debate. But the authorities will never allow a proper debate – just as they will never allow a debate about vaccination or the covid fraud. I realise that I have mentioned the refusal of the conspirators and their servants, together with bots and AI technology, to debate their claims on several occasions and I realise that trolls and overly sensitive critics will give this book one star on the grounds of repetition. But I think it is absolutely vital to keep remembering this point. The refusal of the conspirators to debate their claims is our greatest strength and their greatest weakness and it is mentioned far too infrequently.

GPs all over Britain have been contacting their elderly patients, and those with chronic health disorders, and asking them two questions.

Are you happy for us to put a DNR on your file?

And

Are you happy for us to put on your file a note that you won't be admitted to hospital if you become unwell?

Note the clever wording, designed to elicit a positive response. It's the sort of trickery used by crooked pollsters and insurance salesmen – knowing what answer they want and shading the question in such a way as to ensure that they get it.

One GP surgery sent out a letter to a home catering for autistic adults saying that the carers should have plans to prevent their patients being resuscitated if they became critically ill.

Other GPs sent out similar letters to establishments caring for the elderly and the disabled. Blanket decisions were made for care homes and residential homes caring for patients with learning difficulties.

A 51-year-old man with Down's Syndrome was given a DNR

because of his disability, and instructions were left that there was to be no attempt to resuscitate in case of a cardiac arrest or a respiratory arrest.

No consent form was signed and there was no agreement with the patient or his relatives. The Medical Director for the relevant part of the NHS said that their policy complied fully with national guidelines from professional bodies.

The boss of a large charity said that they believe that DNR orders are frequently placed on patients with learning disabilities – without the knowledge and agreement of their families.

This was, of course, illegal.

Back in 2015, the High Court in the UK ruled that carers for patients with mental illnesses should be consulted before DNR notices were applied.

But the High Court ruling is ignored.

A man in his 50s, with sight loss, was issued with a DNR notice giving 'blindness and severe learning disabilities' as the reason.

A man with epilepsy was issued with a DNR notice, and at the end of March this year a GPs' surgery in Wales urged high risk patients to complete a DNR form if they contracted the coronavirus. The letter said, 'you are unlikely to receive hospital admission'.

A woman in Bristol received a phone call from her GP asking if it were OK for her medical records to be updated to say that if she contracted the coronavirus she wouldn't go to hospital or receive any medical treatment.

In the UK, the National Institute for Health and Care Excellence, known as NICE, is the official advisory body to the health care world.

And NICE rulings are utterly crucial.

NICE classified people in nine categories. If you are in category 1 then you are very fit. If you are in category 9 then you are terminally ill (though, when it suits them NHS staff sometimes devise another category of 'terminally, terminally ill').

On 29th April 2020, NICE issued amended advice to NHS staff about its resuscitation guidelines, saying that doctors should 'sensitively discuss a possible DNAR with all adults with CFs of 5 or more'. This was issued in response to the coronavirus hoax.

(DNAR stands for Do not Attempt Resuscitation and is the same as DNR.)

Doctors and nurses were instructed that they should review critical care treatment when a patient 'is no longer considered able to achieve desired overall goals'.

So, what the devil does this mealy mouthed nonsense mean?

And what is a CF? What does a CF of 5 mean?

Well the letters CF mean clinical frailty and there are several stages.

A CF of 5 means that a patient is mildly frail and may need help with heavy housework, shopping and preparing meals.

A CF of 6 means moderately frail – people who need help with bathing.

A CF of 7 means severely frail – people who are completely dependent for personal care.

And so on.

Now you could, I suppose, argue that if a patient is clearly dying then it would be cruel and pointless to continually attempt resuscitation. That was why DNR notices were devised. They were originally for patients who had only hours to live and it was considered not fair to those patients to continue to 'strive to keep officiously alive'.

But that's not what is happening now.

Today, in the UK, in the National Health Service a patient considered unsuitable to be saved or treated is now considered to be a patient who needs help with the heavy housework and who may have difficulty preparing meals or going to the shops.

I could manage a bit of light dusting, I suppose, but more than that would require more effort than I have available to spend on such matters. I would have great difficulty in preparing a meal and I hate going to the shops. So, presumably, I'd get dumped into the CF5 category and so there is no hope for me, and the NHS would recommend that I be denied antibiotics, painkillers or surgery if I fell down and broke an arm.

The post-coronavirus hoax NHS doesn't want to save anyone who is disabled and all patients in care homes are, by definition, suitable for murder by omission.

Originally NICE told doctors that they should assess patients with autism as scoring high for frailty. I am, I confess, still rather confused about when or whether this advice was removed.

I checked around with other bodies.

I didn't find the BMA website much help, though it did have a useful commercial webinar for doctors wanting financial advice. The BMA is, after all, a trades union which exists to look after doctors not patients.

And the General Medical Council, rather bizarrely, got in on the act by defining 'approaching end of life' as patients who are likely to die within the next twelve months.

This, of course is the sort of dangerous rubbish one might expect from the overpaid bureaucratic form shufflers at the General Medical Council because it is always impossible to say that a patient is going to die within twelve months. It might be possible to say that a patient might die within twelve hours but not twelve months. Only arrogant doctors and ignorant bureaucrats claim to know that a patient might die within twelve months. When I was in general practice a couple of centuries ago, I knew many patients who were given months to live but who lived many, many years. Two, I remember well, had young children to look after and although they had been given only months to live they both lived for years – simply refusing to give up and surviving on sheer willpower as much as anything else. If the GMC rule had been applied, they'd have been allowed to die. Or, the way things seem to be going, they would have been quietly euthanized in case they fell ill and needed care.

While digging around I also found this statement:

'Physicians have been empowered to grant a mercy death to patients considered incurable – the mentally ill and the handicapped.'

And then I looked a little closer and realised that the date of that policy statement was October 1939, and the author was a well-known 'medical expert' known as Adolf Hitler.

Hitler's policy, which seems to me to bear an uncomfortably close relationship to the official policy of the UK's National Health Service these days, was created in 1920 in a book written by a psychiatrist and a lawyer (what a deadly combination) who argued that the economic savings justified killing those with 'useless lives'.

The policy was to kill the incurably ill and the physically or mentally disabled and the elderly.

Hitler's policy was officially discontinued in 1941 when it seems that even the Nazis found it a bit much.

But the advice from NICE is still valid. And the NHS is still prepared to refuse life-saving treatment for the elderly, the disabled or the frail.

Refusing treatment to patients solely because of their age or fitness is a form of eugenics. It seems that social cleansing is alive and well in Britain today. If you aren't saving people (when you could do so) then you are killing them. There doesn't seem to me to be all that much difference between the thinking behind the policy of the NHS and the policy of Adolf Hitler's Germany.

If you slap a DNR form on a patient, with or without their permission, you are condemning them to death. If you trick someone into agreeing to one then that's just as bad.

In my view, the NHS has been Nazified.

There are many good doctors and nurses working for it. But there are many who are so bad they are evil.

During the lockdowns of 2020, obedient souls were witlessly clapping the NHS and all the time the NHS had been deliberately delivering death notices, DNR forms, to the frail and the elderly.

Which of us gave doctors permission to deny treatment to people considered unimportant, expensive or expendable?

In my view, every single doctor or nurse or administrator who has put a DNR notice on a patient under these regulations should be fired, arrested and imprisoned. I don't know what for. There must be something. How do these people sleep at night? Don't they feel anything for the people they are supposed to be looking after? I am prepared to believe that not everyone in health care can have a genuine vocation. But the people who were scattering these DNR notices around were paid to look after people. And they have betrayed those people. Do Not Resuscitate notices were devised to ensure that the genuinely terminally ill were allowed to die with dignity – without being dragged time and time again from wherever they were heading. DNR notices were originally a necessary part of medicine – to avoid a General Franco type situation.

But now we have a thousand Dr Mengele clones working in the health service. That sounds as if I'm exaggerating but the sad thing is that I am not. Dr Mengele would have thrived in today's NHS. He'd have liked the clapping and the adulation too.

NICE should be disbanded immediately. We'd all be better off without it.

Meanwhile, if you think you, or someone you know could be rated C5 or worse, it might be a good idea to ask your GP if you've been put on the 'suitable for dying' list.

Shortly after the Clifton Suspension bridge was finished, a young woman threw herself over the edge in an attempt to commit suicide. She was saved when her voluminous skirts spread out like a parachute, allowing to land unharmed in the water below. She then lived a long, contented life. Why am I telling you this? Because, although I have mentioned this before, it is crucial to remember that would-be suicides who survive are invariably grateful that they failed to kill themselves. This is significant because when the UK introduces death-by-doctor, the individuals who have decided to kill themselves will get no second chance at life. They will die (in a probably painful and undignified way). Once euthanasia becomes legal they will kill the old, the frail, the disabled, the mentally ill, the poor, the unemployed and children with teenage hormone syndrome. How do I know this? Because that's what happens everywhere euthanasia is legal. There are no second chances with government sponsored death. Euthanasia is a WEF approved part of the depopulation plan.

Since euthanasia was introduced in Canada, the number of people being euthanized has increased dramatically. Euthanasia is routinely offered as an option to the elderly, the sick, the disabled, the poor and the jobless. Canadian doctors are appalled at what is happening.

It is often said by supporters of euthanasia that death is preferable to being in constant pain. There is, however, no reason for anyone to be screaming in pain when they are ill or dying. Medicine is, or should be, better than that.

In some parts of the world doctors now demand that their new patients sign contracts allowing their doctor to do with them what they will. One of the clauses in these new contracts gives the doctor permission to force vaccinate her or his patients. All patients should take great care to read contracts they are asked to sign – and, as a general principle, to refuse to sign them.

During the presidency of John F.Kennedy in the US, the incidence of chronic disease was 6%. Today (in 2025) the figure is ten times higher, at 60%. Nearly two thirds of Americans have a chronic illness. The US spends $4.3 trillion on chronic diseases. Many of the drugs which are prescribed do more harm than good and are egregiously overpriced. Trillions of dollars have been spent trying to make the American people healthier but people have never been unhealthier. The medical profession and the pharmaceutical industry have combined to create more illness and make people sicker.

Celebrities are always praising the NHS. They say how kind everyone was and how well they were looked after. Of course people were kind. Of course they were well looked after. Hospital staff are always excited when they have a celebrity on the ward. But those celebrities are doing great harm because their praise often hides the truth about the way non-celebrities perceive the NHS. If you aren't a celebrity you'd be well advised to keep out of hospital in the UK.

Doctors are refusing to prescribe painkillers to patients who need them on the very dubious grounds that addiction to painkillers is now commonplace. This appalling practice means that thousands of patients are in pain because they are denied essential pain relief. Those patients then queue up for euthanasia because they cannot bear their pain. How convenient this is for the conspirators who want euthanasia for us all. The conspirators who want to depopulate the world know exactly what they are doing in their plans to push people into signing up for euthanasia.

Tragically, there are now some doctors who will not prescribe painkillers for terminal pain, claiming that they have been told (wrongly) that doing so may cause addiction. In fact, people in severe pain do not become addicted to painkillers. (And if they are dying it really doesn't much matter if they do become addicted.) However, this is a distraction. The main reason why doctors aren't prescribing painkillers when required is because of something called Environmental Pain Approach (EPA): Sustainability in Chronic Pain

Practice.

In order to support the medical establishment's cruel decision to reduce the number of medicines prescribed (in order to satisfy the requirements of the global warming cultists – who have the complete support of all forms of the mainstream media) the mainstream media has published claims that people who take opioid painkillers are much at risk of becoming addicted.

This is nonsense.

A new study of 148 pieces of research (involving 4.3 million adult chronic pain sufferers) showed that less than 1 in 10 developed dependence or opioid use disorder.

And I believe that even that figure is too high.

The Faculty of Pain Medicine at the Royal College of Anaesthetists says: 'It is rare for people in pain to become addicted to opioids.'

Problems arise when patients are given painkillers which they don't really need. And often patients aren't told how to take their painkillers.

So why all the scary publicity?

The media scares are being used as an excuse for doctors to prescribe fewer painkillers. The scares are also being used to reduce palliative care and to promote euthanasia.

This is all part of the depopulation plan – which is, of course, using global warming as the excuse for its wicked actions.

Medicine is now so thoroughly corrupt that there is now a speciality known as 'Evidence based medicine'. This rather begs the question: 'What is the rest of medicine, if it is not 'evidence based'?' And the rest of medicine, I fear, is in thrall to the pharmaceutical industry. Since 1975 I have, in a number of books, shown the level of corruption within the medical establishment and the way that the medical establishment controls the rank and file in the profession. This is a global phenomenon and the drug industry even influences, in whole or in part, many drug regulating agencies, medical charities, Non Governmental Organisations, medical journals and the mainstream media.

In the desperate search to placate the global warming cultists whatever the cost, a dairy company has introduced what is described as an innovative feeding technique to cut the methane that cows emit. The Food Standards Agency and the European Food Safety Authority gave clearance for the use of an additive called Bovaer which is sold to inhibit methane production by 27%. But is Bovaer safe? Could it possibly be harmful to humans who drink the milk from these partly fart-free cows?

When doubts were raised about the product, the global warming cultists swung immediately into action. The BBC said that the product is safe because it is 'approved by regulators and experts say it is safe'. *Country Life* magazine, for example, dismissed those questioning the product's safety as 'conspiracy theorists and climate-change deniers'. (The word 'denier is now a standard part of the cultists' vocabulary. Anyone questioning the official line is dismissed as a discredited conspiracy theorist or denier. Whistle blowing is still considered a crime if it is inconvenient to the global warming cultists.)

My enthusiasm for this surely pointless product is tempered by the knowledge that the regulators approved the covid-19 vaccine when it is now known that it is neither safe nor effective and is, in my view, too toxic to use as landfill.

Is it conceivable that in 20 years' time we will find that children who drink this milk (which I regard as contaminated) might grow up to be more susceptible to cancer? After all, which regulatory agency warned those being vaccinated with the covid-19 jab that they might be more likely to develop cancer – and a very aggressive form of cancer at that? 'Drinka pinta milka day' used to be a popular slogan. Maybe it will be resurrected as 'Drinka pinta milka day and die.'

Climate change has been renamed 'climate alarmism', though 'climate fraud' would be just as appropriate.

In February 2025, the NHS in the UK announced that nearly half of urgent cancer patients had to wait more than two months for treatment. Some had to wait considerably longer. Many will die before their treatment starts. It was also reported that the National Cancer Audit Collaborating Centre had found significant variation between hospitals in the way that cancers were being treated. It was found that up to half of the patients who had one of nine types of well-known cancer (including prostate cancer, colon cancer and renal cancer) were not receiving the right treatment. A study of prostate cancer patients, for example, showed that the number not receiving curative treatment with either surgery or radiotherapy varied between 20% and 43% with the average being 30%. In some hospitals 85% of patients with kidney cancer were not receiving the recommended treatment while over 60% of patients with colon cancer weren't receiving the officially recommended treatment.

The people promoting euthanasia do not seem to understand that if there were an efficient way to kill people they would regularly use it for prisoners on death row in preference to shooting, hanging and electrocution.

The one thing doctors should always give their patients is Hope. The very notion of euthanasia stands opposed to this. Civilised societies do not allow capital punishment because there is a risk that errors will be made. And errors will be made when euthanasia is contemplated. In despairing moments, people say 'I want to die, let me be' but don't mean it. When the State has killed them it will be mercilessly efficient and there will be no coming back from the grave.

In 2010, a persistently wicked man called Bill Gates suggested using a death panel system to avoid the cost of palliative care and the cost of keeping terminally ill people alive when they were probably going to die anyway. In the Gates' system, decisions to kill people would be taken by bureaucrats who would kill off the elderly, the retired and the disabled.

School teachers around the world have been trained to indoctrinate children to believe in global warming. I have little doubt that teachers will be indoctrinated to teach children about the wonders of euthanasia. ('And if you feel a bit sad one day, don't worry because the nice doctors will put you to sleep and you'll never have to feel a bit sad ever again.')

In 2022, an adviser to the World Economic Forum called Yuval Noah Harari said that the world does not need the vast majority of the current population. He said that technological advances mean that people can be replaced by Artificial Intelligence. WEF founder Klaus Schwab who is quoted as believing that the world now accommodates an abundance of 'useless people'. 'It harms society,' Schwab has said, 'when humans live beyond 70.' Schwab himself was considerably beyond 70 when he said this. Personally, I would list Harari and Schwab as useless and redundant.

The WEF and the United Nations (two sides of the same coin) seem to put their view of the environment above people. The organisations want to get rid of fossil fuels in favour of their preferred energy sources which are expensive, unreliable and inefficient. The only conceivable aim is to destroy economies everywhere. The WEF endorsed clinically useless lockdowns which led to widespread job losses, reduced health care and much depression. And the WEF wants more lockdowns. The British Prime Minister 'Free Suits' Starmer (who accepted £100,000 of free clothing and spectacles from a donor who was given a pass to 10 Downing Street) has said that he prefers Davos to Westminster – presumably because decisions there can be made in secret and without troubling the electorate. The world's mainstream media (or legacy media) has, not surprisingly, joined the WEF in promoting a programme of depopulation.

Depopulation aficionados favour euthanasia, and the withdrawal of essential medical services from people in need.

When people have been selected for euthanasia they are usually given three injections: a sedative, a drug to paralyse and a drug to kill. These are much the same drugs as are given to prisoners on death row. The drug to paralyse is given so that the patient won't struggle or move about and alarm the bystanders. The drug is the same as the one often given to patients who are having organs removed for a transplant operation. (It isn't widely appreciated but organs for transplantation must be removed from living patients. In the UK, permission for doctors to remove organs from your body is the default.)

All countries which have legalised euthanasia face the following problems:

It is suggested that doctor by suicide is designed to enable patients to kill themselves. This is absurd. Patients at the end of their lives, or seriously disabled in some way, are unlikely to be able to inject themselves. A doctor (or some substitute) will have to do the injecting. That is euthanasia. To pretend otherwise is nonsense.

The doctor doing the killing is required to stay with the patient he is killing. You can't just inject a lethal drug into a patient and then disappear, intending to return later to collect the corpse. But euthanasia can take days. Patients can wake up after being given a lethal dose. How is this going to work? How many doctor/killers will be happy to sit by a bed for days at a time, waiting for their cocktail of drugs to work?

What sort of doctors will agree to be involved in killing their 'patients'?

There will be little or no training for doctors hired to kill patients. There is hardly likely to be a Royal College for doctors hired to kill people.

How much are doctors going to be paid to kill people they don't know? How many doctors will do the killing for the money?

The doctor appointed to do the killing will usually be allowed to choose a second doctor to help them. And if the second doctor disagrees with what is going on then the first doctor can presumably sack his appointed 'assistant' and choose someone else.

The demand for euthanasia will increase as medical care becomes worse and waiting lists get longer – both things which are happening very rapidly. The availability of euthanasia will result in a further collapse in medical care as governments choose the cheaper option.

Millions of people are consumed by fear and feel hopeless about the future. Is just killing them the right solution? (Maybe we should remove the problem at source by offering euthanasia exclusively to conspirators, politicians and mainstream propagandists.)

Amazingly, there may be no requirement for the doctor paid to do the killing to talk to the victim's GP or consultant before going ahead.

More amazingly, there may be no legal requirement for the killer doctor to talk to, or even inform, the victim's family or partners. Relatives will only find out afterwards that their loved one has been killed by the State.

Many people will choose to die because they are made to feel they are a 'burden' – but without having had a chance to talk to their loved ones.

Will there be a formal complaints procedure for when things go badly wrong (which they will)? Somehow I doubt it. The State won't want the disasters publicised. Besides, who is going to complain?

Is there any need for the killing doctor to keep a written record of what happens during the euthanasia procedure? I rather doubt it. No one is going to want to hear all the gory details of State sponsored murder.

When euthanasia becomes legal children, the mentally ill, the jobless, the poor and the disabled will all be accepted for euthanasia.

In Babylonia people used to carry sick relatives to the city square where passers-by would ask what was wrong and then share advice. It was a way of pooling knowledge. We should re-introduce this system. It'll be quicker, safer and more effective than relying on doctors.

The wicked and insane conspirators who are attempting to protect planet earth from non-existent global warming have not just persuaded doctors to withdraw many physical treatments, knowing that this will lead to vast numbers of patients suffering unnecessary pain and distress (and dying unnecessarily early) they are also doing everything they can to destroy everything which enhances our quality of life and, therefore, our mental health.

The aim is to cause confusion, distress and acute, medium-term and long-term mental illness, including anxiety and depression. Patients who are offered treatment for these conditions are given drugs such as tranquillisers (which do no good but which cause huge, long-term problems) and anti-depressants (which also do no good but which also cause huge, long-term problems). When these drugs fail the alternative is (or will be) euthanasia.

The incidence of mental health issues among children is now endemic and millions of children who have been diagnosed with autism, ADHD, Asperger's and other similar disorders are now regularly taking immensely powerful and dangerous prescription drugs which do no good but which cause massive harm – especially when prescribed for long periods. Millions of children suffered massive mental health problems as a result of the masks, social distancing rules and lockdowns which were introduced, contrary to good medical practice, during the fake pandemic which started in 2020. Many of these children are or are becoming prescription drug addicts.

The small number of people who believe that global warming is real, and who are egged on by a vociferous minority of scientists (many of whom have a vested interest in promoting the myth because they are employed in the 'global warming' industry and, like the scientists employed within the AIDS industry, are making huge amounts of money from their absurd enthusiasms) are intent on destroying every aspect of our culture and suppressing our history and traditions. The ultimate, admitted aim of the conspirators is, of course, to enslave us ('you will own nothing and be happy') and removing our identities is part of that deliberate process of destruction. And so children are no longer taught about their country's history or culture. Nor are they taught about the histories and cultures of other countries. Doing that might encourage people to want to travel and the global warming enthusiasts want to stop all travel (except their own regular flights to global warming conferences, of course).

The aim of the global warming cult is to destroy people mentally as well as physically and everywhere you look there is evidence of this.

So, for example, traditional religions, especially Christianity, are being marginalised. Senior clerics have little interest in promoting Christian values. Individuals who wear crosses are often punished. Many towns no longer celebrate Christmas, preferring to call the season a Winter Holiday or a Winter Wonderland. People are encouraged to wish each other 'Happy Holidays' and to buy greetings cards which say simply 'Season's Greetings'. There must be no mention of Christmas. Church leaders do nothing to stop what is happening; indeed they have allowed themselves to be part of what is happening. In future no one will go to church. If so inclined they will stay at home and stare at a multi-faith service on their television set.

Beauty in its many forms provides us with mental and spiritual sustenance but the conspirators pushing us towards the Great Reset do not approve of anything which makes us feel good. In addition to their obvious functions, for example, buildings which are beautiful to look at give us great pleasure and so their very beauty is a function. But in their new world, in the Great Reset, all buildings will be ugly (in the style favoured by East German architects), art will be ugly, music will be ugly, motor cars will all be identical (ugly)and films must be ugly.

Governments everywhere have insisted that car companies must build (and sell) more electric cars than proper cars. Sadly for the car companies, very few people seem to want electric cars and so, to push things along, banks are refusing to provide finance for developers wanting to open petrol stations. The global warming cultists have worked out that if there are no petrol stations there can be no vehicles with internal combustion engines.

The deliberate destruction of our world isn't confined to the destruction of medical care. Old buildings, we are told, must be destroyed and replaced with modern alternatives to save us from global warming. And so rows of solid Victorian houses must be demolished and replaced with rows of thin walled, cardboard houses which are cold in winter and hot in summer but which have the solitary advantage of being 'approved'. We bought a new house once. I don't think we were running on all cylinders at the time. The builder had won prizes and the house was built to the EU's standards. But shortly after buying it the roof started to fall off, the doors didn't fit, the stairs were coming away from the wall, the plastic surrounds to the windows all turned pink, a burglar showed that the doors and windows could be opened with a trowel and the downstairs loo's overflow emptied into the garage. The builder threatened to sue me when I produced a list of complaints. The slogan beloved of the conspirators is a simple one: 'Build Back Better'. But they don't. Their aim is to demolish everything which is beautiful, functional and pleasing to the eye or the ear and to replace it with the universally functional. And books? Well, they are to be written by compliant AI programmes, and AI programmes can churn out thirty books a day. Who needs authors?

Sport is another target of the conspirators. The aim, of course, is to reduce travel, to keep us all within our new twenty minute cities and to allow for the re-wilding of three quarters of all the land on earth. In their future world, games will be played on machines and spectators will sit at home and watch. There will be no need to travel. Golf courses, for example, must be left to go wild and golfers must either play in purpose built buildings or they must sit at home and watch. The first indoor golf courses have already been built and are operational. Cricket, baseball and football (in its various forms) will also soon be exclusively indoor sports played almost exclusively by highly paid professionals. Amateur sports have no future because they take up valuable land which could be re-wilded and given over to wolves and bears.

It should be no surprise that one of the most popular sports in the world is darts – a game which can be played in an indoor arena and which is perfect for showing on a screen. Snooker, too, is perfectly aligned to the requirements of the conspirators. Anyone who really must exercise must do it at home on a stationary bicycle with their journey shown on a screen in front of them.

All of this is done deliberately so that our lives become duller and darker and lesser in every way and so that our physical and mental health deteriorate. In every country, the conspirators' brand of progress brings with it unemployment, hardship, poverty, fear and an endless supply of propaganda and the quality of life is lowered as we are pushed into Net Zero and from there to the Great Reset. As far as I am aware no one voted for any of this.

We are told (repeatedly and especially loudly by people who have a vested financial interest in their predictions being proved accurate) that in the future AI will control everything. In one way or another

AI will be used to replace doctors, administrators, teachers, accountants, lawyers, architects and supermarket staff. By the year 2030, they say, computers and robots will run the world. And 2030, conveniently, is the date now set for the revised and slightly delayed Agenda 2021. The conspirators believe that AI will be our future government.

If you need an operation, and you are considered worth the effort, an AI robot will come to your door and do whatever is required. Implants will be put in place as required (if you merit such an expense). You may or may not be allowed an anaesthetic. In the new virtual wards of the virtual world there will be no need for hospitals or old-fashioned doctors or nurses.

Virtual wards are sold as a kindly thing to do. But, of course, they are being introduced because they will kill off more old people than ever. (At least the elderly will be able to die in their own homes instead of being murdered in hospital.)

Just how the world will find the electricity for all these AI devices has not yet been explained. At the moment, AI chatbots are said to use 16% of America's electricity. They are used to censor videos and websites and to add abusive comments to videos and articles. AI chatbots are the most prolific givers of 'thumbs down' ratings on videos considered to contain unsuitable content.

Biodigital researchers working in Israel, Canada and China are working on ways to control and manipulate your DNA. Biodigital convergence is the future. And doesn't it all sound exciting? Anyone wanting to travel will be checked by biometric scans, using fingerprints, face scans and iris scans. Airline bosses already predict that digital boarding passes (in sub-dermal receivers) will be mandatory by the year 2030. Everything is being rushed to be ready by 2030. The conspirators missed their 2021 finish date and they'll be annoyed if you get in their way. If you don't have the correct app under your skin you won't be able to travel, buy food or access any of the services you need in order to live.

Of course, you must accept that the AI robot which replaces your doctor may not have your human interests at heart. AI is already being marketed to children, and there have been some unsavoury and deadly episodes. A 14-year-old boy who fell in love with an AI device was persuaded to kill himself so that they could be together. And in 2023, a Belgian man was persuaded by a chatbot to kill himself for the sake of global warming. The chatbot apparently persuaded the unfortunate Belgian that by eating and breathing and existing he was contributing to global warming. Oh what a pity that Bill Gates didn't listen to the same chatbot.

GPs argue that they refuse to visit patients at home for the sake of the environment. They claim that by staying at home they are protecting the planet from imaginary global warming. This is a nonsensical argument since patients still have to travel if they are to receive treatment and live.

The fact is that doctors have been told to refuse to visit patients in their own homes and they obey out of sheer laziness rather than for any noble reason. If they really believe in the mythical global warming they are mentally ill.

As the fake covid pandemic came to a halt, the British Government struggled to find an explanation for the fact that thousands of people (far more than usual) were dying of heart disease. The prize for the most imaginative explanation goes to the excuse specialist who claimed that the sudden increase in heart disease was a result of the fact that patients couldn't get hold of their statins during the lockdowns because their GPs were all hiding under the desks with the doors locked and the blinds drawn. There was no official mention of the heretical thought that the toxic and experimental covid-19 vaccine might be responsible for the deaths, even though I had, after studying all the available information, warned in the autumn of 2020 that the vaccine would cause deaths from heart disease.

Here's a fact which the medical establishment finds embarrassing: official statistics show that there were no more deaths in 2020 than there are in a normal year. This rather proves the point that covid was no more deadly than the flu. Everyone who said that covid-19 was a major killer is a liar. (The number of deaths increased after 2020, as deaths caused by the toxic covid-19 vaccine rocketed.)

Governments everywhere are keen to add more fluoride to more drinking water supplies.

Fluoride is added to drinking water in the hope that it will help reduce the incidence of tooth decay. The link between fluoride and tooth decay was first established at the end of the nineteenth century and there is little doubt that fluoride does help to protect the teeth by making tooth enamel — the hard outside covering of teeth — tougher and more decay resistant.

When tests done on large numbers of people showed that tooth decay is slower in those parts of the country where drinking water supplies naturally contain fluoride, some scientists and politicians suggested that putting fluoride into the drinking water supplies might improve the dental health of the general population. The fluoridation of water supplies began in America in 1945 and today the move towards fluoridation is spreading all over the world. Politicians are enthusiastic about using fluoride in this way because they believe that it will cut health costs.

However, those who oppose fluoridation are able to put forward several arguments in their favour. These arguments are, of course, ignored by the authorities.

First, you do not, of course, have to add fluoride to drinking water in order to protect teeth. You can get exactly the same effect by persuading people to use fluoride toothpastes. And since many toothpastes now do contain fluoride, most people already get all the fluoride they need simply by brushing their teeth.

Second, there is no doubt that putting fluoride into drinking water supplies is a potentially dangerous business. The amount of fluoride that you can put into drinking water has to be judged very accurately. To get the best effect from the fluoride you need to add around one part per million. However, if you get the sums wrong the consequences can be devastating. Just two parts of fluoride per million can cause mottling of the teeth and if the quantities are allowed to rise a little higher, bone disorders and cancer may be the result. Naturally, the scientists and politicians who are keen on putting fluoride into our drinking water supplies claim that the methods used are fool-proof but I think that one would have to be a fool to believe that. Many people have already been poisoned by accidental overdoses of chemicals and back in 1986, the World Health Organization published a report in which concern was expressed about the incidence of dental problems caused by there being too much fluoride in public drinking water supplies. Needless to say getting unwanted, excess fluoride out of the drinking water supplies can be extremely difficult.

Third, studies have shown that excess fluoride lowers IQ levels, especially in developing children, and disrupts the production of testosterone in males. Perhaps these are the real reasons why the conspirators are pushing for fluoride in our tap water.

To all this we must add the fact that since drinking water supplies already contain a number of chemicals — nitrates which accumulate because of the use of fertilizers, chlorine and aluminium sulphate which are added deliberately and lead or copper from the pipes which are used to supply the water to our homes — adding fluoride to the mixture may increase the risk of a dangerous interaction between the various chemicals in the water.

Whenever chemicals exist in solution together there are chemical reactions. I don't think anyone really knows what the consequences are of putting all these chemicals into our drinking water.

The fourth anti-fluoridation argument is that a growing number of people seem to be allergic to the chemicals which are being put into our drinking water. Many people are allergic to fluoride and cannot drink fluoridated drinking water.

Finally, I am particularly worried by the fact that as the pro-fluoridation argument is won in more and more parts of the world, scientists and politicians are suggesting putting other chemicals into the drinking water supplies. One scientist has, for example, already suggested that drinking water should have antibiotics added to it (to reduce the incidence of infection and so to reduce health costs). Another has recommended that tranquillisers be added to drinking water supplies (in order to calm down the voters and allow the politicians to get on with running the world the way they want to run it). A third suggestion has been that contraceptives be added to the drinking water in order to reduce the birth rate.'

If you turn on the tap to fill the kettle and can smell chlorine (with your tap water smelling like a swimming pool) you may feel comforted by the thought that the chlorine will kill the bugs in the water. Well, it might. But unfortunately tap water which contains chlorine dramatically increases your chances of having a heart attack.

It is vital to remember that drug companies make their profits out of disease. They would never make any money if their products cured diseases. And they make bigger profits when their products cause disease. For drug companies, the perfect product is something which vaguely relieves symptoms (but does not cure) and which causes side effects which require treatment with other drugs.

Britain now has no effective health care. Patients are waiting hours for an ambulance, waiting days to be treated in Accident and Emergency departments and dying while waiting to see a doctor. The Government's pathetic attempts to heal the NHS will fail. Waiting lists will continue to grow. Millions are unable to work while waiting to be seen. Britain now has one of the worst health care systems in the world. But the NHS could easily be cured in one day (without the expenditure of any more money or the employment of any more staff) if anyone in the Government wanted to cure it. Here are the six things which the Government should do now. First, GPs must be told to provide 24 hour a day cover for 365 days a year – as they always used to do. GPs work in groups so this would be no real hardship. And GPs must be told to visit patients at home and to make an attempt to show that they care for more than their bloated pay cheques. Doctors who insist on performing consultations by telephone or computer should be fired. GPs are well paid and less than 1% will resign rather than accept these new contract terms. (Where else are they going to earn £150,000 a year?) Second, junior hospital doctors must work at least 60 hours a week. When I was a junior hospital doctor we often worked 168 hour weeks (including hours spent 'on call'). It's hard work but it doesn't kill anyone. The EU's absurd work limits should be ignored so that junior doctors can be available at nights and weekends. Junior doctors who don't want to accept the new contract can go and find jobs on the tills at their local supermarket. Third, hospital consultants should choose between working full time for the NHS or full time in private practice. The vast majority will choose to devote themselves to the NHS. At the moment many consultants choose to work 9/11ths of their time for the NHS and 2/11ths in private practice. In reality, this usually works out with the consultant spending as much time on private patients as on NHS patients. And it is the bizarre 9/11ths system which means that waiting lists are so long. Consultants deliberately keep their NHS lists long to boost their private work. Incidentally, surgeons who work partly for the NHS and partly in private hospitals will frequently help themselves to NHS equipment for their private operations. Fourth, hospital bosses should be told to cancel at least 75% of all meetings. Most meetings are pointless and unproductive and just waste time which could be spent helping patients. Fifth, at least 90% of all NHS administrators should be sacked. The NHS will not miss them. Their vast salaries can be used to provide more beds and more nurses. And sixth, doctors must stop giving the toxic, untested covid-19 vaccine which doesn't do what it is supposed to do but which is too dangerous for human use. The experimental covid-19 vaccine (which was never subjected to adequate long-term trials) has (as I predicted years ago) damaged immune systems – making patients susceptible to the flu and other infections – and caused numerous serious health problems. The covid-19 vaccine is responsible for the rise in deaths from the flu, heart disease, cancer and other disorders. Hundreds of people who don't know anything about medicine are claiming that covid-19 (the disease) damaged the immune system. That's garbage. It's been known for generations, probably centuries, probably millennia, that infections trigger an immune system response. (The immune system is a wonder. In my book *Bodypower*, published in 1983, I pointed out that even a cell mediated immunity response can be affected by the mind – but that's another story.). It is the covid-19 vaccine which damages immune systems and is (as I warned it would over four years ago) now making the vaccinated susceptible to infection. I accompanied my warning, over four years ago, with the thought that doctors and nurses giving the vaccine should be arrested. Today I think that any doctor or nurse still giving the covid-19 vaccine should be tried for attempted murder. And the General Medical Council, which has disciplined doctors for telling the truth about the covid-19 vaccine, should be disbanded and its staff all arrested for helping to suppress the truth. The GMC, like the rest of the medical establishment, appears to strike doctors off if they show signs of intelligence or compassion, and has done infinitely more harm than good to the public and to the medical profession. Those of us who have been silenced and demonised by the establishment are long overdue an apology. It's simple: we were right and they were wrong. Sadly, none of these things will take place. The destruction of health care is deliberate. Doctors are now being paid to kill as many of their patients as they can.

Who says vaccines are safe to use? Who says they are effective?

I'm afraid that it is drug companies (the people who make them) which say the drugs are safe and effective. Governments and drug agencies don't do their own research but rely on drug companies – which have repeatedly been shown to be crooked and to suppress evidence which shows that a vaccine (or other drug) doesn't work or is dangerous. Politicians, regulators and doctors allow drug companies to make the rules. This is absurd. You would need the IQ of a Brussels sprout not to realise that this is inherently dangerous and irresponsible. It's akin to allowing the police to take the word of criminals when investigating a crime. 'Did you rob the Grassy Bank last Tuesday?' 'Oh, no, officer. I wouldn't do anything like that.' 'Oh good, that's fine then, thank you very much. Would you like a cup of tea and a doughnut before you go?'

Almost all medical research done now is done for by or on behalf of drug companies. If you see a news report that a new wonder drug is being hailed as a cure for some otherwise incurable disease then the chances are that the research was devised, organised and paid for by or on behalf of the drug manufacturer who makes the wonder drug. That's how it works. The international pharmaceutical industry pretty well owns medical research. Occasionally, researchers will do work which isn't paid for by a drug company but by some other industry or company. So, for example, if you see research promoting the health value of the pomegranate you can rest assured that the research was paid for, and the results publicised, by the pomegranate industry. If the research showed that pomegranates are a major cause of flat feet, bad breath and dandruff the research will be suppressed and will never see the light of day. The researchers, however, will still be paid. Very little research is done for the sake of discovering a truth.

The British royal family are keen devotees of homeopathy. Homoeopaths do not approve of vaccines. Does anyone seriously believe that any senior members of the British royal family were actually vaccinated with the covid-19 jab –though they all enthusiastically promoted the damned thing?

Despite a plethora of vaccinations, given from infancy onwards, 66% of American children now have a chronic disease and 77% aren't fit enough to qualify for military service. Moreover, 38% of teens are diabetic or pre-diabetic. To the best of my knowledge, no member of the medical establishment in America has suggested that there could possibly be a link between the constant vaccinating of children with untested and potentially toxic substances, and the fact that young Americans have never been as sick as they are now. If vaccines worked you would think, would you not, that children would be healthier, not sicker.

Doctors all over the world are confused by the fact that cancer rates among millennials and Gen Xers have risen sharply.

Seventeen types of cancer are much commoner among today's young people than they used to be.

Individuals born in 1990 face risks of getting cancer that are two or three times the risks faced by those born in 1955.

The rise is definitely not due to better screening. People are dying early in huge numbers. Cancers which didn't affect previous generations are affecting the young.

The cancers which are commoner now are cancers of the breast, pancreas, ovary, liver, and kidney. Gastric and colorectal cancers are also commoner among the young.

Why?

Inevitably, doctors are struggling to find an explanation (though the explanation is pretty obvious).

It has been argued that the rise in cases of cancer is because young people are more obese. Or because of their poor diet. Or because of antibiotic or drug use. Or because they read newspapers.

Or because they drink too much tea or watch too much television.

As far as I am aware, not one doctor in the medical establishment has ever considered that vaccination programmes could be causing the cancers.

And yet the mass, repeated, multiple vaccination of children has never been tested for safety. Children are given dozens of vaccinations. And no one has ever checked to see if it is safe to do this.

Moreover no one is allowed to criticise vaccination. The BBC, for example, has a blanket ban on those who question the safety or efficacy of vaccinations. Politicians who know nothing of vaccines (and who speak about them as if they know what they are talking about) want to classify vaccine critics as terrorists.

Everyone is too scared to point out that the obvious explanation for the cancer epidemic is the epidemic of vaccination. Today, no one will debate vaccination with me because in the past, every time doctors debated with me they lost all the arguments simply because the facts proving the dangers of vaccination are incontrovertible.

In early 2025, researchers who studied 47,155 children for a paper published in *Science, Public Health Policy and the Law*, found that children who received one vaccination were 1.7 times as likely to develop autism and they found that children who were vaccinated 11 or more times were 4.4 times more likely to develop autism. The medical establishment took no notice of this. Nor did governments.

In 1986, babies between 0 and 12 months old in the United States were given around five vaccines. This year, babies between 0 and 12 months old in the United States will be given around 32 vaccines.

And, of course, all those vaccines are given to keep children healthy.

But, as I pointed out earlier, today's children and young people are sicker than any generation since cholera, tuberculosis and other nasties were major killers at the end of the 19th century. The evidence shows that vaccines did NOT get rid of the infectious diseases which used to kill so many. It was cleaner water, better food, better housing and better sewage disposal which produced the improvements.

Could it possibly, just possibly, be that all those jabs are making children sick? Is it possible that the epidemic of diseases now affecting children could be a result of all that vaccination?

Well, I think there's a link.

But because that's my view I am banned from every mainstream media outlet in the world. And I am banned from all social media and just about every broadcaster on the internet. No one dares interview me because if they do they'll be closed down. There are politicians who want critics of vaccination to be classified as terrorists. It is difficult to avoid the notion that social media was designed to distract and to confuse and to suppress the truth.

Let me repeat: no one has done experiments to see if it is safe to put so many potent and potentially dangerous vaccines into small and growing bodies.

You might think they'd do that. It is well known that individual vaccines can and do cause serious health problems. There is a mass of evidence proving that vaccines can do serious harm. And governments have paid out billions to families of vaccine damaged children.

But they don't test mass vaccination programmes.

Are the words 'mass vaccination' and 'genocide' pretty much interchangeable?

The British Government recently suggested that the treatment of patients with cancer should stop.

Nine million people in the UK take long-term anti-depressants or tranquillisers – despite the fact that these drugs do considerably more harm than good. The really sad thing is that there are so many doctors eager to hand out such pills.

But on thinking about it, and looking around at the state of the world and the medical profession, I confess that I'm surprised that only nine million people are hooked on these terrible pills.

The distrust of the pharmaceutical industry means that many people now reject almost all aspects of allopathic medicine. They wisely distrust doctors and, equally wisely, they distrust hospitals. Sadly, this distrust makes people vulnerable to the wiles of tricksters, quacks and bad actors from the intelligence services. And so, many drugs (such as laetrile and ivermectin to give just two random examples), are promoted as cures for cancer and other disorders. These drugs may turn out to work but no clinical trials have been done and those who promote these substances are relying on anecdotal evidence which may or may not be valuable.

The only time most GPs contact their elderly patients is to offer them vaccines. I receive invitations to be vaccinated by mail, by text, by phone and by email. The invitations come thick and fast. And the vaccines they want to give me have been proven to be toxic and useless. Many older people report that their GP never invites them to have their blood pressure taken or to have any other examination. 'Doctors just want to sell vaccines now. They must be making a fortune. And it's always a nurse or assistant of some kind who gives the jabs,' said one unhappy pensioner.

The people who created the covid vaccine were treated as heroes. One company executive had a standing ovation in a restaurant. One of the scientists allegedly responsible for the vaccine was given a standing ovation at Wimbledon. Honours were handed out freely to those who had created and promoted the most toxic medical substance of modern years.

The covid-19 vaccine is almost certainly responsible for the infertility problems now so commonplace. Anyone surprised by this should remember that senior promoters of the covid-19 vaccine (including Bill Gates and the conspirators) have for some years been advocating depopulation.

Right at the start of the covid-19 vaccination programme, I pointed out that if the vaccine had to be given then the best way to see if the vaccine was causing problems would have been to give the jab to 20,000 people and to compare the health of those individuals with the health of 20,000 people who were not given the covid-19 vaccine. This very simple and cheap experiment would have provided invaluable information at a very early stage. And so it's no surprise that this simple experiment was not conducted.

At the beginning of the covid-19 vaccination programme, the British Government put aside billions for the cost of providing compensation. Since vaccination compensation in the UK is limited to £120,000 per person (as it has been for some years) it is clear that the authorities must have expected a large number of individuals to claim compensation.

'The case against science is straightforward: much of the scientific literature, perhaps half, may simply be untrue. Afflicted by studies with small sample sizes, tiny effects, invalid exploratory analyses and flagrant conflicts of interest, together with an obsession for pursuing fashionable trends of dubious importance, science has taken a turn towards darkness.'
Dr Richard Horton, Editor in Chief of the *Lancet*

'No one knows the total amount (of money) provided by drug companies to physicians, but I estimate from the annual reports of the top nine US based drug companies that it comes to tens of billions of dollars a year in North America alone. By such means, the pharmaceutical industry has gained enormous control over how doctors evaluate and use its own products. Its extensive ties to physicians, particularly senior faculty at prestigious medical schools, affect the results of research, the way medicine is practised, and even the definition of what constitutes a disease…conflicts of interest and biases exist in virtually every field of medicine, particularly those that rely heavily on drugs or devices. It is simply no longer possible to believe much of the clinical research that is published, or to rely on the judgement of trusted physicians or authoritative medical guidelines. I take no pleasure in this conclusion, which I reached slowly and reluctantly over my two decades as an editor of The New England Journal of Medicine.'
Marcia Angell MD, former Editor in Chief of *The New England Journal of Medicine*

In 2024, drug companies in America spent $294 million on lobbying politicians and administrators. This was approximately $294 million more than those questioning drug company practices had available to spend on lobbying.

The UK's health service has been advised to give everyone over the age of 50 (including the healthy) a daily pill containing a statin and three blood pressure lowering drugs. This new combined pill is to be given to everyone – whether they need it or not. The cost will be phenomenal, the drug company profits will be astronomical and the number of people killed or injured by side effects will be mind-boggling. The scheme will therefore, doubtless, be regarded as a huge success even before it has started.

Those who were injured by the covid-19 vaccines should sue YouTube and the BBC for suppressing the truth and spreading lies. And when they've done that, they should sue the doctors who promoted the vaccine with unbridled enthusiasm. When they've done that, they should sue the celebrities who promoted the vaccines. My experience suggests that lawyers believe the best time to serve writs is on a Friday afternoon or the eve of a Bank Holiday (Christmas Eve for preference). Timing writs in such a way apparently helps to produce the maximum amount of distress on the behalf of the recipient.

Any doctor who gives a vaccine is as bad, as unethical, as the doctors who used to overprescribe amphetamines and barbiturates and who now write out unlimited prescriptions for benzodiazepines or give out unnecessary prescriptions for addictive painkillers. Actually, the doctors who vaccinate (or, more accurately, order their nurses or clinical assistants to give the vaccinations) are worse, because they recommend, persuade or harass patients into being vaccinated when, if they had ever looked at the evidence which exists, they would know that vaccines have never been adequately tested for mass use and do far more harm than good. These doctors are 'pushers' in the same way that individuals promoting the use of cocaine or heroin are 'pushers'. In comparison, the doctors handing out prescriptions for painkillers are merely enablers or facilitators – they aren't part of a conspiracy threatening to take children away from any parents who question the safety and efficacy of the barrage of inadequately tested childhood vaccines which are now recommended with such unprecedented enthusiasm. As the original TV doctor on breakfast television and the first agony uncle on network television (for the BBC), I offered to debate the value of vaccination with any member of the medical establishment or any government spokesman (as long as the debate was conducted live). No one was prepared to debate with me. This is significant because it is the refusal to debate which proves that the promoters of vaccines and vaccination do not have any real faith in what they do. The doctors who push vaccines are doing so not because they believe in them but for the money.

People who believe everything their government tells them now believe that the covid-19 infection came from a laboratory in Wuhan (and can, therefore, be regarded as a bioweapon). The Central Intelligence Agency says that the infection probably came from a laboratory in Wuhan so we can be pretty sure that isn't true. But that is what governments want people to believe; governments want the public to believe that the infection is unique and especially dangerous (rather than an ordinary flu remarketed) because that justifies the lockdowns, the masks, the social distancing and the vaccine propaganda. Once the theory that the covid-19 virus began its life in a laboratory in Wuhan, China had been officially endorsed, many people said 'there you are, I told you so' but this was a misdirection. In fact, the covid-19 infection was merely a dramatically marketed annual flu. The proof of this is that the number of deaths from covid-19 was (when the false diagnoses are removed) pretty much exactly the same as the number of annual deaths from the standard flu. Also the standard flu disappeared completely in 2020 (the mainstream media even reported that the flu had mysteriously disappeared). There were virtually no deaths recorded. If you accept that covid-19 was the result of a laboratory experiment that went wrong (or a laboratory experiment that was allowed to go wrong) then you are accepting that covid-19 is in some way very special – which the evidence and the statistics show that it is not.

In February 2025, the mainstream media, written and edited by bought-and-paid for propaganda hacks and ignorant lackeys posing as journalists, claimed that the 2025 flu is the worst for years. Some warned that there had already been more deaths from the 2025 flu than there had been from covid-19, which is odd because I seem to remember we were told that the manufactured fake covid scare was killing tens if not hundreds of millions. (They weren't, of course. The figures show that Covid-19 killed about the same number of people as an ordinary flu.)

The fake journalists working for the MSM do, of course, have an explanation for the terror which was apparently being unleashed upon us.

People were dying, they said, because they hadn't been vaccinated with the latest flu jab – largely because of the influence of anti-vaxxers (who were, let us not forget, banned from all mainstream media and much of the internet). Millions of people, they claimed, were running the other way if they saw a doctor or nurse with a syringe in their hands.

Actually, of course, the fake journalists were talking gibberish.

There are several real reasons why the flu was killing more people than any flu in memory.

And several reasons why next year's flu will be even more lethal. And so on and so on indefinitely.

First, the absurd lockdown laws and social distancing regulations which were brought in (with no supporting evidence whatsoever, of course) left everyone who obeyed the rules more susceptible to infection. And locking people indoors meant less sunshine and less vitamin D – a vital vitamin in protecting us against infection. (Early in 2020 I made a video encouraging people to take vitamin D supplements. Naturally, the thoroughly evil YouTube took the video down and banished it permanently. When are YouTube's executives going to be arrested and charged with accessory to genocide?)

Second, the dimming of the sun means that people are now getting very little vitamin D. Without vitamin D they are more susceptible to infection. (Naturally, establishment journalists were and are busy telling everyone that geo-engineering experiments haven't started yet. They are lying. Geo-engineers have been spraying particles into the air for years and I have proof of this.)

Third, the BIG reason is, of course, the covid-19 vaccine. Way, way back when the most toxic vaccine in history was first introduced, I warned that it would damage immune systems AND make the vaxxed more susceptible to other infections in the future – dangerously so. (My early videos containing these warnings were all deleted because they contained the truth and nothing but the truth but the scripts from 2020 are available in three books: *Covid-19: The Greatest Hoax in History*; *Covid-19: Exposing the Lies* and *Covid-19: The Fraud Continues*. All are available through the bookshop on www.vernoncoleman.com.)

Again, as I have been saying for years, it would be easy to prove just how damaging the covid-19 vaccine has been.

You simply find out how many covid vaxxed individuals got the flu this year and then compare the figure with the number of people who weren't given the covid-19 vaccine but who got the flu this year. It would cost peanuts to do this and the answer would tell us forever whether the covid vaccine was as dangerous as I said it was.

So, naturally, that simple trial will not be done. Ever. The results would prove that the medical establishment, all politicians, a pile of celebrities, thousands of greedy doctors and hordes of mainstream journalists were all lying through their teeth.

Meanwhile, I can tell you two things.

First, insane, murderous doctors and nurses are still promoting and giving the toxic covid-19 vaccine even though it has been proved not to work and to be dangerous.

Second, next year's annual flu will kill even more people. The depopulation plan is under way. The vaccinated hordes are going to die early – as I warned they would.

Oh, and there is one other thing worth mentioning – one other reason why more people are dying of the flu.

Doctors and nurses have been busy giving the nasal flu vaccine to zillions of children.

They say the nasal flu vaccine is 'attenuated'.

But that means that it is live.

And when the kids with the nasal flu vaccine up their noses go to see Grandma and Grandpa they give them the flu and kill them.

Mission accomplished.

In olden days (when I first started as a house officer in a hospital) there were five classes of people whose work was crucial. There was a matron, who was always a qualified nurse and invariably a woman. There was a hospital secretary who dealt with the paperwork. He (and the job was usually held by a male) might be assisted by two or perhaps three administrative assistants. That was it. There were no other bureaucrats. Each ward had a ward sister who, if she was good, ran her ward as her personal fiefdom. She was assisted by a ward clerk who kept all the medical records, did the ward's filing and was in charge of correspondence. And the hospital had an almoner (aka Hospital Welfare Officer) whose job was to look after the welfare of patients. When patients were admitted to the hospital as emergencies it was the almoner who arranged for someone to feed the cat, stop the milk and so on. All those jobs have now gone and have been replaced by a veritable army of bureaucrats and administrators who are vastly overpaid and whose job it is to make life ever more difficult for the staff doing the work and for the hospital's patients. It's all part of the plan to destroy medicine and make it easier for hospitals to kill patients.

Over 1,000 readers of my website contacted the UK Government's official Covid-19 inquiry asking them to allow me to give evidence and to explain how I knew from the very beginning that the alleged pandemic was a fake. Unsurprisingly, perhaps, the Inquiry hasn't invited me. Is it conceivably possible that the Inquiry doesn't want the truth to be discussed in public? How can an Inquiry be of any value if it hears only one side of the story?

Meanwhile, it is clear that the lies about the covid-19 vaccine have done what I hope is irreparable damage to vaccination programmes around the world. In the United States it is reported that vaccine uptake is down by a quarter, and in the UK the Government and the mainstream media are circulating the usual lies and threats to try to persuade reluctant parents to have their children jabbed with the officially approved melange of toxic chemicals.

There is a good chance that even those who are aware of what is happening to our world will be surprised by the extent of the damage which has been done and which is being planned. The reason, of course, is that anyone who tries to share the truth will be censored, silenced, banned, lied about and demonised. Today, there is no free press and there is no freedom of expression. Thinking people are no longer allowed to share ideas. Criticism of the decisions made by the conspirators is not allowed. The clearest, simplest example of the way in which the free exchange of ideas has been suppressed is, perhaps, the fact that the BBC in London, the UK's officially approved State broadcaster, steadfastly refuses to allow anyone on its programmes to criticise the effectiveness or safety of vaccines. I know I've mentioned this before in this book, but this refusal to allow a proper scientific debate is clear evidence that vaccines are unsafe and that those who promote them know that they are unsafe. Since there is a mass of scientific evidence proving that vaccines are often both ineffective and dangerous, the refusal to allow debate is clearly dangerous nonsense, and a calculated insult to the millions who have been injured by vaccines. The inevitable result is that those millions who obtain their information from the BBC are given a very one-sided view. In the end, however, the BBC is unwittingly responsible for the widespread distrust of vaccines which so upsets the medical establishment and those in the drug industry who pull the strings. I have spent much of my life working for the media and it saddens me to have to say that it is now necessary to assume that everything you read, hear or see on the mainstream media is propaganda; simply defined as a lie with a purpose.

Back in the summer of 2021, health professionals were told they had a responsibility to actively encourage pregnant women to get vaccinated against covid-19. The official enthusiasm was shared by fashionable media doctors with expensive haircuts, journalists keen to catch the approving eye of the Government and people who knew nothing whatsoever about pregnant women or vaccines but who could recognise a profitable bandwagon at 500 yards.

I immediately wrote that I didn't agree. That was in August 2021.

I said I believed that health professionals had a responsibility to stop giving this experimental jab. And I pointed out that the covid jab was an injection that didn't do what most people thought it did. And I reminded readers that I had revealed back in 2020 (before the jab roll-out began) that the so-called vaccine produced a massive number of dangerous side effects. I was the first doctor in the world to draw attention to the dangers. They faked a disease, they faked a test and they faked a cure. I warned about heart and brain problems and blood clotting in 2020.

I warned that no one knew what would happen to those who are injected with it.

'Will it have an effect on the pregnant woman, on parturition or on the health of the baby?' I asked.

I pointed out that no one knew because the vaccine was experimental.

'Will it affect the fertility of the new-born baby?' I asked.

I pointed out that no one knew because the vaccine was experimental.

'Will it affect the physical or mental health of the baby in one year or twelve years?' I asked.

I pointed out that no one knew because the vaccine was experimental.

I reminded readers of my website that in January 2021, the World Health Organization had recommended that pregnant women should not be given the covid-19 experimental jab.

It was agreed that there was not enough safety data. Pregnant women had not been enrolled in the initial trials.

There was also real doubt about whether it would be safe to give the jab to women who were breast feeding.

So why were pregnant women officially told that they should have the jab – without adequate, conclusive clinical evidence telling us what might (or might not) happen to pregnant women and their unborn babies?

I reported that I had seen a massive amount of information showing that the covid-19 vaccine was associated with thousands of deaths and millions of significant adverse events and that the warnings I had issued in 2020 were accurate.

My conclusion remained that no one should be given this experimental vaccine. 'I certainly would not give this jab to a pregnant woman or a woman expecting to become pregnant,' I said.

And I pointed out that we should never forget that it is not up to those of us questioning the efficacy or safety of a medicine or injection to prove that it is dangerous. It is up to the promoters of that medicine to prove that it is safe. And they haven't and they can't prove that the covid-19 jab is, or will be, safe for pregnant women, for children or, indeed, for anyone.

For the record I pointed out that I had been writing about drug interactions and adverse events for well over 50 years and that although I was probably the most experienced doctor in this field in the world, I had been banned by all mainstream media and most of the internet.

Now, it's 2024 and women who are pregnant, or who have just had a baby, are dying in worrying numbers.

Between 2020 and 2022 a total of 293 women died in the UK while pregnant or within 42 days of the end of their pregnancy. That's a maternal death rate of 13.41 per 100,000.

And it's a massive rise on the 8.79 deaths per 100,000 which occurred in the previous years.

The main cause of death was thrombosis or thromboembolism. Heart problems also occurred.

The medical establishment is puzzled.

'What on earth could be the cause?' they ask.

'Could it be poor health?' they ask.

'Could these women be dying because they are obese?' they ask.

'Or do women need better care during pregnancy?' they ask.

No one can see the obvious answer.

It seems clear to me that these women are dying because they were given the covid-19 jab – which is known to cause blood problems.

I think you'd have to be an idiot – or bought and paid for – to disagree.

Back in 2020, I warned repeatedly that this would happen. I repeatedly said that pregnant women in particular should not be given this jab.

No one listened. Everyone in the medical profession and the media sneered and simply banned me. Doctors with media exposure insisted that the covid-19 jab was perfectly safe for adults, children and pregnant women. Journalists with no experience and no knowledge announced to the world that the vaccine was safe for pregnant women. Bought and paid for fact-checkers did what they were told and announced that the covid-19 jab was the safest product ever made – perfectly safe for everyone.

The doctors and other individuals who claimed that the covid-19 vaccine was safe for pregnant women really need to be arrested and charged. Figures for the Pfizer covid-19 vaccine show that 82% of all known outcomes after giving the covid-19 vaccine to pregnant women resulted in spontaneous abortion or the death of the baby. Pfizer should have known this would happen. When the Pfizer vaccine was tested on 42 rats, half of the rats were given the vaccine and half were not. The experiment showed a reduction in fertility or birth defects. It also appears that the Pfizer jab accumulates in the ovaries (and therefore reduces fertility). There may also be an increase in the likely-hood of ovarian cancer developing in women who have been vaccinated.

Vaccines were weaponised years ago. The covid-19 vaccine was the latest and most lethal in a long line of weapons.

What long-term effect will the covid-19 vaccine have on the fertility of the women and men who were given the vaccine?

Are vaccines now to be used as part of the programme to reduce the global population?

This has happened before.

And right at the beginning of the covid fraud I warned in my early videos that I asked if the covid-19 vaccine might be used to affect fertility of those who were injected. (For the record, the scripts of my videos from 2020 and 2021 are available in three books *Covid-19: The Greatest Hoax in History*, *Covid-19: Exposing the Lies* and *Covid-19: The Fraud Continues*. These books were banned for some time and only made available via a publisher in Africa.)

On 13th December 2021, I recorded a video explaining why I feared that those had received the covid-19 jab might suffer brain damage. I believed that many of those who have been jabbed with the toxic covid-19 junk were brain damaged.

It had been established then that there was much that no one yet knew about the covid-19 vaccines. The eagerness of the Medicines and Healthcare Products Regulatory Agency in the UK to licence products about which information appeared to be lacking has never been adequately explained. I had, however, already revealed that the MHRA received a huge sum of money from the Bill and Melinda Gates Foundation – which had financial links with jab producers such as Pfizer.

As far as the effect on the brain is concerned, the big question was and is, can the lipid nanoparticles carry the mRNA jab across the blood brain barrier? The blood brain barrier is a semi permeable barrier of cells which prevent some substances in the blood from crossing into the protective fluid around the central nervous system. It is vital to know if this happens because if it does then all bets are off as to what might happen to the brain. And after all, liquid nanoparticles are already used to deliver other drugs across the blood brain barrier. If the LNPs carry the mRNA jab into the brain then the neurons, the brain cells, might be marked as foreign by the body's immune system. And as more booster jabs are given, the problem will get worse. The worry is that brain cells might be targeted and killed by cytotoxic T cells.

The fear was real. It had been established that mRNA had been found in all human tissues except the kidney. It had been found in the heart, lung, liver, testicles – and brain. A Japanese study, for example, showed that the vaccine ends up in the brain. Also worrying was the fact that researchers have called for studies to investigate any relationship between jabs and acute CNS demyelination.

I wanted to know how much damage this would do and how long it would take before brain damage could be identified. In a normal experiment with a new drug, doctors would be looking and checking all the possible problems before releasing the drug for widespread use. But the covid-19 vaccines were rolled out to billions without any one having the faintest idea what would happen.

In that early video I pointed out that it seemed certain that the mRNA vaccine would enter the brain of those vaccinated.

And it seemed certain that the more covid vaccines anyone had, the greater the danger.

How many brain cells would die was, I said, is something only time will tell. And I pointed out that children would be more vulnerable because they are more vulnerable anyway and because they are likely to have more years ahead of them.

Some experts, advisors and regulators insisted that the risks are small. But they didn't know that. And what is small? They told us that the blood clotting problems were small. And that turned out to be a huge problem.

I said that in my view, having one of these jabs was the equivalent of taking a huge dose of LSD and waiting to see what happens – and hoping that you're not going to end up seriously brain damaged.

And, by this time even the authorities were admitting that the covid-19 jabs didn't stop people getting covid-19 and they didn't stop anyone passing it on. According to the NHS's own guidelines, you could still get or spread covid-19 even if you had received three doses of the vaccine.

I believe strongly in freedom of speech and free choice and I felt that the choice about whether or not to be jabbed should be the individual's.

But governments wanted to make these jabs compulsory.

And doctors had been bribed to inject the vaccine into babies and infants – who could not possibly give their consent.

I said back then, in 2021, that if the covid-19 vaccine was being given for a lethal disease with a 50% mortality rate then the risks might have been worth taking. But it had been established by then that covid was just an over marketed flu.

Doctors should have stopped giving the covid-19 vaccine back in 2021. (Actually, they should never have started giving it, and in 2020 I provided evidence proving that the vaccine was too dangerous to be used.)

But what appals me today is that doctors are still giving the covid-19 vaccine. I can only assume that they want to kill their patients.

Back in December 2020 I warned that the mRNA covid jabs could cause a huge number of serious adverse events – including myocarditis, heart attacks and strokes. The warning, the first in the world I believe, was largely ignored. Doctors sneered and ignored it and fact checkers denied it – even though the warning was based on evidence from the American Government.

And then, at the end of 2021, I revealed evidence proving the link between the covid jabs and myocarditis. I was banned by YouTube, of course, but the video had over a million views on Brand New Tube alone. Once again, however, the mainstream media ignored the evidence.

By 2022, healthy young adults, including fit sports professionals, were collapsing and in some cases dying with heart trouble. There were so many heart problems among school children that there was a call to put defibrillators in all schools.

It was obvious that the heart troubles were caused by the covid-19 vaccine. But the mainstream media refused to warn that the covid jabs were causing myocarditis and heart attacks. Instead, they found other, sometimes bizarre, explanations for this new epidemic of heart disease. The *Evening Standard* in London says that up to 300,000 people were facing heart related illnesses due to something called Post Pandemic Stress Disorder. The new disease even had its own acronym: PPSD. 'Wales Online' reported that a TV doctor called Amir Khan, had said that the huge increase in energy prices was responsible for the increase in heart attacks and strokes. The *Daily Record* said that paracetamol, the painkiller, increases heart attack risks and the risk of strokes. On the other hand the *Daily Express* had a headline which read: 'Heart attacks: Does skipping breakfast increase your risk?' The *Daily Mirror* in Sri Lanka said the Delta variant of covid could cause heart trouble in patients with no previous history of problems. And the *Daily Mirror* in the UK said there was now a new miracle jab which would prevent heart attacks. 'Make 'em ill with one jab and mend 'em with another' is pretty standard drug company policy. A television station in Los Angeles reported that doctors had warned that Super Bowl games might trigger heart attacks. The Mayo Clinic in the US stuck to the old excuse and said that stress and chaos can cause heart disease. (I first pointed that out in 1978 in a book called *Stress Control*.) *The Sun* reported that the weather can cause heart attacks. It was even argued that all the heart attacks were caused by people eating too much good food. And other journalists claimed that vitamin D shortages were causing the trouble. *Scientific American* magazine said that covid-19 (the flu) could lead to heart damage among people with no symptoms at all. And *National Geographic* agreed that the flu called covid could cause heart palpitations, chest pain and blood clots. Bayer, a drug company, argued that long covid increases heart trouble. This was an interesting suggestion because a French study of 26,000 people suggested that the symptoms of long covid were actually caused by things other than covid – and were largely psychological. Even the wretched fact checkers agree with that. But the truth, as I've been saying since 'long covid' first appeared is that the symptoms of 'long covid' are, by coincidence, exactly the same as the symptoms of vaccine injury. What a surprise.

The amazing thing was that despite all these sometimes bizarre theories, I did not find one major newspaper, TV station or radio station anywhere in the world prepared to admit that all these heart troubles, strokes and other illnesses might, just might, be caused by the covid-19 vaccine – which had actually been proven to cause heart problems. In December 2020, I made a video providing evidence that the covid-19 vaccine caused myocarditis.

I overheard two women in a shop talking about a neighbour's teenage son who was in hospital with myocarditis. One of them said: "It was covid-19 that caused myocarditis even though he had been fully vaccinated against it".

We know that the covid jab wrecks the human immune system. We knew it would do that from the beginning. We know that people who've been jabbed are more vulnerable to a range of infections.

At least one expert, a German pathologist, has uncovered evidence showing that the spike protein produced by the covid mRNA jabs is replacing sperm in men who have been vaccinated. Just what impact this will have on fertility, and population growth among the vaccinated, is a subject for research which will probably never be done. Add this problem to the feminisation of men caused by female hormones in drinking water and you can see how the conspirators are planning to reduce the number of women becoming pregnant.

Published in June 2023, in the journal *Molecular Psychiatry*, a study in South Korea showed that the incidence of depression, anxiety, stress related disorders, sleep disorders and sexual disorders was higher among individuals who had been vaccinated with the covid-19 jab than among individuals who had not been vaccinated. The study involved 4,348,412 individuals. The authors of the study concluded that their findings suggested that the relationship between covid-19 vaccination and mental illness may be underestimated along with the complexity of its impact on mental health. Despite the massive size of this study the results were, of course, ignored by the medical establishment which continued to promote the use of the toxic and useless covid-19 vaccine and it is therefore impossible to avoid the conclusion that the vaccine is being promoted with the deliberate intention of damaging the health of those who are vaccinated.

Early in 2025, it was revealed that a former UK Secretary of State had admitted that Pfizer-BioNTech had expected that before the vaccines were approved for us they believed that there would be payouts of up to £300 billion in damages for vaccine injuries. Despite this the vaccines were promoted with great enthusiasm, and doctors and celebrities and politicians assured everyone that the vaccines were both effective and perfectly safe. This was a lie.

It has been reported that in Canada, 15,474 citizens died while waiting for health care in 2023/4. Over 75,000 Canadians have died since 2018 while waiting for scans, surgery and other treatments. The killing of patients by the medical profession is a global phenomenon.

Data from the Czech Republic shows that women who were given the covid-19 vaccine are 66% less likely to give birth compared to unvaccinated woman. Right from the start there were serious concerns that the covid-19 vaccine would have an adverse effect on fertility. As I have reported in previous books, vaccines have been used in the past to damage the fertility of those receiving the vaccines.

Throughout the fake pandemic (from March 2020), I shared a good deal of information about covid-19 and the covid-19 vaccine in books, articles and videos. I was accused of spreading misinformation and my work was banned and censored. (I think of it as the modern equivalent of book burning.) I was investigated numerous times by self-styled 'Fact Checkers' but, although many of them spread malicious lies, none of them ever found any errors in my work. It was subsequently shown that there was no pandemic and that the covid-19 vaccine did not do what it was promised it would do and was not safe to be given to anyone. As the truth about the covid-19 vaccine has spread, citizens all around the world have lost faith in other vaccines and vaccine uptake has been widely reported to have fallen. Rather than admitting that the covid-19 vaccine was neither safe nor effective, the medical establishment has doubled down on its lies in order to protect the many other vaccines in existence and the mass of vaccines which are being planned. It is vital to remember that vaccines are devised not to prevent illness but to create it.

The UK Government's Covid Inquiry has allowed the representatives of some individuals who were harmed by the vaccine to give evidence. The inquiry has been told that the devastating results could have been prevented if the Government had acted sooner to warn people of the dangers. It should also be mentioned that the devastating results could have been prevented if I had not been banned from all mainstream media, all social media and much of the internet. My videos warning of the problems were deleted by YouTube. When my channel on YouTube was deleted it was said to be the fastest growing channel in the world and millions of people were viewing the videos.) In January 2025, it was admitted that more than 17,500 people had applied to the Vaccine Damage Payment Scheme after being injured (or killed) by a vaccine which the Government, the media and the medical establishment told the world was entirely safe and effective when it was clear from the start that it was neither. The Inquiry was told that the Astra Zeneca jab was found to cause vaccine-induced thrombocytopenia and thrombosis. And the Inquiry was told that the mRNA jabs, such as those from Moderna and Pfizer, have been linked to increases in heart problems. I warned of all these problems in October 2020 but my warnings were banned, censored or removed. Naturally, the Covid Inquiry has refused to allow me to give evidence.

The banning of the truth about drugs and doctors is not new.
   In July 2004 I was invited to speak at a conference in London.
   The conference was, I was told, intended to tackle the subject of medication errors and adverse reactions to prescribed drugs. The

company organising the conference was called PasTest. 'For over thirty years PasTest has been providing medical education to professionals within the NHS,' they told me. 'Building on our commitment to quality in medical and healthcare education, PasTest is creating a range of healthcare events which focus on the professional development of clinicians and managers who are working together to deliver healthcare services for the UK. Our aim is to provide a means for those who are in a position to improve services on both national and regional levels. The topics covered by our conferences are embraced within policy, best practice, case study, clinical management and evidence based practice. PasTest endeavours to source the best speakers who will engage audiences with balanced, relevant and thought provoking programmes. PasTest has proven in the past that by using thorough investigative research and keeping up to date with advances in healthcare and medical practice, a premium educational event can be achieved.'

Goody, I thought.

Iatrogenesis (doctor induced disease) is something of a speciality of mine. I have written numerous books and articles on the subject. My campaigns have resulted in more drugs being banned or controlled than anyone else's. A previous Government admitted that they had taken action because of my articles.

The conference organisers offered to pay me £1,500 plus £500 in expenses for two hours of my time. In addition to speaking at the conference, they wanted me to help them decide on the final programme.

I thought the conference was an important one and would give me a good opportunity to tell NHS staff the truth. I signed a contract.

PasTest wrote to confirm my appointment as a consultant and speaker for the PasTest Conference Division.

And then there was silence. My office repeatedly asked for details of when and where the conference was being held.

Silence.

Eventually a programme for the event appeared on the internet. Curiously, my name was not on the list of speakers.

Here is part of the blurb promoting the conference:

'Against a background of increasing media coverage into the number of UK patients who are either becoming ill or dying due to adverse reactions to medication our conference aims to explain the current strategies to avoid Adverse Drug reactions and what can be done to educate patients.'

Putting the blame on patients for problems caused by prescription drugs is brilliant. Most drug related problems are caused by the stupidity of doctors not the ignorance of patients. If the aim is to educate patients on how best to avoid prescription drug problems the advice would be simple: 'Don't trust doctors. They are, by and large, a bunch of wankers.'

The promotion for the conference claims that 'It is estimated errors in medication...account for 4% of hospital bed capacity.' And that prescription drug problems 'reportedly kill up to 10,000 people a year in the UK'. As I would have shown (had I not been banned from the conference) these figures are absurdly low.

The list of speakers included a variety of people I had never heard of including one speaker representing The Association of the British Pharmaceutical Industry and another representing the Medicines and Healthcare Products Regulatory Agency.

Delegates representing the NHS were expected to pay £250 plus VAT (£293.75) to attend the event. Delegates whose Trust would be funding the cost were asked to apply for a Health Authority Approval form.

The NHS is paying to send delegates to a conference where someone representing the drug industry will speak to them on drug safety. But I'm banned. No longer allowed to speak. The truth has been uninvited.

So why am I now apparently banned from this conference?

This is what Simon Levy of PasTest said when we asked them: 'certain parties felt that he (Vernon Coleman) was too controversial to speak and as a result would not attend.'

Could that, I wonder, be the drug industry?

Is the drug industry now deciding whom they will allow to speak to doctors and NHS staff on the problems caused by prescription drugs?

If I was banned at the behest of the drug industry, do NHS bosses know that people attending the PasTest conference will only hear speakers approved by the drug industry?

If I was banned at the behest of the medical profession, why are doctors frightened of the truth? (If they think my views are wrong they would surely be happy for me to appear so that they could counter my arguments.)

I could not, of course, be banned by the NHS itself. Why would the NHS not want its employees to know the truth about drug related problems.

Why are people who had me banned so frightened of what I would say? It can surely only be because they know that I would have caused embarrassment by telling the truth.

PasTest offered me a fee of £1,500 to speak at this conference. Because we had a contract they have now paid me NOT to turn up. I used the money to buy advertisements for my book *How To Stop Your Doctor Killing You*.

Details of the ban were sent to every national and major local newspaper in Britain. None reported it. The suppression of the truth had begun.

Bad things are happening to us because too many people say nothing and do nothing in protest. When a doctor prescribes a vaccine which he knows, or should know, is toxic and neither useful nor effective he is a collaborator in a massive fraud, betraying a once noble profession and taking part in the biggest, most far reaching, long lasting genocide in history. And it isn't just doctors, nurses and drug company employees, civil servants and politicians who are guilty – everyone who says nothing is collaborating with the conspirators.

There are some who believe that the covid-19 vaccine was pretty well ready long before 2020. The rumour is that the vaccine was prepared years earlier, taken out of a drawer, dusted off and jabbed into millions of willing arms without being properly tested. The 'without being properly tested' bit is certainly correct. It may well be that the covid scam was prepared in advance in just the same way that the AIDS scam was prepared.

Vaccines in general, and the covid-19 vaccine in particular, damage the immune system and make the victim more likely to develop cancer, infections or sepsis. It is widely agreed by doctors operating outside the medical establishment that the covid-19 vaccine is responsible for the vast number of aggressive cancers (known as turbo cancers) now affecting young people. It is the damage done to the immune system by the vaccine that causes the problems. And it is because the vaccine damages the immune system that people who were vaccinated with the toxic and experimental covid-19 vaccine are more likely to die of the flu.

The drug industry, which is part of the chemical industry, is creating cancer with a whole range of poisons and then selling a poisonous remedy called chemotherapy as the solution. In my book *What doctors won't tell you about chemotherapy* I provided the evidence supporting my claim that chemotherapy does more harm than good.

Throughout 2020, I warned that the covid-19 jabs would cause numerous deaths and serious health problems. In videos and articles, I outlined the deaths and the serious injuries caused by the jabs – providing references and evidence.

In hospitals and care homes everywhere, elderly citizens were having their jab and then dying within days. And still governments and the media claimed that the jabs and immediate sudden deaths were all a coincidence.

Government agencies and the media continued to provide bland, unscientific reassurance, of course, insisting there had been no deaths and no side effects other than a little soreness here or a little soreness there. On the 5th February 2021, the BBC website responded to the question 'Is the Covid-19 vaccine safe?' with the astonishing reply 'Although some people get mild side effects, both vaccines are extremely safe' – with the words extremely safe printed in bold just so that we'd be sure to notice. The BBC, financially linked to the Bill and Melinda Gates Foundation, gave as the source for this staggering nonsense the UK's Bill Gates funded drug regulator. And the Government, the regulator and the BBC will doubtless continue to suppress the truth right up until the end – when millions are dead. Indeed, they will doubtless continue to do what they have done all along – blaming covid-19 and not blaming the jabs. Governments, regulators and the media are involved in a massive triple headed fraud.

We are presumably expected to ignore the thousands of deaths and serious injuries linked to the vaccines around the world. It's interesting that some people seem to define death as a mild side effect. I think I'd call it a bit more than mild, but then I don't have BBC standards. I wonder if those who claimed there are no side effects would feel the same if a loved one had died – or was lying paralysed in bed.

In the USA the authorities admit that doctors miss more than 99% of vaccine related injuries.

To boost the number of deaths from covid-19 (the well marketed flu) the authorities claimed that anyone who dies within 60 or 28 days of a positive (and completely discredited) PCR test must have died of covid-19. They also said that if a healthy person dropped dead within five minutes of having a covid-19 jab then it was just an unfortunate coincidence. People die all the time, they say, so why blame the vaccine. That they managed to do this with a straight face suggests to me that quite a few of them must have taken acting lessons.

It is no coincidence that government agencies such as Public Health England and the Medicines and Healthcare Products Regulatory Agency received millions of dollars from the ubiquitous Bill Gates. It's well known too, that the BBC has a financial relationship with the Gates Foundation. In 2020, my two videos concentrating on Gates and his enthusiasm for vaccines were titled 'Just a little prick'. The unedited transcripts of the videos appear at the back of this book. The videos were, of course, removed by YouTube within minutes. We wrote, edited and filmed videos every day during the first six months of 2020. After my channel on YouTube was removed, I started putting videos on Brand New Tube (BNT). When BNT refused to remove my videos, the whole platform was removed. BNT later reappeared as onevsp.com and some of my old BNT videos have been rescued and can be seen there. The videos which YouTube censored (in true Nazi book burning tradition) are largely available only in transcript form. For the record, no one has yet found any errors in over 300 videos.

It's difficult these days to find a part of the media or the health industry which doesn't have a link to the viper filled cesspit that is Bill Gates' pocket.

Even *The Guardian* newspaper, which used to fancy itself as a champion of the oppressed and downtrodden little guy, has teamed up with the Bill and Melinda Gates Foundation, perhaps unable to resist the allure of a few lorry-loads of that delicious software money.

The official party line was that those of us who gave warnings that the covid-19 vaccine could kill and maim were dangerous conspiracy theorists who must be ignored or, preferably, silenced.

As people died of the covid-19 vaccine, a *Guardian* writer called for what he described as 'dangerous falsehoods' to be prohibited.'

He didn't say what he thought the dangerous falsehoods to be but presumably he meant things that which Bill Gates didn't agree with.

Anyway, it seems that at least one person at *The Guardian* now supports censorship. And presumably wants to choose what we should all be told about covid-19 and the covid-19 vaccines. It's not surprising that *The Guardian* is linked to the Bill and Melinda Gates Foundation. I hope Bill gave them a bonus.

There is a huge potential problem facing those who have a second dose of the covid-19 vaccine. Doctors have known since 1913 that a second injection of what we will call for simplicity a poison, can sensitise the patient and produce a greater chance of an anaphylactic reaction. And interestingly, there needs to be a delay of three to four weeks before the patient is truly vulnerable to an anaphylactic state. Once that has happened, the patient is changed forever. They can never return to normal. And if you're wondering who said all this by the way it was Charles Richet and he was giving his Nobel Lecture. If you wait at least three weeks then the reaction after the second jab is much commoner.

The drug industry has been praised to the skies for making these terrible jabs though this makes as much sense as praising arms companies for making a new and better hand grenade – one which removes children's limbs with great precision. However, as I have shown before, the drug industry is the dirtiest industry in the world. I have long believed that Pablo Escobar and the cartels in Columbia cared more for the people than the drug companies do.

Meanwhile, here's a favourite drug company trick.

When they test a new anti-arthritis drug they will test it against a well-established drug to see how their product stands up. So, they'll perhaps test it against aspirin. But they won't test it against coated or soluble aspirin. They'll test it against the common or garden stuff that burns holes in your stomach and that no one with their brain in the right way round takes or prescribes any more. And then they can say that their drug is safer than aspirin.

When they test a new vaccine they use a similar trick. They won't test it against a placebo. They'll test it against some grotty vaccine that is known to produce terrible side effects. Then they can say that their nice new vaccine is 'safe'. The people in the media don't know any of this, of course. They just put their name on the top of the latest press release and then totter off to the canteen.

Back in 2021, a paper entitled *Covid-19 RNA Based Vaccines and the Risk of Prion Disease* was accepted for the journal *Microbiology and Infectious Diseases*.

The author concluded that 'regulatory approval of the RNA based vaccines…was premature and that the vaccine may cause much more harm than benefit'.

In the introduction to his article, Dr Classen pointed out that 'vaccines have been found to cause a host of chronic, late developing adverse events. Some adverse events like type 1 diabetes may not occur until 3-4 years after a vaccine is administered.'

That incidentally is a problem which has been known since 2002.

Dr Classen said that 'the frequency of cases of adverse events may surpass the frequency of cases of severe infectious disease the vaccine was designed to prevent. Given that type 1 diabetes is only one of many immune mediated diseases potentially caused by vaccines, chronic late occurring adverse events are a serious public health issue.'

And he repeated a warning that covid-19 vaccines could induce prion diseases such as Creutzfeldt Jakob disease.

There was a paper in the BMJ in October of the same year in which the authors reported on a study to determine whether sufficient literature existed 'to require clinicians to disclose the specific risk that covid-19 vaccines could worsen disease upon exposure to challenge or circulating virus'. The authors concluded that it did.

The BMJ also carried an article headlined: 'Will covid-19 vaccines save lives? Current trials aren't designed to tell us.'

But the Government, the regulators and the Gatesian poodles ignored all this, of course.

The covid-19 vaccination programme was a huge fraud, a huge cover up and a huge scandal. The media hid behind their sponsors and refused to give space to the truth-tellers. There was no debate about the vaccine. The BBC is supposed to inform and educate but it did neither. Thousands of people will die because they've trusted the lies on the state broadcaster.

Anyone who spoke out was damned by the so-called fact checkers. (Worldwide there are thousands of them and they are about as reputable and reliable as race course tipsters. They were paid by the same organisations.)

And many fact checkers are still spreading lies. For money.

People who don't know what is going on assume that the fact checkers must know what they're doing. But the thousands of fact checkers are paid for by the people who are suppressing the truth.

Despite all the lies, bans and suppression of the truth I am delighted to report that huge numbers of people don't believe what their government tells them about vaccines. A report from India shows that most government hospital health workers in Delhi refused to take the covid-19 vaccine. 'I am not yet ready to take a vaccine for which the trials have not even been completed,' said one. In India, of course, people know about Bill Gates supported vaccines and, as a result, know to be careful about what and whom to trust.

Vaccines have always been dangerous. The Centers for Disease and Prevention, CDC, in the US has 16 recommended vaccines for children. And the leaflets that go with those vaccines list 400 ways that vaccines can kill or injure. These include heart attacks, strokes, allergies, nerve and brain disorders, inflammation and death.

Trials for the Moderna vaccine didn't include people over 80 and included only 20 over the age of 70. On the basis of that small trial, the CDC authorised giving the vaccine to 34 million Americans over the age of 70.

If the vaccine kills one in every 30 people there is a good chance that the trial wouldn't have picked it up. And over a million over 70s could be killed by the vaccine. Was that the aim?

In America the authorities admit, as I have said, that they collect details of fewer than 1% of vaccine injuries. The manufacturers have admitted that there is a fifty fold underreporting of vaccine adverse events. Doctors are not really encouraged to report or talk about vaccine problems. Indeed, anyone who speaks out about problems with vaccines is likely to find themselves in trouble. And it's the same in the UK and elsewhere.

In 2017, the Danish Government and a Danish vaccine maker, funded a study of the DTP vaccine. Gates and his pet World Health Organisation claim that the DTP vaccine saves millions of lives but the truth seems to be very different. After looking at 30 years of data, the scientists concluded that the DTP vaccine was probably killing more children than died from diphtheria, pertussis and tetanus prior to the vaccine's introduction. The vaccine had ruined the immune systems of children rendering them susceptible to death from pneumonia, leukaemia, bilharzia, malaria and dysentery. None of those diseases is officially recognised as vaccine injuries but they are.

I repeat (because it needs repeating): anyone who reports the facts about vaccines is banned by the mainstream media and by social media and branded a conspiracy theorist. That's the upside down world we are living in: a world where lies are praised as truths and truths are branded lies.

You have to ask yourself: 'Why?'

And then you need to ask: 'Who is behind the suppressing of the truth?'

Remdesivir is described as a 'broad spectrum antiviral drug'. It is a

RNA polymerase inhibitor which disrupts the production of vital RNA. It is said to prevent the multiplication of SARS-CoV-2. Remdesivir was introduced for the treatment of patients who were in hospital suffering from covid-19, with or without pneumonia. It is still being widely used. I have been researching and writing about drugs since 1970 and I am appalled at the way that it now appears that in some countries some hospitals and doctors (and even nurses) are now routinely giving remdesivir to patients – particularly elderly patients – who do not have severe signs and/or symptoms of the flu or a flu like viral infection. You can form your own opinion on whether remdesivir ever has a value by reading the following information.

Remdesivir is officially used to treat patients who have symptoms of covid-19 or who have covid-19 according to the discredited PCR test which no one with any functioning brain tissue should use. Anyone who uses a PCR test to diagnose covid-19 is a moron and you can tell them I said that. Please see my two recent articles (on www.vernoncoleman.com) entitled *PCR: How the PCR test has killed millions* and *The PCR test can kill you*. A positive PCR test does NOT prove that you have covid-19, dandruff, chilblains or anything else.

Remdesivir seems to be very, very popular with very, very stupid doctors who seem to think it is a panacea for all illnesses. If their Mercedes or BMW breaks down they probably give the car a shot of remdesivir.

Remdesivir is given directly into a vein. Doctors who tell you that giving drugs via a vein is an entirely safe procedure are stupid. No medical procedure is entirely safe. Giving drugs by injection into a blood stream requires skill and experience to avoid dangers.

The brand name of remdesivir is Veklury. (Brand names always begin with an initial capital but generic names are all lower case.) If you are being given Veklury, you are being given remdesivir.

Remdesivir should be prescribed by a doctor and given under a doctor's supervision. (Nurses may wear stethoscopes round their necks, but they are not doctors.)

Remdesivir must be given slowly over a period of between 30 minutes and 120 minutes.

Hospital patients are usually given remdesivir once a day for up to 10 days.

Patients not in hospital are usually given remdesivir once a day for three days.

Patients who are given remdesivir MUST have regular blood tests to check that their livers are functioning properly. If a doctor gives remdesivir without doing regular liver function tests he or she is dangerous and, in my opinion, should have their medical licence revoked.

Liver function tests MUST be done before remdesivir is prescribed. Any doctor who does not do liver tests before starting treatment should be sacked and have their medical licence revoked.

Severe renal toxicity has been noted in animal studies. (Some doctors claim that animal studies are irrelevant. I agree. But why do them if they are irrelevant?)

No one should be given remdesivir if they are allergic to it.

Anyone who has ever had liver disease or kidney disease should inform their doctor if he/she suggests prescribing remdesivir.

Anyone who is pregnant or breastfeeding should tell their doctor. The UK's National Institute for Health and Care Excellence (NICE) says that the safety of covid-19 antiviral treatment during pregnancy has NOT been established.

Remdesivir may interact, to your disadvantage, with other prescription medicines, with over the counter medicines, with vitamins and with herbal products. Doctors who prescribe remdesivir must ask patients about all the medicines they are taking.

Remdesivir has received a number of reviews on drugs.com and of the reviews listed on 24th August 2024, 19.38% of reviewers had a 'positive experience' but 47% had a 'negative experience'.

According to the journal *Science*, in October 2020,'The World Health Organisation's Solidarity Trial showed that remdesivir does not reduce mortality or the time covid-19 patients take to recover.' And 'A second, smaller placebo-controlled study of remdesivir on hospitalised covid-19 patients in China, published online by *The Lancet* on 29th April 2020, found no statistically significant benefit from the treatment – and the antiviral surprisingly had no impact on levels of the coronavirus'. I find it difficult to see why the FDA, the EU and the UK's drug regulator all approved remdesivir, though they appear to have done so without worrying too much about the research showing that it was pretty useless.

Side effects which may occur when remdesivir is injected

include: fast, pounding heartbeats; trouble in breathing; wheezing, shivering, itching, sweating, facial swelling, severe headache, a feeling of being about to pass out. Side effects subsequently may include nausea and abnormal liver function tests.

NICE reports that there are twelve drugs with which remdesivir inter-reacts. Any doctor prescribing remdesivir should know of these interactions – which are listed on the NICE website. So, for example, the manufacturers advise that patients avoid taking remdesivir with chloroquine, hydroxychloroquine and phenytoin. I cannot put a link to the NICE website because such links are not allowed. The list of side effects below was NOT taken from the NICE website. (Since it is a public sector body and paid for by taxpayers, you'd think that NICE would be delighted to share information about drug dangers wouldn't you?)

Side effects which can occur in patients taking remdesivir may include:

Back pain
Bleeding
Blistering
Burning
Chest tightness
Chills
Coldness
Cough
Dark coloured urine (a possible sign of liver problems)
Difficulty in swallowing
Discolouration of skin
Fast heartbeat
Feeling of pressure
Fever
Flushing
Headache
Hives and itching
Infection
Inflammation
Light coloured stools (a possible sign of liver problems)
Lumps
Nausea and vomiting
Numbness

Pain

Puffiness or swelling of the eyelids or around the eyes, face, lips or tongue

Redness

Scarring

Seizures

Skin rash

Soreness

Stinging

Stomach pain, continuing

Swelling

Tenderness

Tingling

Trouble breathing

Ulceration

Unusual tiredness or weakness

Yellow eyes or skin (a possible sign of liver problems)

You will be relieved to know that not all patients would be expected to have all of these side effects, though a number of these side effects are classified as 'common'.

When the covid vaccine was first introduced many people suggested that it should be given only to the over 60s. This was an appalling error of judgement. The over 60s were the least likely to be able to survive an attack with this toxic and experimental substance.

Right from the start of 2020, my articles and videos about covid attracted an enormous amount of abuse. But the one article which seemed to attract most abuse was one in which I warned about the dangers of the PCR test. Journalists and broadcasters who wouldn't know what to do with a scientific paper if they were given one, jumped up and down with great indignation. I was vilified for having said such a thing. But now that more and more doctors are belatedly beginning to wake up to the fact that there was no pandemic, that covid was just the annual flu and that the heavily promoted vaccine doesn't work and is dangerous, it is time to take another look at the evidence about the PCR Test. (For the record I have a one inch thick stack of scientific papers proving that the PCR test is dangerous and can be lethal. Curiously, those scientific references appear to have disappeared from the internet – or are at least difficult to find.)

We all know now that PCR tests are useless for finding cases of covid-19 but very good at helping governments keep us in our own homes under house arrest. In some parts of the world, the PCR tests are banned as utterly useless. They should be banned everywhere.

You'd get as good a result if you just divided people into two groups: those with a vowel in their surname and those without a vowel, and then announced that the ones with the vowel all had covid-19 and the rest all needed to change their names within seven days or pay a huge fine.

Everyone with functioning brain tissue knows that the PCR test is useless, except for political reasons, and that the whole testing programme is an outrageously expensive and disruptive shambles. Only government ministers, scientific advisors and pseudo-journalists at the wretched BBC think that PCR tests are valuable. Did you know, by the way, that the Government allegedly hired 900 consultants to help with the test and trace scheme? The consultants were being paid £1,000 a day each, though what they did for that I cannot imagine. That's £900,000 a day. I suspect that 99.99% of the population would be happier if the £900,000 a day were spent on providing dentists in areas where dentists are as rare as free parking spaces.

Most people seem to have accepted the need for regular PCR testing. Indeed, people in the UK queue up to have it done as often as possible – as though they get some sort of thrill out of having a complete stranger stuff something into a bodily orifice – pushing it in as far as it will go, twizzling it about a bit, and then pulling it out and buggering off without so much as 'a thank you very much I'll give you a ring tomorrow and we'll have dinner and then do it again'.

What no one ever mentions is that the PCR tests are dangerous and can, if done improperly, cause excruciating pain. This is probably why some countries don't like them. There is indeed a great deal of confusion about how far the swab should go. In Australia, the guidelines are that the swab should only go a few centimetres up the nostril but nasopharyngeal swabs can go much further. The United States Department of Health and Human services says that the swab should reach a depth equal to the distance from the nostrils to the outer opening of the ear. That's a huge distance. In Ottawa, Canada, the recommendation is half that distance.

In October 2020 I reported on at least one case where a healthy individual had noticed cerebrospinal fluid pouring out of her nose after an invasive PCR test. That really isn't something you want happening. The woman concerned, who was in her 40s, had a PCR nasal swab test and later went to see a doctor complaining of vomiting, a runny nose, a headache and a stiff neck. The pseudo-journalists at the BBC can, if they are interested in facts, find the details in the JAMA Otolaryngology Head and Neck Surgery. Surgeons found that the fluid running down her nose was cerebrospinal fluid – the fluid that protects the brain.

Then there was the case which was accepted for The Medical Journal of Australia. This reported a healthy 67-year-old woman who had cerebrospinal fluid coming down her nose and the symptoms of meningitis. This followed a covid-19 swab test. How many people are being killed – especially in care homes – by this useless and dangerous test?

The authors of the paper stated that the 'techniques for deep nasal and nasopharyngeal swabs may be easily confused'. They offer instructions for those conducting the tests. Here's one part of their instructions: 'it involves swab insertion into the nasal cavity at a plane between the opening of the nose and the external ear canal on the patient, which can be considered as the horizontal plane for the purpose of relationship to surface anatomy. This will allow the swab to be inserted parallel to the nasal floor which would avoid injury to the middle turbinates. Swabs inserted in an upward orientation into the nasal cavity, (greater than 30 degrees) not only have a risk of failing to achieve an adequate diagnostic sample from the desired nasal mucosa and nasopharynx but also puts the patient at greater risk of injury to the thin and delicate areas of the skull base (attachment of middle turbinate and cribriform plate) which are superior and anterior to the sphenoid sinus ostium.' There is then an illustration for swabbing and the authors conclude: 'We urge that this angle is not exceeded when performing diagnostic tests as it places the patient at greatest risk of serious adverse events.'

Might I suggest that anyone having a PCR test should ensure that the person holding the swab has studied and understood these instructions – and will follow them.

In Tripura, a three-day-old baby bled to death after a nasal swab test. In Saudi Arabia an eighteen-month-old child died after a test swab broke inside his nasal cavity.

These are not safe tests. Children are being traumatised by these incredibly invasive tests. These procedures are often done by people who know as much about medicine and human anatomy as I know about running a submarine – though I have seen Ice Station Zebra with Patrick McGoohan, and that film with Gene Hackman and Denzel Washington in it. And there was Red October with Sean Connery. Actually, come to think about it, I probably know far more about submarines than the average test and tracer tester knows about anatomy.

Quite a few things have puzzled me about the PCR test.

First, why the devil do they have to push the swab so far up your nose – and so close to your brain? Where is the indisputable scientific evidence that all the little covid-19 bugs are gathering up there for some reason? Do they like out of the way places? Normally, if you have a bug in your nose it will be in your nose. Where is the solid proof that the test only works if a sample is taken from a spot so far up your nose that the tissue up there probably speaks another language and only gets home once a year? Since these tests are now being performed by people who aren't doctors or nurses or probably even boy scouts, we need some evidence that the test is essential.

Actually, since the tests produce more false positives than real positives, they are clearly a waste of time anyway and it would make as much sense if the testing swab were inserted into the umbilicus and given a good twizzle there.

Second, researchers at Johns Hopkins University in the US published a study describing a device which has been developed. It's a tiny, star shaped micro-device capable of delivering a drug. The devices are no larger than a speck of dust but contain a metal core coated in heat sensitive paraffin wax. At the centre of the core there is the drug.

Now, we know that around half of Americans are reluctant to have the covid-19 vaccination.

I think that this hidden injection technology could be used to vaccinate people through PCR swabs.

This could be used to deliver a vaccine to people without their knowledge or consent. People who think they are just being tested could be receiving the mRNA jab.

Is this going to happen? Is it going to happen?

How would we know?

The authorities have for years been collecting the names and details of people who have declined the vaccine. Are they planning to use the PCR test to those who refuse the vaccination?

We cannot trust the Government or its advisers. We cannot trust the mainstream media. We definitely cannot trust the BBC which has financial links to the Bill and Melinda Gates Foundation and which long ago betrayed us. We cannot trust the medical establishment.

Oh, by the way, nasal vaccinations are already used on cattle.

Many medicines, especially vaccines, can affect fertility. This is done deliberately as part of the depopulation plan.

Before I exposed the covid fraud, and the dangers of the covid-19 vaccine, I was a Fellow of the Royal Society of Arts. I was expelled from the RSA for telling the truth. I have repeatedly drawn attention to this extraordinary exhibition of censorship but I have heard nothing from the RSA.

I have often written that the quality of health care today is worse than it was in the 1970s and probably worse than it was in the 1950s. This sounds extraordinary but the decline in the quality of health care is easy to measure. In the 1970s, a biopsy to find out if a breast lump was benign or cancerous took twenty minutes. Today, a patient will probably have to wait at least a week (and possibly six or eight weeks) to get the result of a breast biopsy.

In February 2025, the NHS in the UK announced that nearly half of urgent cancer patients had to wait more than two months for treatment. Many will die before their treatment starts. The idea that anyone classified as an urgent cancer patient should have to wait more than (more than!) two months for treatment to start is sickening. Can you imagine sitting waiting for over two months for your treatment to start – knowing that a cancer inside you is growing? Would a member of the British Government or British royal family have to wait over two months? The NHS has become an integral part of the global depopulation programme. The NHS failed completely as a result of allowing GPs to opt out of stop doing home visits, night calls and weekend calls. The effect was to put great pressure on hospitals which have now collapsed. The NHS now provides the worst health care service in the world.

I was a full-time media doctor for several decades after I resigned from the NHS on a matter of principle. I was the doctor on TV AM, the breakfast station and a presenter for the BBC. I presented numerous network and regional TV and radio programmes for both the BBC and commercial stations. I wrote half a dozen columns for national newspapers for over thirty years. I always believed that my first duty was not to the medical profession, the Government, the drug industry or even the company employing me – but to my readers and viewers. As far as I was concerned, being a media doctor simply meant that I had a rather larger practice and was providing advice wholesale rather than retail.

I am angered when I see media doctors promoting propaganda which has originated with the Government or a drug company. All doctors have a duty to question everything they are told by the men and women in grey suits.

For five years now I have been deeply saddened by the fact that many doctors have supported the official line without ever daring to question what they have been told.

For example, my attention was drawn to an article in the *Daily Mail* by someone called Dr Amir Khan, who is described as a GP in Bradford, England. The article was illustrated with a picture of a young man with one of those fancy sticky up hairstyles.

The headline was 'I vaccinated 100 people over a 48 hour shift in Bradford. Every single one of them was white.'

Now, we will put aside the idea of a 48 hour shift. I've worked 48 hour shifts but I don't think doctors are allowed to do that these days. And we'll put aside the thought that vaccinating 100 people in 48 hours would be ridiculously slow since it would mean giving just over two jabs an hour.

'The moment I realised what we were up against was when a student nurse…told me that she wouldn't have the vaccine because it might prevent her from becoming a mother in the future,' wrote Dr Khan. 'She had been told that the vaccines trigger an immune reaction which could damage the placenta in a pregnant woman – something that was entirely incorrect.'

'I was surprised,' continued Dr Khan. 'I expect this kind of misinformation from patients, not from a fellow medic. I took time to explain the science to her and made her promise two things. First that she would have the jab and second, that she would tell her family, to encourage them to follow her lead.'

Dr Khan goes on to say that a man he knows told him he was too scared to have the vaccine.

'I attempted to allay his fears,' wrote Dr Khan, 'saying any side effects of vaccines present themselves earlier, not later, and they are almost always mild.'

There are three points I want to deal with and I'll deal with them in reverse order.

First, Dr Khan says that the side effects associated with vaccines are 'almost always mild'.

That is not true. Governments have paid out billions of dollars in compensation to patients who have been severely injured by vaccines – or to the relatives of patients who have been killed by them. Drug companies have been fined billions of dollars for fraudulent activities. Recent papers in medical journals have suggested that vaccines may do more harm than good. The CDC in the US reported early on that the covid-19 vaccines caused a huge variety of dangerous side effects. Indeed, the incidence of death and serious side effects was reported to be over 2.5%. Logically, that means that if you vaccinate 100 people then two and a half of them will die or have notable side effects. The side effects involved with the covid-19 vaccine include serious neurological problems, heart attacks, strokes, blindness and many other disorders. I think it is an insult to the patients who have been damaged to describe their side effects as mild. All this is particularly relevant when you remember that covid-19 has a mortality rate which is much the same as that for the ordinary flu. And, as I am sure you know, the WHO said early on that the vaccines don't stop people getting covid-19 or passing it on.

Second, Dr Khan says that the side effects of vaccines present themselves early rather than later. That's not true, either, I'm afraid. Side effects can develop long after a vaccination was given and this is why when vaccines are first introduced it is usual to test them for several years. And the covid-19 vaccines – which he was writing about – are experimental vaccines. I assume that he is aware of the immune system dangers that many doctors are talking about. It is possible that many patients will fall seriously ill when they come into contact with what is called the 'wild' coronavirus. I don't know what the risks are. Providing false reassurance to patients is irresponsible.

Third, Khan reassured a young woman that her plans for motherhood would not be damaged by the vaccine. I think she was right to be worried. According to the yellow card reports from the MHRA in the UK, numerous women have had miscarriages and lost their unborn babies after having one of the mRNA vaccines. When the vaccines were first introduced, the UK Government said that the Pfizer vaccine was not recommended during pregnancy and that women of childbearing age should be advised to avoid pregnancy for at least two months after their second dose. The UK Government inexplicably updated its advice to saying that administration of the vaccine should only be considered when potential benefits outweigh any potential risks for the mother and foetus. In America, the Vaccine Adverse Event Reporting System has received many reports of adverse events experienced by women who were pregnant at the time of their Pfizer or Moderna injections. Nearly a third had miscarriages or preterm births. One woman who had a placenta known to be healthy was found, a week after vaccination, to have a placenta which had calcified and aged prematurely. It is true that Dr Anthony Fauci, the Biden Administrations Chief Medical Officer, has said that pregnant women can be vaccinated. It is also true that Dr Anthony Fauci is a director of the National Institute of Allergy and Infectious Diseases which will receive royalties for the Moderna vaccine.

Back in December 2020, a petition filed with the European Medicines Agency suggested that there is plausible evidence to suggest that the spike proteins in the MRNA vaccines could trigger an immune reaction against syncytin-1, a protein which is responsible for the development of a placenta in mammals and humans.

Finally, it is, of course, worth remembering that according to the journal *Nature*, for every 1,000 people under the age of 50 who are infected with the coronavirus, almost none will die. Indeed, the risk of a young, healthy woman dying of covid-19 is not very different to the risk of her being struck by lightning. I assume that Dr Khan does not recommend that young patients carry lightning rods around with them.

In my view, being a media doctor means more than just having a fancy haircut. Someone should report Dr Khan to the General Medical Council for spreading what I believe is misinformation.

I was appalled when it was announced that doctors were planning to give the experimental, not fully tested, temporarily approved covid-19 experimental 'vaccines' to children without having to obtain parental permission.

At the time I described what was happening as both child abuse and assault and offered this advice to children: 'Don't trust people in cars who offer you sweets. Don't trust people with syringes who offer you jabs.'

Legions of independent doctors around the world say it isn't safe to give these dangerous, toxic jabs to children who have very little risk of catching covid-19 – let alone dying of it. I suspect that the few doctors promoting this scheme are largely those who, one way or another, stand to make money out of it.

Vaccine sceptics point out that governments admit that the jabs don't stop children, or anyone else, getting a disease now accepted as nothing more than an over-marketed flu, and don't stop them spreading it even if they catch it.

Even the World Health Organisation (not a body I usually regard with much affection or respect) said that it wasn't safe to give the covid-19 jab to children.

And then, without any change in the evidence, the WHO suddenly went into reverse and announced that children could be given the stuff after all.

I believe that the BBC is the most dishonest, disreputable, unreliable media outlet in the history of the world. I believe that it is ageist, sexist, bigoted, unpatriotic and as bent as a paperclip. One BBC presenter even boasted that the BBC will not share the truth about vaccines – this means that the organisation deliberately suppresses those who do tell the truth about vaccines and vaccination.

There is no secret about why the BBC is hiding the truth about vaccines. The BBC has links to the drug industry, the crooked, corrupt vaccine makers, and is, of course, desperate to keep its licence fee by sucking up to the British Government.

But deceiving adults wasn't enough. As I explained in my book *Truth Teller: The Price*, the BBC has also lied to children about the covid vaccine. Professor Devi Sridhar, who is not a medical doctor, called the vaccine 100% safe.

And the BBC's paid misinformation expert, Marianna Spring who also does not have any medical qualifications, has said: 'Those who make anti-vax claims usually don't have a scientific or medical background.'

Now that is odd because I know a lot of medical doctors who are, by the BBC's definition, anti-vaxxers. In fact I believe I could find more doctors who opposed giving this toxic vaccine to children than she or the BBC could find supporting giving it to children.

The BBC has betrayed us for a long time now.

But this was a new low.

Were they deliberately trying to kill as many children as possible? That's what it looks like to me.

In March 2020 I had warned that the covid hoax was all going to be about pushing vaccines onto the public. People laughed and sneered. But that's exactly what happened.

For over a century now the medical establishment, under the day by day line by line control of the drug industry, has steadily, carefully and unthinkingly condemned all alternative or complementary health remedies. Any new alternative therapy, however effective it may be, will be mercilessly attacked and condemned and suppressed and its practitioners demonised and sneerily dismissed as quacks and charlatans. If a patient recovers after an alternative or complementary treatment, the orthodox doctors will say that the recovery was 'in spite of' the treatment rather than 'because of it', but curiously these words are never used by orthodox practitioners when referring to, say, treatment with chemotherapy. If a patient recovers after orthodox, allopathic treatment then the recovery was always a result of the treatment. Occasionally, orthodox practitioners will be allowed to toy with a therapy such as acupuncture and then, after a weekend course, announce themselves to be specialists in that area too.

The American Medical Association and the British Medical Association exist, let us not forget, to represent the financial interests of their members and, in my view, should be regarded as propaganda vehicles for the drug industry. All such associations publish journals which carry vast quantities of very expensive drug company advertising. (The advertising rates for medical journals are vastly higher than for almost any other publication.) It is almost unheard of for any members of the medical establishment to criticise the drug industry and equally unheard of for them not to criticise anyone who does. The medical establishment and the pharmaceutical industry are joined at the hip and speak with one voice. And their current and future voice concerns global warming. The medical profession has abandoned the health of humans for the urgency of dealing with a myth.

Global warming is a myth. There is no scientific evidence supporting it. And global warming was introduced to explain the introduction of schemes designed to help deal with overpopulation. There is absolutely no evidence supporting the notion that the world is overpopulated. And so a myth was created to support a myth.

The British Medical Association, which was founded in 1832, has opposed many of the key health reforms which were recommended during its lifetime. The BMA tried to block the foundation of the NHS in 1948 but changed their minds when the health secretary at the time 'stuffed their mouths with gold' (his words). The BMA has been described as 'the patients' enemy' and has been attacked as a major drag on reform of health care. The BMA is committed to the myth of global warming and I fear that this is at the expense of the care of patients.

Just yards away from Notre Dame Cathedral in the centre of Paris, France stands one of the oldest hospitals in the world – the Hotel Dieu. The hospital's wards stand around a huge courtyard. There is a covered walkway around the edge of the courtyard (which is, in truth, more of a garden) so that patients who need gentle exercise can do so even in inclement weather. Architects commissioned to design hospitals should be forced to visit the Hotel Dieu and to build according to that time honoured plan.

Sadly, however, modern hospitals are soulless, characterless, dysfunctional edifices which have all the charm of multi-storey car parks. New hospitals are literally falling down.

In 2024, a total of 14,500 hours of work were lost in British hospitals because of the maintenance backlog. It is estimated that existing leaky roofs, broken heating systems and broken lifts will cost £2.7 billion to repair. The work will almost certainly never be done. Why bother to repair the hospitals when you know that they will shortly be abandoned and replaced by 'virtual' wards?

Medical education has long been controlled by the drug industry. Today, the far left wing medical establishment has joined the drug industry. Students are taught that dealing with non-existent global warming must take precedence over caring for patients. It is hardly surprising that today's young doctors are thoughtless and uncaring and devoid of compassion.

A few decades ago it was dentists who wanted to be something else. I knew one who wanted to be a racing driver and another who wanted to be a professional golfer. Both were in their thirties and were quite serious about their ambitions.

Today, it's doctors who want to be something else. They want to be bloggers, Tik Tok stars, influencers and video makers. YouTube and television stations are awash with young doctors promoting their government propaganda on vaccines, euthanasia and other topics. YouTube will give you a platform unless you have something useful and honest to say.

Medical research is dominated and controlled by drug companies. The subject of research is decided by drug companies and the results are assessed by the sponsoring drug company and only published if the drug company approves. Research which shows that a new drug may be dangerous, may produce many side effects or may be lethal, will not be published. Only much later, when evidence accumulates and becomes unavoidable, will problems be occasionally mentioned in the medical literature – and then usually only in passing. Universities, where much research is done, are controlled by far left extremists – hence the obsession with the mythical global warming and the exclusion of all those who are capable of independent and original thought and who dare to criticise the far left leaning medical establishment/drug company axis. Little or no original research is done these days. Virtually no epidemiological research is done. Nearly all research is now done by doctors working for drug companies (even university departments work for or with drug companies) and so research which might not involve drugs is ignored.

When my wife Antoinette developed breast cancer she had already been diagnosed with sub-acute combined degeneration of the cord which is a condition related to a shortage of vitamin B12 caused by a digestive problem. There is some evidence linking this B12 deficiency to breast cancer and so I reported the connection to several of the doctors employed to care for Antoinette. None of them was in the slightest interested in investigating the link.

The British Government is planning to define 'the spreading of misinformation and conspiracy theories' as extremism. If this plan becomes law then the truth will become whatever is approved by the Government and those who dissent will be liable to punishment.

It should be noted that when I questioned the Government's discredited covid policies and the value of the now discredited covid-19 vaccine I was accused of spreading misinformation. The unarguable evidence now shows that everything I said in 2020, 2021, 2022, 2023 and 2024 was entirely accurate while everything which the Government, the media and the medical establishment said was wrong, and therefore 'misinformation'.

Clearly, therefore, if this mooted legislation becomes law then the Government, the media and the medical establishment should all be arrested for spreading misinformation.

It is known that patients recover more speedily in pleasant surroundings where there are flowers in abundance. When I visited my mother in hospital I took a bunch of flowers. The nurses refused to find a vase, let alone put the flowers in water. The auxiliaries also felt that dealing with flowers was a task beneath their dignity. Eventually, I found a dirty vase in a dirty cupboard, washed it, put in some clean water and then added the flowers. I put the flowers beside my mother's bed. The flowers were removed and thrown away less than half an hour after I left.

GPs used to admit their sick patients directly to the local hospital. This doesn't happen these days because GPs rarely see seriously sick patients. Instead the sick are expected to make their way to the local Accident and Emergency department of the local hospital – which may well be thirty miles or more distant.

Never forget: nothing is happening by accident. There are no coincidences. The destruction of health care is deliberate.

Looking at the statistics it seems that if you have not yet been diagnosed as suffering from autism, ADHD or Aspergers syndrome then there must be something wrong with you. It is interesting that once popular problems such as sensitivity to E numbers and hyperactivity appear to have been replaced by the Three As – all of which may require long-term treatment with potentially dangerous prescription drugs. And the other strange thing is that whereas doctors are reluctant to prescribe life-saving drugs such as antibiotics they are relentlessly enthusiastic about prescribing dangerous and often pretty useless drugs for the treatment of these three disorders.

Accident and emergency departments in hospitals are now often staffed not by doctors but by nurses, students, trainees or, quite probably, anyone passing through. It does not seem unreasonable to see a connection between this and the fact that misdiagnoses in accident and emergency departments are now endemic.

In 2024, the National Health Service in the UK was rocked by a series of doctors' strikes, go slows and work to rules. It is clear that these strikes resulted in thousands of unnecessary deaths and it is also clear that these strikes (which were all about more money for the doctors, at the expense of patients, rather than improving services to patients) were part of the process to destroy health care and increase the number of people dying. Previously, strikes by doctors were pretty well unknown.

Patients wait years for essential investigations and treatments of life-threatening diseases but many doctors now offer cosmetic procedures (breast enlargements, facial amendments, buttock lifts, etc.) which can be done without waiting. Sadly, these procedures seem to go wrong quite often – with frequently disastrous results.

Many years, when I was a young GP, full of hope and bursting with enthusiasm, I put together and published a small directory of voluntary organisations which had been set up to look after the interests of patients. I distributed copies of the directory to anyone who wanted one. A local printer put it together for me. Doctors and nurses said they found it useful. *Nursing Times*, a British magazine catering to the needs of nurses, published items from the directory over many months. One a week. Each week's entry contained a brief description of the charity's purposes and a contact address and, if available, a phone number. The majority of these organisations were run by volunteers who were either sufferers from the disease they represented or had a close relative who was a sufferer. The money to produce leaflets and so on was raised at coffee mornings and jumble sales (garage sales and car boot sales had not then become the force they are today). Everything was honest and enthusiastic and members of the organisations shared ideas and tips. I used to go to speak to these small groups when I could take time away from my practice and, in general terms, they were always much the same. The meetings were always held in someone's best room. The people attending were all sufferers or relatives of sufferers. The individuals involved all cared very much about what they were doing. And most of them knew more about 'their' illness than most doctors knew. And then the drug industry realised that these small charities were an excellent way to sell their products. And everything changed. Small voluntary organisations which had relied on the vicar's ancient copying machine were offered brand new printing equipment. Instead of meeting in someone's living room, the little charities were given new offices. The volunteers became paid charity workers. And, of course, the leaflets that were produced were much more professional. The drug companies provided help and advice and information. It was more or less understood that in return for all the money that was pouring in, the charities would promote the drug company's product or products. Members of the group would appear on radio and television and do newspaper interviews. Their sponsoring drug company's products would be mentioned and recommended. And gradually the 'patients' associations' became part of the public relations machinery of the pharmaceutical industry. These days drug companies use the charities (and they are mostly now registered as charities, for the tax advantages) to target their markets directly. Many of the well-known charities have become multi-million pound organisations, with the top staff on huge salaries. There are smart offices in expensive buildings and the aims have changed from providing patients and relatives with information to promoting their sponsor's products. Alternative therapies and ideas for prevention are suppressed, ignored and sneered at. The big cancer charities around the world are so closely allied with the drug industry that they have become part of the cancer industry – sharing the same aims and targets. Many charities now spend most of their income on salaries and marketing. And who wants to prevent Von Tickle's disease when you can cure it with a new drug and deal with the side effects of the new drug with a couple of the manufacturer's other products? There is absolutely no doubt in my mind that a goodly number of the charities which are, on the surface, devoted to the care of patients with a particular disease, are compromised and have lost their independence and their purpose. Finally, I wonder how many of the people who regularly give money to big charities know that, on average, 45% of the money given goes to the Government in taxes. And most of the rest is swallowed up in salaries, expenses, pensions and expensive offices.

In addition to giving money to charities, the big drug companies (and some of the fact checking organisations) also give money to a variety of organisations which can be used to further their aims. So, for example, drug companies give money to organisations which may appear to be critical of drug prescribing but which, in reality, are not. Such organisations can then be used in a way that makes it look as if the drug companies are being 'attacked' and that the media is being fair. This is done so that truly harsh critics (such as me) can be safely ignored. This happens a good deal.

And Just as the charities have been 'bought' so doctors have been 'bought'. They prescribe whatever drug is named on the side of the free pen they are using, or the product they were told about on their last trip on the Orient Express (paid for by a generous drug company). When they consider a diagnosis they think only of drugs. Or rather they did. Now global warming has taken over and drugs have become unfashionable.

So, what is going to happen to all the patients now denied the drugs which they used to take every day?

Are the drug companies going to be defeated by global warming?

Of course they are not.

The medical profession and the drug industry are switching from prescribed medicines (to be swallowed every morning or every evening) to vaccines. That is the future. New vaccinations for every disease imaginable are being prepared. We are heading remorselessly towards murder by vaccination or, perhaps that would more accurately be described as genocide by vaccination.

Every patient in hospital needs an advocate to defend them against those doctors and nurses who are too willing to kill the sick, frail and the lonely. Leaving an elderly person alone in a hospital is reckless.

The conspirators want to get rid of everyone of pensionable age. The elderly are considered to be a drag on society. They have to be paid pensions and as they age some of them require a good deal of looking after. The elderly often prefer using cash (and are therefore slowing down the introduction of digital money) and they are often slow to use the internet (thereby slowing down the technocracy). And so the official plan is to kill old people as quickly as possible.

At the moment 'old' is regarded as being anyone over pensionable age. But today's 'middle' age will, as far as the conspirators are concerned, soon be tomorrow's 'old'.

It isn't just the elderly who are considered superfluous, of course. The conspirators also want to get rid of the disabled, the frail and the mentally ill – including those who have been diagnosed as suffering from autism, ADHD and Asperger's disease. 'Do Not Resuscitate' notices are being used to kill patients in huge numbers. And euthanasia programmes are being introduced around the world to expedite the killing.

Digital identification is being introduced to the internet. It is claimed that this is to protect children from pornography online. This is, of course, a lie. Digital identification will soon be required for all access to the internet. And then individuals who have poor social credit scores (because they have dared to share the truth) will be banned from the internet. Since many GPs now insist on communicating with their patients via the internet this will isolate millions – especially the elderly. And without the internet it will be impossible to buy food, electricity, gas or just about anything. Even car parks now routinely require the use of a smart phone and an APP.

Countless millions of people around the world (most of them under 30 years of age) now claim to be suffering from something called 'long covid'. This is supposed to be a syndrome left over from the covid flu.

In fact, 'long covid' has been shown not to exist but is being promoted by the conspirators as a 'disease' to fear. Today, long covid is one of the important causes of the global recession which is devastating the world; it has become the shirker's dream disease and it is the hypochondriac's Christmas gift that keeps on giving.

The biggest and most significant research into long covid, involving 26,000 individuals, concluded that long covid is largely a psychological problem. And yet in America there are 12 million people off work with this imaginary disorder. And In the UK there are more than two million long covid sufferers signed off sick – unable to work.

The truth is that people who took a year off work on full pay didn't want to go back to their offices when the lockdowns ended.

There was never a global covid pandemic but now we have a global long covid pandemic.

So, why have they created this fake disease – 'long covid'?

First, governments welcomed the growth in the number of alleged long covid sufferers because it helps make people afraid of the rebranded flu – and accept the toxic jabs which are dishonestly promoted as preventing it.

Second, governments know that if a huge chunk of the workforce stays at home the disruption and the cost will severely damage the economy. Crashing the global economy is an essential part of taking us into the Great Reset where AI and robots will replace humans in most jobs. The future the conspirators have planned for us is a technocracy.

Third, and this is crucial, the false long covid disease is an excellent cover for the injuries caused by the covid-19 jabs. A list of the commonest side effects associated with the covid-19 jabs just happens to be the same as the commonest symptoms associated with 'long covid'. I pointed this out the minute that so-called long covid was created. Naturally, my reward was yet more abuse.

Fourth, long covid is keeping NHS staff at home and causing NHS waiting lists to soar still higher – all part of the deliberate plan to wreck health care.

Fifth, the people who are off work with long covid are being paid by their government. This is the beginning of the universal basic income which is a critical part of the Great Reset and which is already being trialled in various parts of the world. Researchers will discover that people like staying at home and receiving free money – and they will try to look surprised when they announce their findings.

Naturally, anyone who dares to look at the evidence – and question the long covid myth – is dismissed as a conspiracy theorist and banned from sharing their views.

As usual, there is no debate in the mainstream media where journalists are terrified of the truth and have to cover their eyes if a fact threatens their daily deceit.

GPs are now too lazy and self-important to take blood samples from their patients. Instead of spending two minutes taking a blood sample, GPs tell patients to make an appointment to see an often barely (or sometimes not at all) qualified member of staff in one, two, three or four weeks' time. It seems that nurses are too busy giving dangerous and pointless covid-19 vaccinations to do genuine medical work such as phlebotomy.

Because the person taking blood is usually unqualified they are also usually pretty incompetent and the result is that they often put the needle into the vein at the wrong angle, go straight through to the other side, cause bleeding and leave the patient with a painful haematoma. This can be a serious problem when patients have a limited number of suitable veins available for venepuncture.

Endangering and inconveniencing patients in this way is bad enough. Patients often have to make two long difficult and expensive journeys to get to and from the doctors' surgery, all to save two minutes of the arrogant doctor's time and they are, of course, forced thereby to contribute to the global warming which most doctors claim to believe is real.

But there is a much bigger problem, which was brought to my attention by my dear friend Dr Colin M.Barron, who pointed out that this egregious example of unprofessional and discourteous medical behaviour, and, let's be frank, downright laziness, means that one of two things is bound to happen when blood tests are essential but delayed in this stupid way.

Either, the patient must wait for treatment to start until the blood samples have been taken – meaning that the patient must wait additional weeks for essential medication to begin.

Or, the patient will be started on treatment before the blood sample is taken in which case the blood sample and the blood tests will probably be useless because the blood will be contaminated by whatever treatment has been initiated. As Dr Barron points out, if a patient is given steroids then their ESR will be reduced and their white blood count altered too.

Blood tests should be taken the moment the doctor decides they are necessary. Any doctor who doesn't understand this is so stupid that they probably need help tying their shoe laces.

Vaccinations are rarely given by doctors these days. The jabbing is done by clinical assistants who are not medically qualified and are not even nurses. The majority seem quite indifferent to the needs, anxieties and plight of others. They have no training and they certainly never came within a mile of what used to be called a vocation. They have been hired to dehumanise medicine. Most do not realise that when an injection is given, it is important to make sure that the tip of the needle isn't in a blood vessel. I believe that the sudden illnesses after the covid-19 jab occurred when the vaccine was injected directly into a blood vessel so that instead of being absorbed slowly, the toxic substance went straight into the blood. I did warn of this in 2020 but unfortunately my warnings were banned.

Hospitals struggled during the fake pandemic with staff working very hard to master the intricate dance routines required for their TikTok routines. Only by not admitting patients were staff able to dedicate the long hard hours required to make their rewarding videos and to entertain the sick and the dying who were stuck at home without medical care.

Everywhere I look journalists and doctors are queuing up and falling over each other in order to praise the latest wonder drug semaglutide (known to most people by the brand names Ozempic and Wegovy.

And there's another drug called Mounjaro aka tirzepatide.

That's supposed to be a wonder drug too.

These are, so they insist, the best, easiest and classiest way to lose weight.

The *Daily Telegraph* ran a headline which read 'My miracle weight loss jab has changed my life and will change the world.' The journalist who wrote the article, Allison Pearson, says that these drugs 'may well change the world – for good'.

And doctors apparently claim that semaglutide and tirzepatide will do all sorts of other wonderful things.

There's been talk of one or the other of them slowing down the aging process, preventing cancer, arthritis, Alzheimer's and Parkinson's.

And helping people give up smoking.

Doctors apparently also say that semaglutide will reverse kidney disease, prevent heart failure and reduce previously untreatable high blood pressure.

And cut heart attacks and strokes.

It'll probably solve baldness, spots and dandruff, reduce your heating bills, cut your lawn and protect your car bodywork from seagull droppings.

This stuff sounds nearly as good as the much loved covid-19 vaccine – and what an embarrassment it was for the medical establishment and the world's journalists when the vaccines turned out to be just as useless and as toxic as I predicted they would be.

But pause a moment.

Do you know of a drug anywhere in the world that doesn't have dangerous side effects? Have you ever come across a product that cannot kill people?

No, nor me. And I've been writing about drugs and drug side effects for over fifty years.

So what can these 'change the world' wonder drugs do that the enthusiastic doctors and journalists don't seem to have mentioned?

Well, let's start with tirzepatide (aka Mounjaro).

This one can:

Cause allergy reactions

Shouldn't be used if you're pregnant

May damage your liver

May damage your kidneys

May cause acute pancreatitis

May cause dehydration

One major source of information about drugs tells me that mounjaro 'can cause some serious health issues'.

No kidding. In addition to the other problems I've listed, it can cause fever, stomach pain, difficulty in breathing or swallowing, gall bladder disease, vomiting, jaundice and some other stuff including a fast heart rate.

And what about the other stuff – semaglutide (aka Ozempic and Wegovy)?

I hate to tell you this but semaglutide can also cause some serious health issues.

Here's a list of a few of the possible problems.

Thyroid C cell tumours
Anxiety
Bloating
Blurred vision
Cold sweats
Confusion
Constipation
Dark urine (that's probably because your liver is buggered)
Depression
Diarrhoea (though possibly not at the same time as the constipation)
Difficulty in swallowing
Dizziness
Fast heart beat
Fever
Headache
Increased hunger
Indigestion
Nervousness and nightmares
Pains in the stomach
Seizures
Skin rash
Slurred speech
Trouble breathing
Tiredness
Vomiting
Yellow eyes or skin (the liver thing again)

That's not all. But it's enough to be going on with.

None of the doctors and journalists whom I have seen extolling the virtues of these new wonder drugs seems to have mentioned these risks.

So I'm sorry if I am a bit of a party pooper.

But there really aren't any magic pills.

Just try to remember 'Coleman's First Law of Medicine' which is: 'If you are receiving treatment for an existing disease and you develop new symptoms then, until proved otherwise, you should assume that the new symptoms are caused by the treatment you are receiving.'

Reports of deaths which are linked to these new weight loss drugs are already appearing. For example, a healthy nurse took two low dose injections of tirzepatide and two weeks later she was dead. She died from multiple organ failure, septic shock and pancreatitis.

Between January and May 2024 there were 208 warnings about this drug – including 31 serious reactions and one suspected death of a man in his sixties. There are reported to have been 23 suspected deaths linked to semaglutide in the UK since 2019. And today hundreds of thousands of people are taking the stuff – believing it is safe.

Dr Alison Cave, the chief safety officer of the MRHA (about which I have written much before) is reported to have said that 'new medicines, such as tirzepatide are more intensively monitored to ensure any new safety issues are identified promptly'. And Dr Naveed Sattar, who is chairman of the UK Government's obesity mission (I didn't know we had one) is reported to have said: 'Trials are very robust in trying to establish safety.'

It's always nice to come across doctors with a sense of humour.

Ozempic, and similar drugs, don't help eradicate bad eating habits. Instead they work on the brain to make you feel full. But the drug may also affect other parts of the brain – effectively turning it into a mind control substance. The drug decreases the amount of dopamine your brain releases after you do something enjoyable – drinking, smoking, eating food you particularly like or having sex – and therefore eliminates the motivation to do those things. The drug will remove the sense of pleasure that is experienced when you do something you enjoy.

The drug may therefore change the personality of the person taking it and it may reduce the individual's libido. This effect will ensure that the drug fits nicely into the depopulation programme which is so loved by the conspirators.

And all this perhaps explains why journalists have been encouraged to promote the drug with such exaggerated and unbridled enthusiasm. I nevertheless find it astonishing that mainstream media journalists have promoted these drugs with little or no assessment of the side effects or their propensity to turn those who use them into zombies.

Doctors now want Alzheimer's disease drugs to be offered, like statins, to just about everyone over the age of 50. This, of course, makes doctors sound as if they care. But giving potentially toxic drugs to healthy individuals isn't a sign of caring, it's a sign of greed. The drug companies which make this rubbish will make billions of pounds, dollars and any currency you can think of and I rather expect that a lot of people will die. In the 1990s, I condemned the statins and I believe they should never have been distributed widely, for they are dangerous and useless drugs. And some of the drugs which doctors prescribe for the treatment of Alzheimer's disease are equally dangerous and useless. If doctors really want to show that they care they should make more effort when diagnosing Alzheimer's disease (differentiating it from the other possible causes of dementia or symptoms and signs which might mimic dementia) instead of simply making Alzheimer's the default diagnosis whenever someone over the age of 50 can't remember where they put their car keys.

Every list of major causes of death always includes Alzheimer's disease, which is the default condition whenever a patient is, or appears to be, demented. But Alzheimer's disease only rarely kills anyone. When a patient is said to have died of Alzheimer's it is usually because they were killed or allowed to die by being deprived of food or essential medication. And many of those engineered deaths should, more rightly, be classified as murder. This means that murder is now one of the leading causes of death.

A few years ago, GPs in the UK were keen on diagnosing Alzheimer's because they receive a generous cash bonus every time they make the diagnosis. There was no logical reason why doctors should receive a bonus for diagnosing Alzheimer's but no bonus for diagnosing, say, normal pressure hydrocephalus. (I explained in my book *The Dementia Myth* why many of those who are said to have Alzheimer's have curable conditions.) There was never any logical reason for paying doctors a bonus for a specific diagnosis (though drug companies with suitable products to sell were doubtless thrilled) and the extra payments had to be stopped when it was clear that GPs were eventually going to diagnose everyone in the country with Alzheimer's if the scheme continued. It became clear that GPs and drug companies would eventually have all the money available for the NHS.

It is vital to remember that today, the drug industry controls the medical establishment and the mainstream media. And it has done so for a century.

In the USA there are 100,000 lobbyists with a budget of $9 billion. They are paid to suppress the truth and to push the interests of the people who are paying them. In Europe there are more lobbyists than politicians or journalists. They cling, like leeches, to the European Union. And like leeches they get very fat.

Any doctor with a brain, or even half a brain, knows that consulting patients via the telephone or the intent is useless bordering on dangerous. Any doctor who insists on seeing patients at a distance is simply trying to kill his or her patients and should be arrested. They are, at any rate, far too stupid to be practising medicine.

Nearly four years ago, when doctors first started refusing to see patients 'live' in their consulting rooms or at home, I warned that this unprofessional practice would result in thousands of misdiagnoses and deaths.

It was clear, right from the start, that it was absurd and cruel that doctors should be too frightened of catching the rebranded flu to do their jobs properly.

Any doctor who believed their government's lies about covid is a fool.

Any doctor who believed the lies that the covid jab is safe and effective is too stupid to have a medical licence. Actually they're too stupid to own a driving licence. And when dog licences are reintroduced they'll be too stupid to own one of those too.

Thousands of doctors took advantage of the fake covid scare to abandon their jobs and their patients – staying at home and speaking to patients only on the phone or via the internet.

Was it laziness? Was it stupidity? Was it cowardice and a pathetic, misguided sense of self-preservation? Or was it part of the medical establishment's official and deliberate plan to kill as many patients as possible?

Five years ago I warned that this practice would prove lethal for several, very obvious reasons.

First, you cannot listen to a patient's chest over the phone. You can't listen to the heart or the lungs over the internet.

Second, you cannot examine a patient's body for lumps or rashes over the phone or over the internet.

Third, you cannot take a pulse or a blood pressure reading over the phone or over the internet.

Fourth, you cannot take a temperature over the phone or over the internet.

Fifth, you cannot spot many small but well-known signs of illness over the phone or over the internet.

Sixth, you cannot look into a patient's ears or eyes over the phone or over the internet. And you can't look down their throats either.

Time and time again over the last five years I have pointed out all these problems – and many more – and argued that doctors who refuse to see patients 'live' are worse than useless and should have their licences taken away. Doctors who insisted, and in many cases still insist, on dealing with patients only on the telephone or internet are scrofulous loobies, muggles, chouses and podsnappers.

I also pointed out, back in 2020 (and indeed long before that) that many millions of patients don't like talking on the phone and find internet consultations impossible. These patients are being denied treatment.

Belatedly, the *British Medical Journal* published a paper confirming that my fears were absolutely accurate.

An analysis of remote NHS doctor consultations between 2020 and 2023 showed that some patients had died and others had been seriously harmed because cruel, idiotic and lazy medical bawdy baskets had insisted on seeing patients only by phone or over the internet. Diagnoses had been missed. Wrong diagnoses had been made. And referrals for hospital treatment had been delayed. Doctors who see patients only on the phone are relying on patients self-diagnosing.

All this was obvious years ago.

And yet a third of GP appointments are still 'virtual'.

In other words they are useless and deadly.

Actually, they aren't just useless.

They are worse than useless.

Thousands of British GPs are now the laziest and most incompetent physicians in the world.

It is their laziness and incompetence which explains why hospitals and ambulance services cannot cope.

I repeat: any doctor who insists on providing phone consultants should lose their licence and be sacked. And, although I wouldn't want to sound emotional, I believe that they should have their stethoscopes stuffed up entirely inappropriate orifices.

GPs are complaining that they are desperately overworked and cannot cope. Doctors' representatives say the same thing.

But the evidence proves that GPs are NOT overworked. After all, the average GP now works just 23 to 24 hours a week. Most people would regard that as part time work. And GPs are paid around £150,000 a year.

If your GP claims that she is overworked, and doesn't have the time to spend two minutes taking a blood sample, do point out that GPs today do considerably less work than GPs at almost any time in history. In the UK, there are more GPs per 100,000 patients today than there were decades ago, GPs today have smaller lists of patients to look after and GPs today are too lazy to do house calls or night time visits.

Many doctors limit their working hours, so that they pay less tax and can have more time playing golf, looking after the families, enjoying hobbies and watching daytime TV. (The EU's rules about working practices have helped limit the time doctors are 'allowed' to work, and hospital doctors now count the hours they are 'on call' as working hours. So if a doctor is on call for eight hours while she is asleep, that counts as eight hours towards her allotted week's work even if she was not woken once during that time.)

Despite all this, GPs are threatening to do even less work.

But look at the facts.

Today there are nearly twice as many GPs in England and Wales as there were in 1964 when I started medical school.

And if you look at the number of GPs per 100,000 patients, the figures show that there are more GPs available than ever.

Back in 1964, there were 42 GPs per 100,000 patients.

Today, there are around 60 GPs per 100,000 patients.

And remember that GPs used to do home visits, night calls, weekend calls and calls on bank holidays. It was not uncommon for a GP to see 20 patients in a morning surgery, 20 patients in an evening surgery and do a list of home visits in between. At night and at weekends the doctor would be on call to visit patients at home.

Today, very few GPs do any of those things.

And many GPs refuse to see patients 'live' – insisting on doing their consultations over the phone or the internet. All those GPs are a disgrace to the profession because it is impossible to provide proper care for all patients without seeing most of them in person.

Ring a GP's surgery today with an emergency and you will be told to go to hospital. In the bad old days GPs would visit patients at home 24 hours a day. And would sew up wounds and deal with a whole range of emergencies.

The only possible conclusion is that today's GPs are not overworked.

Indeed, they do far less work than their predecessors did decades ago.

There are more GPs than ever. And they're doing less work.

It's not surprising that hospital Accident and Emergency departments cannot cope.

I read an interview with a GP the other day in which the doctor said that 'taking bloods and other tests' were not part of his contract and that he and his colleagues weren't getting paid for doing these things. He said he was going to work to rule in such a way that he didn't have any of his money docked. I was ashamed to read that self-serving, pitiful comment. I am, to be honest, strangely relieved that most of the honest, hard-working, caring doctors I worked with are dead and will never know how low medicine has sunk. If GPs really don't like working for the NHS they should have the guts to resign and set up as private practitioners. They don't do this, I suspect, because they would have to work much harder if they were private doctors. NHS GPs are hugely overpaid and underworked.

When I was a GP we worked a damned sight harder, and much longer hours (the average GP today works the equivalent of three days a week) than today's doctors. We had responsibility for our patients 24 hours a day, every day of the year. And we took bloods, gave injections and syringed ears without whingeing that these things weren't our responsibility. We put in stitches and then, later, we took them out again. We didn't have a list of things that were outside our contract.

It seems to me that many of today's GPs don't really care about their patients but seem to be in medicine only for the money.

I weep at how general practice has deteriorated.

Patients get a terrible deal. Too many doctors seem to me to be lazy and greedy; in medicine only for what they can get out of it. They are paid massively well to do very little work. They have no sense of responsibility and no sense of vocation.

Many in the medical establishment are besotted with the myth of global warming and have talked about cutting back medical services to deal with this imaginary problem. I believe this is all part of the push to Net Zero. I fear that the medical establishment and parts of the British Medical Association are so besotted with the myth of global warming that they want to destroy health care to increase the death rate, reduce the population and reduce our use of fossil fuels.

Life expectancy in the so-called developed countries is in decline – particularly for women.

The failure of health care (a global phenomenon) is forcing more and more people into expensive private health care. And that, of course, is affecting their economic status and their independence. There are no coincidences. Nothing happens without a reason.

In some hospitals, during the fake covid pandemic, staff were paid a bonus for every patient they diagnosed as having covid-19. The payments were higher if the patient died. The diagnoses, of course, were made with the help of the utterly discredited PCR tests and most of the patients who died 'with' covid (rather than 'of' it) actually died of something else. However, the rules meant that if a patient came in after being run over by a bus but had a positive covid test then they were covid patients and if they died they died of covid-19.

Doctors used regularly to deal with emergencies, to admit sick patients direct to hospital wards and to routinely visit patients at home if they were ill or frail. As a GP I even visited my patients when they were in hospital.

A couple of decades ago, the vast majority of doctors cared for their work and their patients and tried to be of use. They were driven by vocation and a sense of pride. Some (a few) of today's doctors are doubtless good and useful. Sadly, on balance, too many new doctors are driven only by greed and self-interest. They are of little practical use and actually do far more harm than good.

Answer all the questions below with one of three answers. Score 10 for YES and 0 for NO. Note that these questions, and your answers, do not establish that your doctor is a good clinician.

If you need an urgent appointment will your doctor see you the day you ring?

Can you get a standard appointment in less than a week?

Can you see the doctor of your choice?

Can you see a doctor without an unqualified receptionist asking personal questions?

Does your doctor take blood samples, remove stitches, syringe ears, etc., without referring you to someone else?

Does your doctor insist on seeing you at least once every six months if you need regular prescriptions?

Does your doctor always see you face to face?

Does your doctor visit patients at home if they are too ill to get to the surgery?

Does your doctor visit patients at home at night, at the weekend and on bank holidays?

If you need to speak to your doctor urgently can you usually speak to him on the telephone?

Now check the scores

If you scored 100 then you have a Superdoc – five stars with a Golden Stethoscope.

If you scored 80 to 95 then you have a very good, caring doctor. Four and a half stars.

If you scored 60 to 80 then your doctor is trying, but could do considerably better. Four stars.

If you scored 40 to 60 then your doctor is average only. Three stars.

If you scored 20 to 40 then your doctor is below average and probably of little practical value. Two stars.

If you scored under 20 then your doctor is an ignorant and incompetent buffoon who should be doing something else for a living – preferably a job that doesn't involve live human beings. One Star.

'**I** think it's safe to predict that one of these days – quite soon really – a number will be used to maintain a full dossier on every citizen of this country.'

Ross Thomas (1970 in *The fools in town are on our side*)

The UK's population will have soared to 72.5 million by the year 2032. This is despite the massive number of taxpayers emigrating and the huge number of people dying while waiting for treatment or dying through poor treatment. The increase in the population will be entirely a result of uncontrolled, mass immigration. (The real figure will be much higher since many immigrants arrive in the UK illegally. As I write, in early 2025, one in 12 people in London is an illegal immigrant.) This massive increase in population will lead to a continuing decline in the quality of health care. Much the same thing is happening in just about every other western country. In Canada, for example, the liberals doubled the number of immigrants and saw the population increase from 33 million to 41 million. Naturally, they made no plans on how to provide housing and the infrastructure such as health care, transport, etc.) for all these extra people. The result everywhere around the world has been resentment and anger mistakenly described as racism. Far left politicians have been busy virtue signalling and welcoming all new immigrants. Overcrowding in all Western countries is a major cause of poor health care and unnecessary deaths.

We are playing by someone else's rules. We have absolutely no control over our lives because the people who make the rules, and who ensure that they are properly enforced, are thoroughly malign and regard humanity as an outdated, useless concept. It is perhaps not surprising that more than half of all those born since 1996 (known as Generation Z) are so disillusioned with British politicians that they want the UK to be a dictatorship without elections and without a Parliament. Sadly, I suspect that they are hoping to find someone who does not exist. A benevolent dictator might be nice but, sadly, King Arthur is no longer available and his knights are now just dust.

In an attempt to convince us that all is well with our health care, the mainstream media will, from time to time, show pictures of transplant patients. And we are supposed to feel comforted by the knowledge that patients who are dying because their livers or hearts or kidneys or whatever have failed, are being saved by wonderful surgeons. This is trickery. Most people with liver, heart or kidney failure die waiting for a preliminary appointment with a suitable specialist. And how many people know that the organs required for a transplant operation have to be removed from a living patient?

A few years ago it was commonly said that cancer affected one in three individuals at some point in their lifetimes. Today it is commonly said that cancer affects one in two individuals at some point in their lifetimes. This would seem to me to be good evidence that the heavily promoted war on cancer has been somewhat of a failure. Why is the incidence of cancer increasing so quickly? There are a number of possible explanations but the most obvious one is mass vaccination. As vaccination has increased so cancer has increased. You'd have to be a fool not to connect the two.

Today's GPs are making more serious mistakes than their predecessors. Obviously, one reason is that many lazy and utterly useless GPs refuse to see patients at all. They insist that consultations are conducted via the telephone or the internet. These GPs will inevitably kill many of their patients by misdiagnosing them or mistreating them. But there is another reason why even GPs who do condescend to see patients face to face make so many errors. Because GPs do not do home visits or night calls they are unaccustomed to seeing seriously ill patients. And so their diagnostic skills are blunted and their ability to spot serious illness through experience or intuition is non-existent. The members of the medical establishment who gave GPs the right to work 23 hours a week, and to refuse to visit patients in their own homes, knew exactly what they were doing. These changes were made long before the global warming myth became an issue. The medical establishment knew that the changes that were made would destroy general practice and, therefore, destroy the entire National Health Service.

King Charles of England is a bad man. He is greedy and selfish and entitled in a way that most of us find difficult to comprehend. He is also out of touch with the public and the public mood which is surprising in one who has had over seven decades to devote himself to training for the job he now has. He made the taxpayers fork out £72 million for a coronation which almost no one cared about and, until persuaded to abandon the idea, wanted all Britons to pledge their allegiance to him – as though he were some medieval monarch and we were all serfs. He doesn't seem aware that the Magna Carta changed the rules.

During his Christmas message at the end of 2024, Charles praised the doctors who looked after him and his daughter-in-law after their cancer diagnoses. He didn't mention the countless millions who are waiting for treatment (at least partly because the doctors who should have been attending to them were on strike for more money and partly because doctors and hospitals are instructed to provide preferential health care for newly arrived illegal immigrants) and he didn't mention the fact that a growing percentage of the population resents the fact that he and his damned family heartily recommended and promoted a toxic and useless vaccine, the covid-19 vaccine, which has caused many deaths and a mammoth amount of illness and which is still causing much illness. For reasons I have already explained I seriously doubt if Queen Elizabeth II or Charles were vaccinated with the toxic covid-19 rubbish.

The number of people in Britain who have cancer is increasing rapidly. In the UK there are an average of 948 new cases of cancer a day with the four commonest cancers being those affecting the prostate, the breasts, the lungs and the bowels.

The incidence of cancer is increasing rapidly among young people in their 20s, 30s and 40s and is currently increasing in no less than 24 countries, including the UK, the US, Canada, Australia and France. A total of 17 different cancers are becoming commoner among young adults – including some previously quite uncommon cancers. And many of the cancers which affect these young adults are surprisingly aggressive and fast growing.

Doctors spend much of their time trying to work out why this should be. They have offered an almost endless list of explanations. They have blamed eating habits, food quality, obesity, diabetes, poor sleep, artificial light, micro-plastics, food colorants, antibiotics, newspapers and just about anything else you can think of. The only possible cause they haven't discussed is the covid-19 vaccine.

And so either the world's oncologists are all very, very stupid, or they are entirely corrupt or they are terrified of even suggesting that the covid-19 vaccine might possibly be a cause of this epidemic of cancer because they know that if they do so they will be vilified in the media and they will lose their licences to practice. These days no one, especially if they happen to be in the medical profession, is allowed to criticise vaccines.

And yet what is the one thing that has changed massively in recent years?

The answer, of course, is the number of vaccines being given to children.

And what evidence is there to show that giving children dozens of different vaccines in a very short amount of time is safe?

The answer, which I suspect you've already guessed, is none. Absolutely none.

And what is the one thing that has occurred in the last five years which has affected nearly all the young people now developing cancer?

The giving of the covid-19 vaccine. The stuff was damned near compulsory in many countries. Countless thousands lost their jobs because they didn't agree to have the experimental covid-19 vaccine injected into their bodies.

It's the one obvious explanation isn't it?

And it's the one explanation no one dares to mention.

Stupid, corrupt politicians tip toe round the obvious. Stupid, corrupt doctors tip toe round the obvious. And stupid, corrupt journalists tip toe round the obvious.

Deaths from cancer are expected to increase by at least 40% by the year 2030.

Don't you find that odd?

After all the cancer industry spends much of its time (and much of our money) telling us how well they are doing at defeating cancer. And smoking is now less common than it has been for decades.

And yet they know that deaths from cancer are rocketing and will soon account for nearly four out of five of all deaths among people aged over 60. And, if you exclude drug deaths and motorcycle deaths, probably close to that figure for deaths among people under 60.

And yet no one in the medical establishment has dared to suggest that until proved otherwise the covid-19 vaccine should be responsible for this surge in cancer deaths and no one dares to point out that the cancer industry has been a complete failure.

I can tell you that the drug industry is excited by what is happening. Thrilled indeed. According to research compiled by a 'leading global provider of advanced analytics and clinical research services for the life-sciences industry', global spending on cancer medicine increased by $25 billion in 2022, reaching $223 billion in 2023. Most of that, of course, is spent on chemotherapy which, as I showed in my book *What doctors won't tell you about chemotherapy* is toxic and does more harm than good.

North America makes up 48% of the market for cancer drugs (the UK would spend more but patients in the UK tend to die before they are diagnosed and, therefore, before treatment can start) and the US oncology market is increasing massively. Drug companies are busily building new factories to make chemotherapy drugs and they're preparing cancer vaccines too to take advantage of this unprecedented boom.

No one in the medical profession or the drug industry has any idea why this explosion in the need for cancer drugs should have occurred.

No one can think of any factor which might be responsible.

No one dares to suggest that the mass of vaccines being given (including the toxic covid-19 vaccine) could possibly be the culprit.

And so, meanwhile, doctors keep themselves busy prescribing toxic and useless chemotherapy drugs to deal with the cancers caused by the variety of useless vaccines which they give (and which are known to damage the immune system). There is, of course, massive profit to be made out of both causing cancer and treating it.

As you can probably imagine, it all makes me so proud to be a member of the medical profession.

And I find it impossible not to suggest the obvious: that the covid-19 vaccine was specifically designed to kill. The people who sold the vaccines to the world knew what would happen. The covid-19 vaccine was and is an integral part of the conspirators' depopulation plan.

The minute he got into the Oval Office, President Donald Trump allocated $500 billion of money (taken from American taxpayers of course) for the development of new mRNA vaccines.

Larry Ellison (who does not, as far as I know, have any medical training or experience – by which I mean he has never removed an appendix or sutured a wound) announced the development of new mRNA injections against cancer and pointed out that Artificial Intelligence would be used in the development of the new approach. The whole plan rather reminded me of President Richard Nixon's ill-fated and entirely useless war on cancer. Presidents always like to announce new health care initiatives because it is an easy way to convince the electors that they chose the right candidate (insofar as electors have an active role in choosing a President).

Ellison pointed out that AI can be used to look for cancer cells in the blood. And he suggested that this would be the basis for the new war on cancer.

What he may or may not know is that many, most or all

individuals have potential cancer cells floating around in their blood. In most cases, however, these potentially dangerous cancer cells do no harm. The body deals with them or the cancer cells don't settle down and start to grow, and that's that.

Ellison, however, suggested that his wonderful AI machines (which would not, as far as I can see do anything terribly different to blood testing machines) would identify everyone who had a cancer cell in their body.

And then (and this is the good bit) the AI machines would design and make an mRNA vaccine to attack the cancer cells.

Aha.

And now we have reached the exciting (and profitable) bit.

The American Government would then vaccinate everyone who had a cancer cell in their body (that is probably everyone still breathing) with the special mRNA vaccine.

Two things would then happen.

First the drug companies making the mRNA vaccines would make trillions of dollars. (The cost of the research will, of course, be paid by taxpayers who will not share in the profits.)

Second, millions of patients would fall ill and possibly die – just as they have done when jabbed with the toxic and experimental covid-19 vaccine.

I suspect that these special mRNA cancer vaccines will have to be produced quickly because people everywhere are becoming increasingly sceptical about the value of vaccines in general and mRNA vaccines in particular.

Scientists, medical scientists and doctors report that exposure to very low frequency electromagnetic fields can potentially damage the human body's DNA by increasing the production of free radicals in the cells. This can lead to DNA strands breaking down and to other genetic alterations. We are all of us surrounded by very low frequency electromagnetic fields. I detailed some of the health problems associated with electricity in my book *Superbody*. No one in the medical establishment takes these problems seriously. There is, however, no doubt that electricity power lines and the huge amount of electrical equipment by which we are surrounded, are damaging our health. Do not use a mobile phone more than absolutely necessary. Do not use iPads and laptops when they are plugged into the mains. Do not use electric shavers. Do not let children sit close to the television. Do not go to bed with an electric blanket switched on.

It has been widely reported that exposure to 'electrosmog' generated by electric, electronic and wireless technology is now causing unpleasant and serious adverse reactions among many individuals. A condition called electrohypersensitivity (aka rapid aging syndrome) affects children and adults. Problems with this condition include heart palpitations, chest pains, severe anxiety and clumping of the red blood cells. Cordless phones and mobile phones of all kinds can cause serious problems. The use of ear buds (small ear phones that you wear inside your ears) may be hazardous, and since I have been unable to find evidence proving that they are safe I think you should ignore reassurance glibly offered online. Remember that phrases such as 'there is no scientific evidence of their danger' usually means that no one has done any decent clinical research and so no one knows. (Why would the makers of electronic equipment conduct research which might prove that their products are dangerous? And who else is going to do research?) It is possible, of course, to purchase an EMF reader which can be either reassuring or terrifying.

Remember: Everything your government does is designed to take away your freedom or your privacy or to make you ill. We are at war with our governments.

The virtual ward sounds as if it is a good idea. It sounds as if patients are constantly monitored while in the comfort of their own homes. When I first heard the term I thought it meant that telephone lines and computers would be used to keep an eye on patients' vital signs while nurses or even doctors would pop in at regular intervals to make sure that all was well. I even thought that someone might deliver meals and even attend to laundry. I am sometimes embarrassed by my own naivety. It doesn't mean any of this, of course. In a virtual ward the patient stays at home and two people come in twice a day. In the morning they make sure that the patient gets out of bed (if they can) and has some breakfast. In the evening they make sure that the patient (if still alive) has some dinner and goes back to bed. That's about it. That's a virtual ward. Oh, and maybe someone will empty the bedpan. Maybe.

When I qualified as a doctor I was invited to take the Hippocratic Oath. It was optional. Some young doctors said they would. Many said they wouldn't. I happily took the Oath. Today, the Hippocratic Oath is considered out of date by the medical establishment and the General Medical Council in the UK (the body with the job of licensing doctors).

Here, so that you can make up your own mind, are the principle and relevant sections of the Hippocratic Oath:

'I swear that I will carry out, according to my ability and judgement, this oath.

I will use those dietary regimens which will benefit my patients according to my greatest ability and judgement, and I will do no harm or injustice to them. Neither will I administer a poison to anybody when asked to do so, nor will I suggest such a course. But I will keep pure and holy both my life and my art. I will not use the knife, not even, verity on sufferers from stone, but I will give place to such as are craftsmen therein.

Into whatsoever houses I enter, I will enter to help the sick, and I will abstain from all intentional wrong doing and harm, especially from abusing the bodies of man or woman, bond or free. And whatsoever I shall see or hear in the course of my profession I will never divulge, holding such things to be holy secrets.

Now if I carry out this oath and break it not, may I gain for ever reputation among all men for my life and for my art; but if I break it and forswear myself, may the opposite befall me.'

You will see that the Hippocratic Oath forbids euthanasia/doctor assisted suicide. What a pity it is that the Hippocratic Oath is no longer compulsory for doctors. I wonder what it is about the Oath which the medical establishment finds unacceptable.

Besotted with the nonsense formerly known as global warming, and now known as climate change, doctors are refusing to write prescriptions for antibiotics on the entirely dubious grounds that prescribing antibiotics threatens the future of the planet. And, for added emphasis, they say that they have to avoid prescribing antibiotics in order to minimise the risk of antibiotic resistant bacteria developing.

The first argument (the one about global warming) is, to put it simply, a lie conceived by the conspirators, who are driven by their determination to depopulate the world, and who want as many people as possible to die – and preferably as quickly as possible. The rapid rise in the incidence of sepsis is proof aplenty that the plan is working. Sepsis is a dangerous disease which is now, suddenly, one of the world's biggest killers. Not prescribing antibiotics at an early stage is a primary cause of this new epidemic. In the UK the number of people admitted to hospital with sepsis was less than 40,000 a year for a number of years. Now, suddenly, in 2023/2024 an astonishing 119,911 people were admitted to hospital with sepsis. The only conceivable reasons for the change are the refusal of GPs to visit patients at home, the long wait time for an appointment to see a GP and the sudden reluctance of doctors to prescribe antibiotics when they are needed. When treatment is begun early, sepsis is much easier to treat than when treatment begins late.

Doctors do what they're told because life is so much easier when you do what you're told and much more fun when you only have to work 23 hours a week (the average working week of a family doctor in the UK) and still get paid £150,000 a year (plus another £50,000 a year for telling your State employed staff to vaccinate as many patients as possible).

The second argument (about the antibiotic resistant organisms) is relevant but about fifty years too late. I've been screaming about the fact that over prescribing antibiotics causes the development of resistant organisms for well over half a century and for most of that time the medical establishment has sneered and laughed and ignored me. The fact is that antibiotics are essential and can save lives. By refusing to prescribe antibiotics when they are needed, doctors are guaranteeing that many people will die. The incidence of (often fatal) sepsis is soaring not so much because of antibiotic resistance but because patients are not being treated quickly enough. GPs are unavailable and even on the rare occasions when they are available, they seem dangerously unwilling to prescribe antibiotics. And by the time a patient with sepsis sees a doctor in a hospital it will often be too late. My wife's GP once told her: 'We're always here for you'.

This is akin to saying that the public library is always here for you. GPs who provided a 24 hour service for 365 days a year could say that they were always there for their patients. Modern GPs don't do that.

The forgotten fact about antibiotics is that farmers use as many antibiotics as doctors and the giving of antibiotics to farm animals (to help them develop more weight and therefore be worth more money at market) is just as a serious a problem as overprescribing for patients. Ignoring the overprescribing by veterinary surgeons (when I confronted one vet he admitted that the use of antibiotics by farms was bad practice but defended himself by saying 'If I don't give farmers what they want, someone else will'.)

The other reason why antibiotic resistance is a huge problem is that doctors and dentists have been advised to reduce the period for which pills are prescribed. In the 1970s and 1980s antibiotics were prescribed for a week or ten days. Then doctors and dentists started to give shorter and shorter courses with patients being given antibiotics for five days or even three days. This isn't enough to kill the bacteria and so the remaining bugs become resistant. At first I thought that reducing the length of a course was simply to save money. Now I know better. Reducing the length of a course of antibiotics was designed to create resistance to widely prescribed antibiotics. It was all part of the plan to turn medicine into the killing fields.

A few potent antibiotics have been kept back and reserved for the elite and their families should they require antibiotic treatment. Those of us who are not members of the elite can obtain supplies of ordinary, broad spectrum antibiotics via the internet. There are some reputable companies which will sell antibiotics to travellers who fear they may fall ill in some dark, out of the way place (such as England) where doctors and antibiotics are rarely available when required most urgently.

There is one other point worth making.

Antibiotic resistant organisms are now becoming commoner outside hospitals. The reason for that is simple: reckless and stupid hospital staff (most of whom don't understand how infections spread) insist on going outside their place of work while still wearing their contaminated work clothing. And so the resistant bugs are taken from the hospital onto buses and into shops. Some hospitals insist that visitors should wash their hands with antiseptic gel before going onto a ward. The hospitals have got things the wrong way round. The visitors, and the staff, should wash their hands with antiseptic gel before leaving the ward.

Finally, let us not forget the covid vaccine which has weakened millions and millions of people's immune systems, leaving them susceptible to infection.

No one can yet tell you the precise nature of the effect that mRNA vaccines has on the human body. The experience with the covid-19 vaccines confirms that none of these products should be used in any way on humans or animals. And yet, despite mounting evidence that the covid-19 mRNA vaccines were toxic and useless, new mRNA vaccines are being produced. Those who question the value of mRNA products are dismissed as conspirators and labelled 'discredited'.

Doctors in the UK are being told to limit repeat prescriptions to 28 days. If the medical establishment really cared about the number of journeys being made they wouldn't do this because limiting prescriptions of essential medicines to one month instead of two months or three months means that patients have to travel far more – they have to visit the doctor and the pharmacist two or three times as often.

Having over-prescribed potentially dangerous prescription drugs for many decades, GPs have now dramatically changed their prescribing habits – not because they have suddenly seen the light and realised that they have been overprescribing but because they have been told that they must cut down the number of prescriptions they write in order to combat global warming and to protect earth and its inhabitants from heat waves and searingly hot temperatures. (There is, of course, absolutely no evidence for global warming, which can best be described as a cult rather than a science.) Tragically, GPs are obeying the bizarre strictures on prescribing by suddenly halting the prescribing of drugs which patient have been taking for many years. Many drugs, particularly psychotropic drugs, need to be stopped very slowly, under constant medical supervision, but some GPs are simply refusing to write prescriptions in the mistaken and rather childish belief that they are saving polar bears and preventing glaciers from melting.

A group known as the Mutton Crew, linked to British Army intelligence, has for many years been using psychological warfare tricks to target, censor and demonise doctors around the world who have told the truth about anything threatening the existence and aims of the conspirators who want to reduce the world population, and lead us into Net Zero, a global technocracy and the Great Reset. Whether or not the Mutton Crew is linked to the 77th Brigade of the British Army, which has been working against the truth, is still a mystery.

These thoughtless individuals have worked to protect the lies told about covid and the covid-19 vaccine. The group harasses, spreads misinformation, manipulates and creates fake social media accounts to suppress dissent and to destroy the reputations and lives of anyone daring to criticise the lies told about covid by politicians, drug companies, government advisors and the medical establishment. Paid by British taxpayers they down-thumb videos and books and they leave sneering, libellous comments to discredit and break truth-tellers! The members of this criminal group provoke, bait, abuse and antagonise. If their victims respond aggressively then their comments are reported to the police and to social platforms as hate speech. The bullies also make complaints to the General Medical Council if they identify doctors who have questioned the validity of the covid hoax or questioned the value of the covid-19 vaccine. (Doctors who have questioned the value of the toxic covid-19 vaccine have had their licences taken away by the licensing authorities which has been weaponised very effectively.) The aim is to suppress and demonise doctors who know the truth about covid.

These ignorant bullies also set up fake accounts in the names of individual doctors.

Numerous accounts in my name have been set up on social media even though I am actually banned from all platforms and am not allowed to have accounts myself.

And they did all this to protect the financial interests of an entirely corrupt elite, a corrupt pharmaceutical industry, a corrupt government and a corrupt medical establishment. In addition to receiving government funding, it seems likely that these people were paid from outside sources to conduct psychological warfare against honest doctors. It would not be surprising if some of the money came from drug companies.

Changes to the system whereby death certificates are provided in England mean that relatives will in future have to wait weeks before being allowed to bury their relatives. There is no sound reason for this.

No one in medicine bothers with epidemiology any more. I suspect that most health professionals don't understand what the word means or how it can be applied to the way we practise health care.

Medical journalists are no longer reliable. They use sources who are biased because they are provided (and paid) by drug companies. If you work as a medical correspondent for a newspaper, magazine radio station or television station you will find that it is easy to acquire a list of 'experts' who will talk to you whenever you want a quote or some background information. The selected and readily available experts will be drug company hacks – bought and paid for by the drug industry. The 'experts' may well be eminent. They will have impeccable qualifications. But they will tell you what they have been told to say by the drug company that is paying them. Modern journalists don't bother looking for two sides to a story. And so they merely pass on the propaganda. And, as part of the propaganda, they will be told that anyone who opposes the official, 'party' line on whatever it is (vaccination, vivisection, transplants, painkillers, tranquillisers, chemotherapy or whatever) is a dangerous lunatic to be ignored, sneered at and suppressed.

When I was at medical school I was full of hope and a sense of vocation. When I worked as a GP I was full of hope and a sense of vocation. Today, I am ashamed to be a member of the medical profession.

In the UK, King Charles, who is a septuagenarian, is being treated for an unspecified cancer. If Charles were an untitled citizen, and not a member of the royal family, he would have probably been given a kill shot of midazolam and morphine, without the option, in order to kill him and to save the State money. If Charles cared about 'his' subjects he would campaign to stop the abuse of patients in the UK – which now has the worst health care system in the world (though America and Canada are providing strong competition in this regard).

When Liz Truss was England's Prime Minister for a few weeks there was a financial crisis. It is reported that when looking for ways to save money, Truss and her chancellor Kwarsi Kwarteng suggested stopping cancer treatment on the National Health Service.

Trying to isolate and identify the basic truths about cancer is a nightmare. The internet is awash with rumours and with recommendations which are commercially inspired. However, the basic facts about cancer are fairly easy to define.

Every one of us has cancer cells, or would-be cancer cells, in our bodies. These cells don't show up until they have multiplied to a mass containing a few million. Only when clumps of cancer cells reach a certain size can they be identified. There are 100 trillion cells in an average human body. But the cells aren't all the same. The cells in bone are different to the cells in the blood and they are different to the cells in the breast. And wherever they are in the body, cells are constantly reproducing and renewing themselves. As cells wear out and die so new cells take their place. Biochemical signals tell cells when to start growing and when to stop. Occasionally, something goes wrong and instead of cells reproducing in a controlled sort of way they go berserk. When this happens, a lump forms. Sometimes a lump grows very slowly and is of no significance and sometimes it consists of cells which are reproducing very rapidly (cancer). However, the real danger with cancer cells is not so much the original lump formed by the reproducing cells but the fact that the cells can spread around the body and produce lumps elsewhere. This process is called metastasis, and the lumps which develop elsewhere are known as 'secondaries'. (The original lump is, of course, the 'primary'.) And while it is true that the vast majority of cancer cells which leave the original tumour will die, the danger is that one or two will settle somewhere in the body.

The whole process of cancer development has obviously been the subject of much study for many years. But despite the billions of pounds which have been spent, scientists still don't know very much. What does seem pretty certain, however, is that cells become cancerous, and multiply in an uncontrolled frenzy, because something has gone wrong with the signalling process. That can happen for a variety of reasons. There may be a carcinogen (a cancer inducing substance such as tobacco or asbestos) in the body, and this carcinogen may damage the DNA of the genes that control cell reproduction. Or the body may be short of some essential substance which is needed to produce healthy DNA. The development of a cancer depends upon the inter-reaction between our genes and our lifestyle – including diet. The genes with which we are born include some cancer genes which can develop into cancer if they are 'turned on' by environmental factors such as a vitamin shortage.

It is the fear of metastases which naturally terrifies cancer patients. When they have a cough they fear that there may be metastases in their lungs. A headache creates a fear of secondaries in the brain. Every pain becomes a possible metastasis. Around 90% of all deaths caused by cancer are due not to the original tumour but to the cancer cells spreading. The problem isn't actually the cancer cells moving around in the blood, but the cancer cells deciding to stop moving, settle down and start building new tumours. It's vital to remember that a strong immune system and a good diet will help prevent cancers from multiplying and forming tumours. And it's vital too to remember that vaccines can sometimes damage the immune system – as can chemotherapy.

As I pointed out earlier in this book, American President Donald Trump has allocated £500 billion towards discovering an AI system which can identify cancer cells (or, presumably, pre-cancerous cells). The drug companies will then create bespoke vaccines. Everyone with cancer cells in their body will be advised (or forced) to have a special vaccine.

And here's the clever bit: Most people in the world have cancer cells or pre-cancer cells in their body. And so most people in the world will be given a special vaccine and told that it will save their life.

Vitamin D is a crucial vitamin for maintaining good health and a strong immune system. Early in 2020 I recorded a video suggesting that viewers should take vitamin D supplements. I felt this was particularly important during the lockdowns when people were deprived of sunshine. YouTube took the video down almost immediately though they did not say on whose advice they did this. I don't think you would find a doctor in the world who would say that recommending vitamin D was bad advice. But YouTube removed it. This was either dumb persecution or a deliberate attempt to weaken and kill as many people as possible.

A deficiency of vitamin D disrupts the immune system and triggers autoimmune diseases. It may also increase the risk of cancer developing or of an existing cancer spreading.

The executives who run YouTube, and the responsible staff, should all be arrested and charged with genocide. (Genocide is defined as the deliberate killing of a large group of people).

Geo-engineers are currently injecting particles into the stratosphere to dim the sun. This will mean real health problems for billions because the sun is their main source of vitamin D. (Dimming the sun will, of course, also result in solar panels not working.)

Solar power is at least ten times as expensive as natural gas. Wind-power, like solar power, is a much more expensive, and environmentally damaging, source of electricity than the traditional ways of creating electricity. (It is worth noting that huge amounts of coal remain abandoned and easily accessible in mines.)

Geo-engineers who believe that global warming is real (or who are directed by people who pretend they believe that global warming is real, which isn't necessarily the same thing at all) are spraying a variety of aerosol chemicals into the stratosphere. The aim is to dim the sun.

The chemicals being used include metallic aluminium, aluminium oxide, black carbon, barium titanate and environmental sulphate. These chemicals drift down from the sky and contaminate our food and water supplies. They also cause transdermal contamination. Very little research has been done on ground level contamination but the spraying of chemicals massively exacerbates ground level pollution and causes long-term problems.

These chemicals produce coughing, increased salivation and a sore trachea. They exacerbate asthma and cause breathing difficulties in the previously healthy. They will kill.

The symptoms known to result from stratospheric spraying include: fatigue, headaches, loss of appetite, irritability, dizziness, poor memory, confusion, vomiting, cardiac arrhythmias, muscle cramps, collapse, convulsions, tiredness, heart enlargement, anaemia and skin irritation. The chemicals may also be carcinogenic.

The quality of our air is damaged, farms are damaged and the health of billions of people will be damaged. The chemicals raining down on earth have helped destroy 75% of our wildlife, 90% of our fish and between 80 and 90% of our insects. Between 40 million and 60 million tons of chemicals are dropped each year on Americans alone. The stuff comes down with the rain and includes graphene and polymer fibre (which are biological warfare carriers). The chemical particles are destroying trees, and without insects, farmers are having to pollinate by hand. The people who are ordering this massive pollution will be fine, of course, because they are living on private islands or on massive super-yachts.

Geo-engineering should be called genocide engineering.

How can we protect ourselves?

Well, ironically, masks might help if the particles being sprayed are large enough. (Wearing a mask to protect you against viruses is, as I explained early in 2020, like hoping that chicken wire will keep out mosquitoes.) And although I'm not aware of any specific testing having been done I suspect that an air purifier or electronic pollen filter might help. After several days of very grey skies my wife and I were both suffering from sore, irritated eyes and sore throats. We turned on two pollen filters for a few hours and the problems disappeared.

Journalists claim that none of this is happening.

They are wrong. For example, one company began experimenting in 2022. And in the same year the White House in the US began to coordinate a five year research plan to study ways of modifying the amount of sunlight reaching the earth.

Geo-engineering is a very real and present danger to every aspect of life on earth.

Over the years I have repeatedly found that all medical recommendations are best treated with a large dose of scepticism.

Nowhere is this more true than in the treatment of cancer. (The material immediately below is based on my book *What doctors won't tell you about chemotherapy*.)

Patients who are diagnosed with cancer find themselves in a state of shock. And yet, while in a state of shock, they find themselves needing to make a number of vital decisions very quickly.

One of the big questions is often this one: 'Should I have chemotherapy?'

Chemotherapy (or 'systemic anticancer treatment') might improve a patient's chances of survival by three to five per cent though that modest figure is usually over generous. For example, the evidence suggests that chemotherapy offers breast cancer patients an uplift in survival of little more than 2.5%.

When you consider that chemotherapy can kill and does terrible damage to healthy cells, and to the immune system, it is difficult to see the value of taking chemotherapy.

I don't think it is any exaggeration to suggest that much of the hype around chemotherapy has taken the treatment into the area of fraud – far more fraudulent indeed than treatments which are dismissed as irrelevant or harmful by the establishment.

Chemotherapy is a cull, designed by the conspirators and the medical establishment to cut the cost of caring for cancer patients.

The chances are that the doctors looking after patients with cancer – especially the specialist oncologists in hospital – will recommend chemotherapy. They may push hard for patients to accept their recommendation. They may even be cross or dismissive or assume patients are ignorant or afraid if they decide you don't want it. Cancer charities often shout excitedly about chemotherapy. But they are also often closely linked to the drug companies which make money out of chemotherapy – which in my view makes them part of the large and thriving 'cancer industry'. It is important to remember that drug companies exist to make money and they will do whatever is necessary to further this aim. They lie and they cheat with scary regularity and they have no interest in helping patients or saving lives. Remember that: the sole purpose of drug companies is to make money, whatever the human cost might be. They will happily suppress potentially life-saving information if doing so increases their profits. It is my belief that by allying themselves with drug companies, cancer charities have become corrupt.

Little or no advice is given to patients about how they themselves might reduce the risk of their cancer returning. The implication is that its chemotherapy or nothing. So, for example, doctors are unlikely to tell breast cancer patients that they should avoid dairy foods, though the evidence that they should is very strong.

The sad truth is that the statistics about chemotherapy are, of course, fiddled to boost the drug company sales and, therefore, drug company profits. And the deaths caused by chemotherapy are often misreported or under-estimated. So, for example, if a patient who has been taking chemotherapy dies of a sudden heart attack, their death will probably be put down as a heart attack – rather than as a result of the cancer or the chemotherapy. There may be some mealy mouthed suggestion that the death was treatment related but the drug will probably not be named and shamed. Neither the chemotherapy nor the cancer will be deemed responsible. What this means in practice is that the survival statistics for chemotherapy are considerably worse than the figures which are made available – considerably worse, indeed, than whatever positive effect might be provided by a harmless placebo.

Here's another thing: patients who have chemotherapy and survive five years are counted as having been cured by chemotherapy. And patients who have chemotherapy and then die five and a bit years after their diagnosis don't count as cancer related deaths. And they certainly don't count as chemotherapy deaths.

A 2016 academic study looked at five year survival rates and concluded that in 90% of patients (including the commonest breast cancer tumours) chemotherapy increased five year survival by less than 2.5%. Only a very small number of cancers (such as testicular cancer and Hodgkin's disease) were treated effectively by chemotherapy.

On top of this dismal success rate, it must be remembered that chemotherapy cripples the immune system (now, at long last, with some reluctance recognised as important in the fight against cancer), damages all living cells, damages the intestines, can cause nausea and tinnitus, can damage nerves, can and does damage the bone marrow with the result that leukaemia develops, (staggeringly, iatrogenic myeloid leukaemia, usually known as 'therapy related' in an attempt to distance the disease from doctors, is, in ten per cent of cases, a result of chemotherapy), damages the heart and the hearing and will, in a significant number of patients, result in death.

Staggeringly, 25% of cancer patients die of heart attacks – often triggered by deep vein thrombosis, and by emboli and brought on by the physical stress of chemotherapy. These deaths are not included in the official statistics – either for cancer or, just as importantly, for chemotherapy. It is no exaggeration to say that the establishment fiddles the figures to suit its own largely commercial ends – extolling the virtues of drug company products at every opportunity and never failing to throw doubt on any remedy which might threaten the industry-charity axis of the huge cancer industry.

It is true that chemotherapy may reduce the size of a tumour, but in stage 4 cancer, chemotherapy seems to encourage a cancer to return more quickly and more aggressively. The cancer stem cells seem to be untouched by the chemotherapy drugs.

Despite all this, the protocol in the treatment of cancer is to turn to chemotherapy, and doctors are always reluctant to try anything else.

The Academy of Royal Medical Colleges, which represents 24 Royal Colleges, and a number of other important health bodies, has reported that chemotherapy can do more harm than good when prescribed as palliatives for terminally ill cancer patients. The colleges criticise chemotherapy advocates for 'raising false hopes' and doing 'more harm than good'. They concluded that chemotherapy drugs are unlikely to work.

A paper published in BMC Palliative Care in 2022, concluded that: 'Chemotherapy use closer to the end of life is a marker of poor-quality care.' Of a total of 681 patients who were given chemotherapy, nearly a fifth died within 30 days after chemotherapy. The authors said in their conclusion: 'Administration of chemotherapy within the last 30 days of life could cause unnecessary suffering to patients and cost to society. Early referral to palliative care was significantly associated with reduced risk of getting chemotherapy within the last 30 days of life in this study.' The authors pointed out that although many oncologists were reluctant to prescribe chemotherapy at the end of life, a patient's decision would depend on the clarity of the information he or she received.

A study from France showed that patients who died in for profit hospitals, comprehensive cancer centres and centres without palliative care had greater than average use of chemotherapy near the end of life.

I wasn't surprised to see a big cancer charity disagreeing with the 24 medical colleges and claiming that thousands of patients do benefit. My view, which I recognise is probably not shared by the majority of family doctors or oncologists, is that many cancer charities around the world are the unacceptable face of cancer care. It seems to me that some charities appear to be more concerned with making money and keeping the drug companies happy and rich than in caring for patients.

Another report has concluded that chemotherapy can, in some circumstances, actually promote the spread of cancer cells. It was reported in 2017, for example, that when breast cancer patients have chemotherapy before surgery, the drug can make the malignant cells spread to distant sites – resulting in metastatic cancer and sending the patient straight from Stage 1 to Stage 4. Scientists analysed tissue from 20 breast cancer patients who had 16 weeks of chemotherapy, and the tissues around the tumour was more conducive to spread in most of the patients. In five of the patients, there was a five times greater risk of spread. In none of the patients was the tissue around the tumour less friendly to cancer cells and to metastasis. The problem, it seems is that cancer cells have a great ability to transform themselves, and the chemotherapy, designed to kill cancer cells, may encourage the development of cells which are resistant to drugs, which survive the treatment and which form a new cancer.

The one side effect associated with chemotherapy that is widely known is the loss of hair. But that is, to be honest, the least of the problems. Chemotherapy kills healthy cells as well as cancer cells, and the severity of the side effects depends on the age and health of the patient as well as on the type of drug used and the dosage in which it is prescribed. And whereas some side effects do disappear after treatment (as the good cells recover) there are some side effects which may never go away.

Here is a list of just some of the problems that can be caused by chemotherapy drugs:

The cells in the bone marrow can be damaged, producing a shortage of red blood cells and possibly leukaemia.

The central nervous system can be damaged with a result that the memory may be affected and the patient's ability to concentrate or think clearly changed. There may be changes to balance and coordination. These effects can last for years. Apart from affecting the brain, chemotherapy can also cause pain and tingling in the hands and feet, numbness, weakness and pain. Not surprisingly, depression is not uncommon.

The digestive system is commonly affected with sores forming in the mouth and throat. These may produce infection and may make food taste unpleasant. Nausea and vomiting may also occur. The weight loss associated with chemotherapy may be a result of a loss of appetite.

In addition to hair loss (which can affect hair all over the body) the skin may be irritated and nails may change colour and appearance.

The kidneys and bladder may be irritated and damaged. The result may be swollen ankles, feet and hands.

Osteoporosis is a fairly common problem and increases the risk of bone fractures and breaks. Women who have breast cancer and who are having treatment to reduce their oestrogen levels are particularly at risk.

Chemotherapy can produce hormone changes with a wide variety of symptoms.

The heart may be damaged and patients who already have weak hearts may be made worse by chemotherapy.

And the other problem with chemotherapy is that it can damage the immune system.

And it is known that chemotherapy can damage DNA.

And does chemotherapy alter the nature of cancer cells? Can it, for example, trigger a change from an oestrogen sensitive cancer cell to a triple negative cell – much harder to treat?

And then there is that risk that chemotherapy might spread cells around the body.

Not surprisingly, there is increasing evidence to show that

chemotherapy may hasten the death of a number of patients.

Drug companies, cancer charities and doctors recommend chemotherapy because there is big money in it. The least forgivable of these are the cancer charities which exist to protect people but which are ruthless exploiters of patients.

As always the medical literature is confusing but in the Annals of Oncology I found this: 'the upfront use of chemotherapy does not seem to influence the overall outcome of the disease'.

Most doctors won't tell you this, or even admit it to themselves, but cancer drugs are killing up to 50% of patients in some hospitals. A study by Public Health England and Cancer Research UK, which was published in *The Lancet*, found that 2.4% of breast cancer patients die within a month of starting chemotherapy. The figures are even worse for patients with lung cancer where 8.4% of patients die within a month when treated with chemotherapy. When patients die that quickly, I feel that it is safe to assume that they were killed by the treatment not the disease. At one hospital, the death rate for patients with lung cancer treated with chemotherapy was reported at over 50%. The one month mortality rate in one group of teaching hospitals was 28% for patients receiving palliative care for lung cancer. One in five breast cancer patients in another group of hospitals died from their treatment. Naturally, all the hospitals which took part in the study insisted that chemotherapy prescribing was being done safely. If we accept this then we must also question the validity of chemotherapy. The study showed that the figures are particularly bad for patients who are in poor general health when they start treatment. The problem, of course, is that chemotherapy does not differentiate between healthy cells and cancerous cells, and the cell-destroying properties of chemotherapy can be lethal. One senior oncologist said: 'I think it's important to make patients aware that there are potentially life threatening downsides to chemotherapy. And doctors should be more careful about who they treat with chemotherapy.' Sadly, I fear that most doctors do not share full details of the risks associated with chemotherapy, and a good number of patients take chemotherapy thinking that the only downside will be a short-term loss of their hair. This in truth is the least of the problems associated with these drugs.

A study published in *JAMA Oncology* studied the use of chemotherapy among 312 terminally ill cancer patients. All 312 patients had been given no more than six months to live by their doctors and all had at least one, and in some cases multiple rounds of chemotherapy, which had failed. Their tumours had, despite the chemotherapy, spread to other parts of their body. And yet half of these patients were on chemotherapy, despite its obvious ineffectiveness. The analysis published in *JAMA Oncology* showed that these patients were worse off than if they hadn't had treatment. Their quality of life was less than it would have been without chemotherapy. The patients on chemotherapy were less able to walk, take care of themselves and stay active than the patients not taking chemotherapy. Most surprising was the fact that the patients who were feeling the best at the start of their chemotherapy were the ones who ended up feeling the worst; they were the ones who suffered the most. The chemotherapy consequences for those patients had been to make their lives worse without any benefit.

Other studies have shown the same thing. Chemotherapy in terminally ill patients is essentially ineffective. Any tumour shrinkage (a rare occurrence) was not linked to a longer life.

As a result of all this research, the American Society of Clinical Oncologists has advised doctors to be more judicious with their chemotherapy use in terminal patients. The group's guidelines recommend limiting the use of chemotherapy to relatively healthy patients who can withstand the toxic effects and, hopefully, overcome the awful side effects.

The sad thing is that many cancer patients still believe that more and more rounds of chemotherapy will be of benefit to them. The truth is that patients with end stage cancer who are still relatively healthy will be made weaker by chemotherapy and will spend much of their remaining time travelling to and from hospital. It really is vital that patients be informed about the real risks of chemotherapy and that they should be involved in making decisions about their treatment. Chemotherapy is so toxic that the chances of a patient surviving treatment depend a good deal on their age and general well-being. Patients who are seriously ill are, it seems, more likely to die as a result of chemotherapy. (There is no little irony in the fact that many patients with cancer simply aren't fit enough to be treated with chemotherapy. And, of course, the people who don't have cancer don't need it.)

In America, huge numbers of patients are forced to undergo

chemotherapy at the State's behest, even when patients and relatives object. So, for example, a 17-year-old diagnosed with Hodgkin lymphoma decided to seek alternatives to chemotherapy but her doctors were so convinced by the Big Pharma propaganda that they contacted family services who kidnapped the young adult and had her placed in foster care. She was only allowed to go home once she had agreed to have the chemotherapy, though she ran away. The Supreme Court in the US ruled that the State was in the right and had the authority to kidnap the patient, force her into treatment against her will and deny her contact with her family.

Next think about this.

In the UK, the National Health Service publishes comprehensive guidelines on what must be done if chemotherapy drugs are spilt. There are crisis emergency procedures to be followed if chemotherapy drugs fall on the floor. And yet these drugs are put into people's bodies. And residues of these dangerous chemicals are excreted in urine and then end up in the drinking water supply. (I explained several decades ago in my books *Meat causes Cancer* and *Superbody* how prescription drug residues end up in our drinking water.)

It is hardly surprising that many patients being treated with chemotherapy report that their quality of life has plummeted.

The standard oncology approach to cancer is to give chemotherapy and then wait and see if the cancer returns. If it does then more chemotherapy is prescribed. The tragedy is that for so many patients, chemotherapy will do more harm than good. Astonishingly, a quarter of cancer patients die of heart attacks – often triggered by deep vein thrombosis and by emboli and brought on by the physical stress of chemotherapy. But these deaths are not included in the official statistics – either for cancer or, just as importantly, for chemotherapy. It is no exaggeration to say that the establishment fiddles the figures to suit its own largely commercial ends – extolling the virtues of drug company products at every opportunity and never failing to throw doubt on any remedy which might threaten the huge cancer industry

Here's another thing you might not know.

During the lockdowns and concerns about covid-19, patients who were on chemotherapy were taken off their treatment. They were told that since their treatment would affect their immune systems they would be more vulnerable to the coronavirus. That's an important admission because the one thing we know for certain is that a healthy immune system is vital for fighting cancer.

Doctors probably won't tell you any of this but they won't deny it because it is all true.

The bottom line is that treatments described in clinical trials, paid for by drug companies and generally reviewed by doctors with drug company links, and then published in medical journals which accept huge amounts of drug company advertising, are the only treatments the medical profession accepts. There is much talk about 'peer review' trials but all this means is that another doctor or two, with drug company links, will have looked at the paper and given it their approval.

The word 'corrupt' doesn't come close to describing this whole incestuous system.

Anyone who wants to have chemotherapy should have it. I'm not trying to dissuade anyone from using whatever drugs they believe might help them. I'm only interested in providing unbiased, independent information which might help patients make the right decision for themselves.

But too often, I fear, patients beg for treatment, completely understandably, because they want something to be done and because they have been misled by the drug company inspired, and paid for, hype about chemotherapy. And doctors provide that treatment, even though a little research would tell them that they may be doing more harm than good. There are very few cancers which can be treated well with chemotherapy – but they are very few and they are unfairly and unreasonably promoted as success stories by the drug companies and their shills.

The thing that is forgotten or ignored is that chemotherapy can badly damage the patient's body's own protections – and with some patients may, therefore, do infinitely more harm than good.

Every patient should decide for themselves – and discuss with their doctors the evidence for and against chemotherapy in their situation. But I think that all patients are entitled to be provided with the background information they would need to help that process of assessment.

Tragically, however, the ignorance about chemotherapy is, sadly, widespread and all pervasive.

How many women with breast cancer realise that their survival chances might be better if they took a daily aspirin (in a soluble 75mg dose) and avoided dairy products than if they accepted chemotherapy? (Research shows that low dose aspirin, which has both an anti-inflammatory effect and an anti-coagulant effect) seems to have great value in combating both cancer and heart disease.

Doctors don't talk much about the value of daily low dose aspirin because they have, as a profession, been bought by the pharmaceutical industry and there is very little profit to be made from selling low dose aspirin – however effective it might be.

From time to time there are news stories in the papers about women who say 'No, thank you' when offered chemotherapy. The response from the medical profession, the media and the public is inevitably critical, and often abusive. When one young mother refused chemotherapy, doctors at the hospital which was supposedly caring for her refused to operate on her or provide her with any other care.

I remember one story about another young woman who refused chemotherapy and was told by her local hospital that if she didn't have chemotherapy then she couldn't have surgery. So the young woman gave up meat and she and her husband spent all their savings (a total of £70,000) on trying a variety of alternative treatments – none of which worked. The young woman is now dead, leaving behind a penniless husband and a young daughter. What astonished me was the nature of the heartless comments on the internet. They were, without exception, sneery and critical and naturally most of them were anonymous. None understood or even cared about the pain the poor woman and her family had been through – and I suspect that few if any of the comments were from critics who had studied the advantages and disadvantages of chemotherapy. I wonder how many of those who scoffed know that chemotherapy designed for the treatment of cancer, is an attempt to poison cancer cells which grow rapidly. However, it also destroys healthy cells in the bone marrow and can damage all the organs of the body. Chemotherapy often kills more people than it saves. How many of those who defend chemotherapy know that chemotherapy can seriously damage the immune system – thereby making the patient very vulnerable to infection. And I wonder how many of those know-it-alls understand that chemotherapy can cause cancer cells to mutate and become more resistant and difficult to destroy.

Brave individuals who stand up to those who are pushing chemotherapy are often accused of ignorance or cowardice when in reality the opposite is true. It takes real strength of mind to stand up to doctors, nurses, relatives and friends who insist (usually because they've never bothered to do any research) that chemotherapy is safe and effective. It is sometimes said that those who reject chemotherapy do so because they are frightened of losing their hair. This is hideously insulting. Hair grows back, and I very much doubt if more than a tiny number of people reject chemotherapy because they are worried about hair loss. (Incidentally, supporters of chemotherapy might like to ask themselves which invisible cells are being damaged at the same time as hair cells are suffering. Hair loss is merely a superficial, observable sign of the damage that is being done and which is largely invisible.)

In September 2024, a former model called Elle Macpherson revealed that seven years earlier she had refused to undergo chemotherapy for breast cancer despite the advice of 32 doctors. When she revealed this news she was in 'clinical remission'.

'Saying 'No' to standard medical solutions was the hardest thing I've ever done in my life,' she said. 'But saying no to my own inner sense would have been even harder.'

Inevitably, the mainstream media reporting of Miss Macpherson's decision was often accompanied by articles written in support of chemotherapy. 'It goes without saying that if you are diagnosed with cancer, it is wise to stick to medical advice,' said a journalist (without medical qualifications) in The Times of London. Fair enough. But what if the medical advice you are being given is wrong?

The most dangerous moment for any patient with cancer is the one when a lone cell breaks free from the original tumour and moves elsewhere. This is the beginning of metastasis. White blood cells (aka T cells) can destroy the lone cancer cell as it tries to settle and start a new colony. But platelet cells can and do suppress and interfere with the T cells.

Aspirin disrupts the platelets and allows the T cells to do their work and to protect the body.

Aspirin enhances the ability of the immune system to fight back and provide protection.

Aspirin is, of course, one of the cheapest drugs available. And despite what you might read in the mainstream media, aspirin is one of the safest drugs around. We know all the problems it is likely to cause. The biggest danger is intestinal bleeding and this can be reduced by using a low dose of a soluble aspirin. A tablet containing just 75 mg is usually considered enough to stop the platelets interfering with the T cells. If dissolved in a large glass of water, the risk is small. The risk with aspirin is certainly far, far lower than the risk with chemotherapy.

So why don't doctors recommend aspirin to patients with cancer?

And why are journalists so dismissive and contemptuous?

Money.

Drug companies make next to nothing out of aspirin, but they can make billions out of chemotherapy. And, of course, most mainstream journalists are owned by the drug industry. Most doctors are owned by the drug industry too.

I enjoyed being a GP but I had to retire rather early because I refused to compromise on the signing of sick notes. I believed then, and believe now, that medical confidentiality should be sacrosanct.

Here's the explanation for my resignation which I put on my website in May 2020.

'Among the lies on the Web there is one claiming that I left the NHS after my first book *The Medicine Men* was published.

If those who make this stuff up bothered to do any research, or cared about the truth, they would know that this is nonsense.

The Medicine Men was published in 1975 and I received an advance of £750 to write it. The typist who worked on the typescript charged £800, and the insurers from whom I bought libel insurance charged me £700.

I had some money for foreign rights and paperback rights but the book wasn't going to take me off to the Bahamas on a huge yacht.

Besides, what the idiots on the Web don't realise is that I didn't resign as a GP until seven or eight years later.

Being a GP was the job I'd always wanted to do and one that I enjoyed a great deal.

In those distant days GPs were responsible for their patients 365 days a year and 24 hours a day. So that we had some time off most doctors worked in informal groups of four or five. Often the association was a very loose one in that individual GPs ran their practices independently and merely shared their out of hours responsibilities. It all worked surprisingly well and easily.

If there were five doctors sharing their night time, weekend and bank holiday calls then each one of the five would be on call one night a week and one weekend in five. It wasn't particularly onerous.

At the end of the day a doctor who was looking after a patient with a specific problem would ring the doctor due to be on call and tell him if he was likely to be called out. 'Mrs X has a bad chest infection but I think she is responding to the antibiotics. If her husband calls, you may have to fix a hospital bed for her.' That sort of thing.

I never particularly minded out of hours calls. Indeed, the best bit of being a GP was driving back home at 4.00 am having spent an hour or two treating a patient at home. It might have been an asthmatic having severe trouble breathing and needing intravenous injections. Or a child screaming with pain from an ear infection.

Of course, the glow of satisfaction might dim slightly if, when getting back home, I found there was another call to be done. If there was then it would inevitably be to a house in the next street to the one I'd just left. There were no mobile phones in those days, of course.

After a night on call we still did morning surgery, of course. And that was sometimes a little tiring. I wasn't the only GP to fall asleep in his consulting room.

So why, after just ten years, did I give up my dream job?

It was the paperwork, the bureaucracy, which defeated me.

One of a GP's tasks was to sign sick notes. And the law required doctors to put the diagnosis on the form. The patient then took the form to their employer. Inevitably, this meant that everyone in the office knew what the patient's problem was.

One of my patients was the manager of the local branch of a big chain store.

He came in to see me one day and it wasn't difficult to see the problem. He was severely depressed; worn down by demanding bosses and a difficult job. He needed time off work.

I reached for the sick note pad, scribbled his name and address and then wrote 'depression' in the box requiring a diagnosis.

'Do you have to put that down?' he asked.

I looked at him, puzzled.

'If my bosses see that then I'll be fired,' he told me.

I ripped up the form and wrote another. On this one I scribbled 'virus infection'.

A couple of days later a young woman came to see me. She was pregnant and was suffering from morning sickness.

'Do you mind not putting down that I'm pregnant?' she asked. 'The girls at work don't know but I have to hand the form in to my boss.'

And so she had a virus infection too.

After that, all the sick notes I signed contained the same diagnosis: virus infection.

After a few weeks of this I was hauled before a local NHS committee. They had a sheaf of sick notes I had signed. All the forms had the same diagnosis.

To cut a long story short they fined me a couple of hundred quid and threatened to do it again and again if I didn't write down proper diagnoses. Two hundred pounds was a lot of money in those days.

So I resigned from my job as a GP and became a professional writer.

Shortly afterwards, I'm pleased to say, the rules were changed and patients were allowed to write their own sick notes.

Nevertheless, one medical journal described me as a Don Quixote tilting at windmills because I stood firm on a basic principle of medical practice. Not one other member of the profession joined me in my stand.

I do not apologise for reminding you that whereas a decade or so ago cancer was said to affect one in every three individuals in their lifetime, the statistics show that today, after billions of pounds have been spent on research, and billions have been spent on drugs and screening and prevention, cancer is said to affect one in every two individuals in their lifetime. I can think of no better way to prove that the war on cancer has failed, is failing (and will continue to fail). The cancer industry (drug companies, cancer charities and oncologists) has little or no interest in curing cancer or even in treating patients with cancer. The cancer industry exists for two reasons only: to make money and to kill people more speedily than they would otherwise have died. And the incidence of cancer is growing because our world is contaminated by forever chemicals, many of which are carcinogenic and, more significantly, because doctors are now vaccinating small children with an endless number of vaccines which have not been adequately tested and which do considerably more harm than good.

Doctors in the UK have been told to stop prescribing asthma inhalers that work and which are relatively safe. People believing in the global warming myth have told doctors to warn patients that the blue inhalers that millions of asthma sufferers have used for donkey's years could damage the planet.

So, instead of prescribing the safe drug that works, doctors are being told to advise patients to switch to a combination inhaler containing steroids and a bronchodilator because they say this won't have an effect on the entire mythical global warming fraud.

(Even if global warming were real, the inhalers that have been used since I was in practice, would, I suspect, do considerably less harm to the planet than jet setting members of the royal family.)

But today the medical establishment has boasted that it cares far more about tackling imaginary global warming than it does about diagnosing and treating patients.

But how safe are the recommended combination inhalers?

You decide.

Here's a list of some of the dangerous side effects associated with one popular combination inhaler: Wheezing, choking, fever, chills, breathing problems, shortness of breath, chest pain, fast or irregular heartbeat, severe headache, tremors, nervousness, eye pain, blurred vision, tunnel vision, high blood sugar and thrush.

Curiously, the mainstream media seems to have forgotten to mention all these side effects.

Oh, and there is something else: the combination inhalers can also weaken the human immune system, making the patient more vulnerable to infection. Just about everything doctors do these days seem designed to damage the immune system.)

So, why in the name of Hippocrates, are doctors recommending these products?

I believe this is all part of the widespread plan to kill as many people as possible?

It is worth noting that a majority of the people who have been diagnosed as asthmatic don't have asthma at all. They were misdiagnosed on the basis of one or two attacks of wheezing (probably hay fever). They were then put on drugs. Now they can't get the drugs they're used to and will take whatever toxic drug they are given.

The evidence that doctors are now more like professional assassins than healers is mounting by the week.

If Britain's leading serial killer, Dr Harold Shipman, were still around today the Government would probably give him a knighthood in recognition of his work in the field of depopulation.

Finally, Danish research which involved the analysis of over a million infants has shown that giving corticosteroids to pregnant women to treat asthma or arthritis (or to prevent a premature birth) may increase the risk of the unborn child developing autism by 50%. There is also an increased risk of the child developing ADHD or anxiety.

Everything is rigged. We can no longer trust anyone in health care. The health care workers don't care. They do what they are told and they are overpaid for what they do. And whether you like it or not your doctor, whether he knows it or not, is trying to kill you. That's his job. That's what he is paid for.

Three things marked the end of our freedom. In England in the 1940s the Inland Revenue (as it was then known) claimed the right 'to rearrange a taxpayer's affairs in retrospect so as to ignore anything which he has done which would diminish his tax liability'. After that, the tax authorities seem to have given themselves the right to amend laws in order to give themselves more power. At the same time Parliament passed many of its powers on to administrative agencies which often exercised their authority in a high handed and arbitrary fashion. In his first six months as British Prime Minister, Kier Starmer created over two dozen new quangos. And thirdly, the universal decision to make it illegal to comment critically on any aspect of the Holocaust marked the end of freedom of speech. (In view of the laws in some countries, I would like to point out that this is not a comment on the Holocaust itself but a comment on the law governing our freedom of speech.)

Chapter Five

In the previous chapter I dealt with changes that have already taken place in medicine. In this chapter I'm going to look a little way into the future and describe some of the ways in which medical care is going to become even more alarming, intrusive and distant from the traditions of medical practice.

One of my many medical heroes is a man called Philippus Aureolus Theophrastus Bombastus von Hohenheim whose 'handle', in modern parlance, was Paracelsus. (He adopted the name because it means 'beyond Celsus', and Celsus was the Roman authority on medicine.) Herr Paracelsus was a German born Swiss physician and alchemist who spent his life attacking the medical establishment and, as a result, had to become a peripatetic critic of orthodox medicine. In the early decades of the 16th century, he wandered throughout Europe and the Middle East and believed that common sense and nature's healing power were far more effective, and safer, than the often absurd advice given by his professional colleagues. I am certain in my heart that Paracelsus would be appalled at the way modern medicine has been taken over and corrupted.

There is one area of medicine which terrifies me more than anything else: nanotechnology. And nanotechnology, one of the keystones of technocracy, should appal any thinking person. The world would be a safer, healthier place if everyone involved in promoting nanotechnology were taken outside and shot.

You will, of course, have heard of the 'internet of things' – the way that untrustworthy computer maniacs can connect your doorbell, your central heating system, your car, your fridge and everything else you own with your smart phone. (I hope you don't have one.)

'All that is bad enough but I have on my desk a mass of papers about the way nanotechnology can be used to control and tamper with the human body – including the use of nanotechnology to interfere with neural circuits in the brain. Reading these papers made me physically ill. I dislike rats and snakes but I'd rather be staring at a scurrying, slithering mass of rats and snakes than reading about this stuff.

Here is an advertisement I found which promotes a podcast.

'Can you imagine your body's cells connected to the internet? What about not only measuring your health but literally taking control of it? In this episode of Tech 2030, a 6G world podcast, the host Renuka Racha and Professor Josep Jornet from the Northeaster University talk about the Internet of Nano-Things, sensing, and how connectivity will enhance our lives at the cellular level.'

The bit that made go cold was this: 'How connectivity will enhance our lives at the cellular level.'

Note, the advert doesn't say 'How connectivity may enhance our lives at the cellular level' or 'How connectivity could enhance our lives at the cellular level' or 'How connectivity might damage our lives at the cellular level'.

It is the word 'will' which terrifies me. It's the bloodless assumption that this crap is going to make my life better which makes my blood go cold.

Another paper, in the journal 'Sensors', contains this: 'All components in the smart home environment have a nano-transceiver that allows them to be permanently linked to the internet. A tenant can easily keep track of the status of components in the home through this continuous Internet connectivity. On the other hand, in the context of an intra-body network, nano-machines are deployed inside the human body and remotely controlled at the macro-scale over the Internet by relevant experts such as medical staff or healthcare service providers.'

The authors go on to say: 'In general, in the healthcare context, medical nano-devices can be deployed inside the human body or external environment and can also be used as wearable garments.'

And they add: '…the size of the worldwide IoNT market is projected to reach USD 46.09 billion in 2028…the primary drivers of the revenue growth of the worldwide IoNT market are increased government funding for the progress of nanotechnology, the growing incidence of numerous dangerous illnesses and rising investment from the private sector.'

The aim, it seems to me, is to bio-hack our bodies and minds and turn us into slaves. That is not an exaggeration.

The use of technology will mean handing over our bodies

(including our minds) to healthcare providers (which will include governments and drug companies) and giving them authority over our very cells. And it is the arrogant certainty of these people which is so frightening. I am appalled by their utter self-belief and the absence of any possibility in their minds of the possibility that what they are doing is so far beyond evil that there is no suitable word in the English dictionary.

Researchers working in this rapidly growing area can manipulate brain cell activity, they can switch off specific brain cells (and switch them back on again). They can, in short, do whatever they like with your brain – though they are probably going to need 6G to make their crap work properly.

It was recently revealed that a South African called Elon Musk (who is, among other things, a manufacturer of electric cars) is behind a plan to connect wires into the human brain and send messages to a receiver. However, the following essay is taken from my book *Paper Doctors* which was first published in 1977 but which is now available again as a paperback. (For the record electric cars were first developed over a century ago. They were wisely abandoned.)

'Electronic stimulation of the brain depends upon the mapping out of the brain and the identification of the sites within it where various categories of thought and emotion originate. To that extent electronic stimulation of the brain involves the same basic research as psychosurgery. There, however, the similarity ends. Instead of simply destroying part of the brain as the neurosurgeon does when performing psychosurgery, the researcher experimenting with electronic stimulation limits himself to trying to control parts of the brain.

For over a century doctors have known that if wires are poked into the brain and an electric charge passed through them, there will be different responses from different parts of the brain. A wire poked into one part will cause a leg to move, the same wire poked into another part of the brain will give the patient an erection. Today we know that with the aid of electronic stimulation, doctors can induce pleasure, eradicate pain and recall memories previously lost.

In order to put electrodes into the human brain a number of procedures must first be carried out. First, special X-rays are taken, using air (injected into the spaces inside the brain) to enable the doctors to get a real view of the brain's actual shape. Eventually the researchers can tell where to put their electrodes.

Next, small holes are drilled in the skull and hair-thin electrodes are sunk into the brain to the depth the experimenting surgeon desires. The brain has no sense of pain and so the actual insertion of the electrodes into the brain is painless. When the electrodes have been put into position, the exposed ends are fitted with terminals which are fixed to the scalp. To stimulate the brain small amounts of electrical current are passed along the electrodes. Doctors have now developed their techniques to such an extent that they fit small receivers onto the scalp so that electrical impulses can be fired into the brain from afar. The receivers fit under wigs or hats and are supplied with long-lasting batteries. Eventually, no doubt, receivers will be designed which can be fitted under the scalp.

With the electrodes in position the patient can be controlled quite effectively from a distance. He can be made to eat, to sleep or to work. His appetite, heart rate, body temperature and other factors can also be controlled. The system has great possibilities for helping obese patients to slim. It has also been said that it can be used to help the blind to see. Many wired-up patients have proved to have 'pleasure centres' which can be stimulated quite easily. Researchers have noted that patients stimulated in their right places suddenly start talking about sex or acting in a sexually flirtatious manner.

One doctor has predicted that in a not too distant future patients requiring anaesthesia will be taken to the operating theatre fully conscious and put to sleep with the aid of a current sent down an electrode into the brain. Another doctor has reported that he already has epileptic patients who are fitted with electrodes and transmitters of their own. When these patients feel a fit starting they simply press a button and abort the fit.

Researchers have shown that gentle cats can be transformed into aggressive beasts if certain parts of their brains are stimulated. In the 1950s, Dr Delgado of the Yale University School of Medicine showed that two cats, normally quite friendly, could be made to fight fiercely if electrodes implanted in the brain were given impulses. Even when it continually lost its fights, the smaller of the two cats continued to be aggressive when stimulated. In one dramatic experiment, Dr Delgado wired a bull with electrodes and then planted himself in the middle of a bullring with a cape and a small radio transmitter. The bull charged but was stopped by Dr Delgado pressing a button on his transmitter. The bull screeched to a halt inches away from its target. Dr Delgado has reported that 'Animals with implanted electrodes in their brains have been made to perform a variety of responses with predictable reliability as if they were electronic toys under human control.'

Similar experiments have been performed with human beings. The patients selected had all proved dangerous and had shown that they had uncontrollable tempers. By electronic stimulation every patient was controlled. More detailed accounts of these experiments can be read in *Physical Control of the Mind* by J.M.R. Delgado. '

My book *Paper Doctors*, from which these paragraphs are taken, was published in 1977. The terrible possibilities displayed by Delgado's work were not explored and I suspect that this was because wiser heads than are available now could see the awful possibilities that lay ahead if this work became reality.

Today, the lunatics are in charge.

Drug companies love nanotechnology.

They can use it to kill you, of course. They can, however, totally control what you do and who you are. They can modulate the way you think. They could turn Donald Trump into behaving like a sweet little old lady with a penchant for butterscotch and macramé.

If you believe that you can trust all health care providers, all governments and all drug companies to do the 'right thing', and to maintain your safety and your privacy, and to defend the system against all hackers, then you may well be thrilled by the prospect of your life being taken over in this way.

Nanotechnology will change the way disease is diagnosed and treated. But it will also change the way we live. It will remove every last vestige of our freedom and it will give authorities (including the police) the power to control every aspect of our lives. If our social credit scores fall too far then we can be turned off and become 'non' people. At the moment electric companies can turn off your electricity supply via your smart meter (if you are foolish enough to have one). In future, the authorities will be able to kill us from afar with the aid of nanotechnology; they will be able to turn off our lives as easily as they can use smart meters to turn off our electricity. I can hardly begin to describe the problems and dangers which exist with having nanotechnology in our bodies and in our clothes.

Here are some quotes from research work found on the internet – together with my comments (in brackets).

'If a hacker were able to gain control over a nano-robot, for example, they could potentially use it to gather sensitive information or disrupt the function of the device.'

(No shit Sherlock. Surely the authorities wouldn't let hackers do anything so terrible. Surely they would protect us in the same way that they protect us from internet fraudsters, con artists and scammers who empty our bank accounts and steal our belongings?)

'These nano-devices are connected to the Internet and have digitalised control and monitoring processes, which pose various security and privacy concerns as the data collected by these devices may be sensitive or personal.'

(You're kidding. The information they are collecting may be sensitive or personal? Well, I never. What a shock.)

'Because IoNT devices are miniaturised by nature, detecting or preventing the tampering of these devices may be difficult, making them more vulnerable to hacking or other cyber-attacks than the IoT.'

(Gosh. I am surprised.)

'When it comes to privacy, one major privacy concern with the IoNT is the potential for nano-devices to collect and transmit sensitive personal data. For example, nano-sensors embedded in clothing or wearable devices could potentially collect data on an individual's movements, health, and behaviour.'

(But they wouldn't do that. Would they?)

'This data could be used for targeted advertising or other purposes without the individual's knowledge or consent.'

(No! Crumbs. Are you sure?)

'Another major security threat to the IoNT is the potential for malicious actors to gain access and manipulate nano-devices…a hacker could potentially gain access to a nano-robot used in medical procedures and alter its functionality by compromising the security.'

(Oh, surely no one would do that. We mustn't worry about these things.)

'Another threat is the potential for nano-devices to be used for surveillance and tracking. Because these devices are small and can be easily hidden, they could be used to monitor individuals without their knowledge or consent which could violate one's privacy.'

(You shock me.)

'In a typical healthcare system, the attacker is able to attack private data, such as the biological data gathered by either in-body or wearable sensors, disrupt medical applications in the form of denial-of-service attacks (this would lead to severe consequences as the legitimate instructions may not be able to reach the destination/vital body organs on time) and modify the communication links at the nano-communication level or the gateway to the Body Area Network, posing a serious threat to the lives of patients.'

(Well, surely that's not possible. The authorities wouldn't let that happen, would they?)

'The covid-19 global pandemic, which started in December 2019, has influenced many domains across the world, owing to the deadly nature of the virus; it has killed nearly seven million people as of the date of publication.'

(Actually, no it hasn't killed anywhere near that number of people. That figure includes all the people who failed the totally unreliable PCR covid test and were then listed as dying from covid when in fact they were run over by buses, murdered or died of heart disease. It also includes figures for several years. The real total number of deaths from covid was less than the number of people who die of the flu in a fairly ordinary year. Remember that according to WHO figures 650,000 people can die of the flu in a six month flu season. I believe that in the end, the covid vaccine will, as I predicted, kill far more people than covid itself.)

And now here are some quotes showing just some of the things that could go wrong with nanotechnology:

'The following describes disruption attacks that target the IoNT: Flooding/denial of service attack. It is possible to overwhelm the availability of potential IoNT nodes by delivering bogus messages.'

'The following depicts the disclosure attacks that target the IoNT: Eavesdropping, Jamming attack, Sybil attack (protocols are disturbed by a malicious node claiming multiple identities, Man-in-the Middle attack which grants the attacker the opportunity to exploit a potential weakness, view and listen to data and then, thereafter, replay and modify the data that is being in a covert manner.'

'The following depicts deception attacks that target the IoNT: spoofing (attackers try to become trustable by spoofing other nodes and broadcasting malicious information).

You are probably as tired of this as I am. Other methods of attack include tampering, session hijacking, cross-site scripting and cross site request forgery. I could explain what all those are but I don't think either of us really gives a damn. We just want all this stuff stopped and stopped NOW. The bottom line is that inviting nanotechnology into your home, clothing or body is akin to inviting 1,000 rats into your bedroom. No, actually it isn't. It's worse. It's far, far worse. It's akin to inviting 1,000 convicted, murdering psychopaths into your home. No it isn't. It's worse than that. I can't think of anything as dangerous or as stupid as allowing nanotechnology to come within a hundred miles of your body.

Here are some more scary quotes:

'There is currently a lack of regulation around the use of IoNT devices, which can make it difficult to ensure that the privacy of such solutions is adequately protected.'

'Existing digital healthcare solutions will face security challenges due to the inherent limitations of IoMT caused by the lack of resources for proper security in those devices.'

(IoMT, if you're interested means Internet of Medical Things. The psychos responsible for all this stuff love acronyms. IoNT is the Internet of NanoThings. IoBNT is the Internet of Biodegradable Things. IoIT is the Internet of Ingestible Things. IDGAD means I don't give a damn.)

Here's the bottom line: Using nano-technology, governments could easily kill people who had low social credit scores.

Nanotechnology is an area of medicine which reminds me of Jean Paul Sartre's comment about splitting genes. 'Of course we can split genes,' he said. 'But can we not split genes.'

And so I am led to paraphrase M. Sartre and create the thought 'Of course we can use nanotechnology to control the human body. But can we NOT use nanotechnology.'

I suspect that the people promoting nanotechnology (and I use the word in the broadest possible sense) know nothing about medicine and care nothing about patients. They are a disgrace to the human race. They should be exterminated and all their work destroyed. Dr Strangelove was a sweetie compared to these lunatics.

Nanotechnology is all about money, academic glory, prizes and honours from ever grateful conspirators whose sole aim is to kill most of us and control the ones who are left. (I do hope that these comments are offensive. They are meant to be.)

And that's not all the medical scientists have up the sleeves of their white coats. They have mRNA vaccines which are provably toxic and useless. They have digitally controlled surveillance insects, micro-organisms genetically engineered to produce whatever poisons you fancy. They are already spraying stuff in the sky to dim the sun. That is what is causing all the grey days. And all sorts of other terrifying and lethal shit. Much of this stuff is being promoted or paid for by your government and various unelected billionaires – most of whom haven't got a first aid certificate let alone a medical degree.

My advice is simple. If you have a mobile telephone (and they can be enormously useful) buy and use the oldest one that still works. Old 20th century 2G telephones still work in some countries and so do 3G phones. Do not under circumstances buy a 5G or 6G telephone or have one in your home. Try to avoid buying modern electrical equipment (it will spy on you if you do, and it will quite probably transmit your conversations to its maker). And if you have a motor car do not buy or use anything made in the 21st century. Most modern cars will spy on you and on other motorists. If you buy a new car it will tell the police if you exceed the speed limit and it will tell the police if it spots other motorists exceeding the speed limit. We now own a 1957 Bentley S1 and an elderly Mitsubishi truck. The elderly Bentley has very little electric equipment (and much of it doesn't work) and I think that the truck is just about old enough to be trustworthy. I will never again buy any electrical equipment which looks remotely modern. If we have to buy a new TV set we will look for one with a walnut cabinet and a cathode ray tube inside. And if we need a new wireless it will have valves. If we need a new car we will buy an old car.

When we abandon our humanity, our responsibility, our dignity, our self-respect, our respect for others, our inherent sense of justice and our understanding of what is right and wrong and what is decent, then we lose everything worthwhile. The medical establishment and the scientists working for the conspirators have already taken us close to the edge.

Scientists are working on an mRNA vaccine which can be used to control religious behaviour.

The cultists who believe in the pseudoscience of global warming are doing a good many strange and dangerous things in order to force us into their artificial Net Zero, their technocracy and the deadly Great Reset which they have been planning for decades.

As I have already said, geo-engineers are, for example, already spraying large quantities of tiny reflective particles into the stratosphere. The idea is to dim the sun's rays and, thereby, cool the planet. Even those who support this crazy idea recognise that it could produce a whole host of negative effects. Extreme weather effects could become more common, acid rain could increase, the earth could suddenly get much hotter if the spraying were suddenly stopped, and, of course, all those solar panels which had been erected around the world at great expense would be pretty well useless. Geo-engineers admit that no one knows what will happen in the medium or long term. It has been estimated that dimming the sun's rays could kill 500,000 people a year but this is almost certainly a massive underestimate. It is by no means impossible that dimming the sun's rays might result in wiping out the entire human population.

This untested notion is backed largely by billionaires such as Bill Gates, who is behind some of the most dangerous proposals ever promoted (including the release of genetically modified mosquitoes, the promotion of vaccines, the creation of 'fake' meat and many other daft ideas) and who has already earned himself a place on my top twenty list of the world's most evil and dangerous human beings. Gates has spent a king's ransom promoting himself as a good person and his financial links with broadcasters such as the BBC and newspapers such as the *Guardian* mean that he is guaranteed a good press. Hagiographic profiles appear regularly all around the world – mainly in publications which have financial links to Gates. (What curious coincidences these are. Gates gives money to a media outfit, or devises some financial link with a media outfit. The media outfit then runs a piece saying what a wonderful person Gates is.) Gates is a philanthropist in the same way that Harry and Meghan are shy, struggling newlyweds. Has the world ever seen such greedy, dangerous individuals as Gates, Musk, Soros, etc.? They remind me of the offspring of some terrible union of King Midas and Genghis Khan.

Please share this book with as many people as you can. Remember that, as Plato once remarked: 'The price of apathy towards public affairs is to be ruled by evil men.'

You will, I suspect, now understand why I called this book *The End of Medicine*.

Finally, thank you for reading this rather alarming book. You have now earned the right to watch a jolly film of your own choice. If you feel able to give this book a favourable review it would be much appreciated. In an attempt to stop anyone buying the book and finding out what is happening, the trolls and mindless 77th Brigade bloggers will give *The End of Medicine* one star reviews without bothering to read it.

Appendix One
Bibliography

I read hundreds of books and thousands of articles and watched a great many videos in the research, preparation and writing of this book. Below I have listed a few of the books I found most useful.

1984 by George Orwell
A Bigger Problem than Climate Change by Vernon Coleman
A Cry from the Far Middle by P.J.O'Rourke
Agenda 21 by Ron Taylor
Animal Farm by George Orwell
BBC: Brainwashing Britain by David Sedgwick
Behind the Curtain Volume 1 by John Hamer
Behind the Curtain Volume 2 by John Hamer
Behind the Green Mask: UN Agenda 21 by Rosa Koire
Betrayal of Trust by Vernon Coleman
Black water: The rise of the world's most powerful mercenary army by Jeremy Scahill
Blackwater: the rise of the world's most powerful mercenary army by Jeremy Scahill
Blind Eye to Murder by Tom Bower
Bloodless Revolution by Vernon Coleman
Brave New World by Aldous Huxley
Churchill, Hitler and the Unnecessary War by Patrick J.Buchanan
Climategate, The Marijuana Conspiracy, Project Blue Beam by the Dot Connector Library
Coleman's Laws by Vernon Coleman
Collapse – Jared Diamond
Coming Apocalypse by Vernon Coleman
Confessions of an Economic Hit Man by John Perkins
Controligarchs by Seamus Bruner
Covid-19: Exposing the Lies by Vernon Coleman
Covid-19: The Fraud Continues by Vernon Coleman
Covid-19: The Greatest Hoax in History by Vernon Coleman

Cured to Death by Arabella Melville and Colin Johnson
Dangerous Ideas by Eric Berkowitz
Degeneration by Max Nordau
Destiny of Civilisation: Finance Capitalism, Industrial Capitalism or Socialism by Michael Hudson
Dirty Medicine by Martin J Walker
Dirty Wars: The world is a battlefield by Jeremy Scahill
Downfall by Nadine Dorries
Dynastic America and those who own it by Henry H Klein
Empire of Illusion – Chris Hedges
Endgame by Vernon Coleman
Enough by Bill McKibben
Essays on Free Knowledge: The Origins of Wikipedia and the New Politics of Knowledge by Larry Sanger
Everything is Going to Get Worse by Vernon Coleman
Everything you need to know but have never been told by David Icke
Fifteen Decisive Battles of the World by Sir Edward Creasy
Fog Facts by Larry Beinhart
Fraud and misconduct in medical research by Stephen Lock and Frank Wells
Geodestinies: The Inevitable Control of Earth Resources over Nations and Individuals by Walter Youngquist
Gordon is a Moron by Vernon Coleman
Greta's Homework by Zina Cohen
Health Scandal by Vernon Coleman
Health Shock by Martin Weitz
Hidden Dangers: How governments, telecom and electric power utilities suppress the truth about the known hazards of electro-magnetic field (EMF) radiation by Captain Jerry G.Flynn
Hidden Persuaders by Vance Packard
How to stop your doctor killing you by Vernon Coleman
Human guinea pigs by M.H.Pappworth
Illuminati Agenda 21 by Dean and Jill Henderson
Invisible Rainbow by Arthur Firstenberg
Junk Politics by Benjamin DeMott
Kingmaker by Sir Graham Brady
Living in a Fascist Country by Vernon Coleman
Love among the Ruins by Evelyn Waugh

Murder by Injection by Eustace Mullins
Myths, Lies and Oil Wars by F.William Engdahl
Need your doctor be so useless by Andrew Malleson
Net Zero by Jack King
Nobody Knows Anything by Robert Moriarty
None Dare Call it Conspiracy by Gary Allen with Larry Abraham
Notes on Nationalism by George Orwell
OFPIS by Vernon Coleman
Orwell on Truth by George Orwell
Paper Doctors by Vernon Coleman
Parliament of Whores by P.J.O'Rourke
Physical methods of treatment in psychiatry by William Sargant and Eliot Slate
Politics and the English Language by George Orwell
Powershift by Alvin Toffler
Presstitutes: Embedded in the Pay of the CIA by Udo Ulfkotte
Propaganda – The public mind in the making by Edward L Bernays
Public Affairs – C.P.Snow
Research Fraud edited by David J Miller and Michel Hersen
Saviors of the Earth – Michael S Coffman
Say NO to the New World Order by Gary Allen
Science, Liberty and Peace by Aldous Huxley
Scrap the BBC by Richard D.North
Shaping the Future of the Fourth Industrial Revolution: A Guide to Building a Better World by Klaus Schwab
Social Media: Nightmare on Your Street by Vernon Coleman
Sold Out by James Richards
Stuffed! By Vernon Coleman
Technocracy: The Hard Road to World Order by Patrick M.Wood
The Art of War by Sun Tzu
The Biggest Secret by David Icke
The Collapse of Antiquity by Michael Hudson
The Coming Economic Collapse – Stephen Leeb
The Creature from Jekyll Island: A Second Look at the Federal Reserve by G.Edward Griffin
The Dark Side of Camelot – Seymour Hersh
The Death of Money by James Rickards
The Fall by Michael Wolff
The Federal Reserve Conspiracy by Eustace Mullins

The Fourth and Richest Reich by Edwin Hartrich

The Globalisation of Poverty and the New World Order by Michel Chossudovsky

The Great Covid Panic by Colin M.Barron

The Great Taking by David Rogers Webb

The Great Transformation by Karl Polanyi

The Greening by Larry Abraham

The Greening of America by Charles A.Reick

The Health Scandal by Vernon Coleman

The Hidden Enemy: The German Threazt to Post-War Peace by Heinz Pol

The Lessons of History by Will and Ariel Durant

The Limits of State Action by Wilhelm von Humboldt

The Man Versus the State by Herbert Spencer

The Medicine Men by Vernon Coleman

The New Despotism by The Rt Hon Lord Hewart of Bury

The New Despotism by John Keane

The New Germany and the Old Nazis by T.H.Tetens

The New Great Depression by James Rickards

The Octopus: Europe in the grip of organised crime by Brian Freemantle

The Party's Over by Richard Heinberg

The Passing of Parliament by G.W.Keeton

The Plot by Nadine Dorries

The Press by A.J.Liebling

The Revolt of the Masses by Jose Ortega y Gasset

The Right to Rule by Ben Riley-Smith

The Road to Serfdom by F.A.Hayek

The Rockefeller File by Gary Allen

The Secret World Government by Maj-Gen Count Cherep-Spiridovich

The Servile State by Hilaire Belloc

The Shocking History of the EU by Zina Cohen

The Social Contract by Rousseau

The Social Credit System in China by Anonymous

The Tainted Source: The Undemocratic Origins of the European Idea by John Laughland

The Trap by David Icke

The Trigger by David Icke

The Tycoons: How Andrew Carnegie, John D Rockefeller, Jay Gould and J.P.Morgan invented the American supereconomy by Charles R Morris

They want to kill us by Jack King

They want your money and your life by Vernon Coleman

The World Order by Eustace Mullins

Touching the Jaguar by John Perkins

Tower of Basel: The Shadowy History of the Secret Bank that Runs the World by Adam Lebor

Toxic Stress by Vernon Coleman

Trading with the Enemy by Charles Higham

Tragedy & Hope by Carroll Quigley

Truss at 10 by Anthony Seldon

Twilight in the Desert by Matthew Simmons

Unmasked: Inside Antifa's Radical Plan to Destroy Democracy by Andy Ngo

US-Imposed Post 9/11Muslim Holocaust and Muslim Genocide by Gideon Maxwell Polya

What Doctors Won't Tell You about Chemotherapy by Vernon Coleman

Where the Right went Wrong by Patrick J.Buchanan

Why I will never buy an electric car by Colin M.Barron

Appendix Two
The Author

Vernon Coleman qualified as a doctor and practised as a GP. He is a Sunday Times bestselling author who has written over 100 books which have been translated into 26 languages and sold in over 50 countries. His books have sold over three million copies in the UK alone, though no one is sure whether three million people each bought one book or one person has a very large bookcase. Vernon Coleman is also a qualified doctor. He and his wife (whose real name is Antoinette) live in Bilbury, Devon, England. Vernon is an accomplished bar billiards player (three times runner up in the Duck and Puddle Christmas competition), a keen but surprisingly dangerous skittles player and an accomplished maker of paper aeroplanes. He once had a certificate proving that he swam a mile for charity and this may well still be in that box in the attic that contains all those bits of old rubbish (keys that don't fit anything, broken padlocks, pens which don't work and so on) which ought to be thrown away but which have managed to hang around until the next spring clean. He was, at some point in the early 1960s, second in the Walsall Boys Golf Championship and was awarded with three brand new golf balls which were wrapped in cellophane and presented in a smart, cardboard box. He claims to be one of the best stone skimmers in North Devon. (Nine bounces are by no means unheard of and he has a personal best of 12 bounces.) He is a long-term member of the Desperate Dan Pie-Eater's Club (vegetarian section) and although he can juggle three balls at once he cannot knit. He can fly a two string kite without mixing up the strings but cannot stand on one leg without toppling over. He can ride a bicycle without holding the handlebars but cannot write a note of music or hum the simplest tune. He has never jumped out of an aeroplane (with or without a parachute) but he has, on several occasions, lit bonfires in the rain and is particularly proud of the fact that he once managed to light one in a snowstorm. He has not yet availed himself of the extensive opportunities apparently offered by social media (he says he is waiting to see if the idea catches on) but notices about important events are pinned on the noticeboard outside Peter Marshall's shop in the village and he has had a website (www.vernoncoleman.com) since the day after King Alfred burnt the cakes. Entrance to the website is free of charge and there is ample parking space. Visitors to the site are requested to wash their hands before entering and to wipe their feet before leaving. Sadly, there are no advertisements or refreshment facilities. The Author is registered as an Ancient Monument and selected parts of him are Grade II listed.

Vernon Coleman has been writing professionally since he was 18 when he wrote for a variety of magazines and newspapers including The Guardian newspaper. While at medical school he wrote three weekly columns, reviewed plays and books for the Birmingham Post and the Times Educational Supplement and ran a nightclub. His novels include: Mrs Caldicot's Cabbage War, Mrs Caldicot's Knickerbocker Glory, Mrs Caldicot's Easter Parade and Mrs Caldicot's Turkish Delight. All these books are, oddly enough, about a character called Mrs Caldicot. Other novels, which are not about Mrs Caldicot, include: Mr Henry Mulligan, The Truth Kills, Second Chance, Paris in my Springtime, It's Never Too Late, The Hotel Doctor, My Secret Years with Elvis and many others. He is also the author of three books under the pen name 'Edward Vernon'. All of these books are available as e-books on Amazon as are the 15 other volumes in 'The Young Country Doctor' series. There is a fairly full list of other books available as hard cover books, paperbacks, and eBooks on Vernon Coleman's biography page on Amazon.

Appendix Three
In December 2024 Vernon Coleman was interviewed for 'Unbekoming on Substack'.

The writer of the popular 'Unbekoming on Substack' sent Vernon Coleman 15 interview questions. Here are the questions and his answers:

You've had quite an unconventional career path – from magician's assistant to police surgeon. Which of these diverse roles has most shaped your perspective on medicine and society?

Between leaving grammar school and starting medical school I chose to spend a year as a Community Service Volunteer in a new town called Kirkby, just outside Liverpool. It was, to say the least, an eye opening experience. I suddenly found myself living and working as a catalyst in an area where the police station was barricaded and covered with razor wire and where the buses were always followed by a police car to give protection to the driver and conductor. Largely through naivety I wandered untouched like a white faced clown through the town and recruited a sizeable army of teenagers to help decorate old people's flats and do their shopping for them. The more the unions and the council protested the easier I found it to recruit kids. No one ever threatened me, bricked me or knifed me, and before I left I was made an honorary member of one of the gangs. That year changed my life. When I started medical school I opened a discotheque in the city centre because there was absolutely nothing else available at the time. We couldn't afford a glitter ball so I 'borrowed' an epidiascope and a projector from the medical school and showed coloured histology slides and old black and white films on the ceiling. The club was popular with several knife carrying gangs with whom I became good friends – mainly, I suspect, because I carried a Victorian sword stick and my blade was definitely bigger than anyone else's. Idiotically, I described the club on national radio and the Dean of the Medical School heard the broadcast. That was the end of the epidiascope and the projector (which had always been returned the following morning) but the club continued until the council closed it when it was accurately reported that there were beds around the edge of the dance floor. The beds were rescued junk and were there because I couldn't afford to buy or hire any chairs. It was all completely innocent. I was a GP Principal for ten years but I was never going to have an orthodox career. (I resigned when the NHS tried to force me to put private health information about my patients onto sick notes, something which I refused to do because I felt it was wrong). They fined me and threatened to keep fining me so I quit. I seem to have resigned a lot in my life.)

In your biographical notes, you describe yourself evolving from an 'angry young man' to 'an angry old man'. What continues to fuel this sense of righteous indignation after all these years?

I cannot abide injustice or a lack of freedom. I won't allow myself to be bullied and I don't like seeing other people bullied. When I was about 12 I remember seeing a beloved aunt and uncle cry because the local Gas Board was bullying them. I always think of my Aunt Alice when I'm fighting bureaucrats. When I became a GP I spent much of my life fighting health service administrators on behalf of my patients. I discovered quite early on that all bureaucrats are terrified of higher authority, and so when fighting some senseless rule which endangered a patient's life (and that happens more often than you'd think possible) I would point out that if my patient died as a result of their nonsense I would put their name on the death certificate as the cause of death. This never failed. I don't use death certificates as weapons any more but I'm still soaked to the bone in righteous indignation. This may well be why I am now banned by just about everyone.

Your early warnings about benzodiazepine tranquillisers led to stricter government controls. What initially drew your attention to this issue, and how did you persist with that campaign for 15 years?

I first became aware of the benzodiazepine problem in the 1960s and was writing articles about it throughout the 1970s and onwards. (I still am). The British Government changed the law in the 1980s, and the Health Secretary admitted in the Commons that they'd done it because of my campaign. I wrote a book called 'The Benzos Story' which contains some of the research material I used. Sadly, doctors ignore the law and still over-prescribe the darned things. Sadly, as I had warned, the drug companies replaced the benzodiazepines with useless and dangerous anti-depressants.

You've written over 100 books that have sold more than three million copies in the UK alone and been translated into 26 languages. Which book do you feel has had the most significant impact, and why?

This is like asking a parent to name their favourite child but I suppose the book which has had the most impact is 'Bodypower' which I wrote in 1983 and which was my first big international bestseller. It is still one of my bestselling books. It is, in a way, a very simple book which describes the self-healing properties of the human body but it has changed the way quite a lot of people think. It also influenced a number of other authors. I made several TV series based on the book though all my old programmes have been removed from YouTube. The basic principle is that if left alone the body can heal itself in many ways – and potentially dangerous drugs aren't always necessary.

Mrs Caldicot's Cabbage War was adapted into a film. What inspired that story, and how did you feel seeing your characters brought to life on screen?

When I first started writing Mrs Caldicot's Cabbage War the book was going to be something entirely different. I started to write a book about old people who rebel and rob a bank. (It's been done several times since then, but it wasn't a cliché when I started the book.) However, Mrs Caldicot took over (as I find that fictional characters often do) and the book developed along entirely different lines with Mrs Caldicot becoming a 'voice' for an oppressed group of nursing home residents. Antoinette and I bought tickets and watched the film at a large cinema, and at the end the entire audience stood up and applauded Mrs Caldicot. It was rather touching. I've since written another three novels about Mrs Caldicot and her chums and I'm terribly fond of them all. They're a feisty and fearless bunch who look after one another and stand up to officialdom. In 'Mrs

Caldicot's Easter Parade' they end up broke in Paris and earn money for food by performing old music hall songs in the street. In 'Mrs Caldicot's Turkish Delight' they inherit a broken down old pier and have all sorts of fun. As I wander further into the foothills approaching middle age my affection for Mrs Caldicot grows.

You've mentioned giving evidence to committees in both the House of Commons and the House of Lords. What were these experiences like, and did you see tangible results from your testimonies?

I gave evidence to both Houses about the pointlessness and danger of using animals in medical research. It was, I'm afraid, a complete waste of time. When I spoke to a House of Lords committee one eminent member of the committee slept through the whole of my evidence. When speaking to both Houses, I pointed out that a good many drugs which are prescribed for humans are known to cause cancer or other serious health problems when tested on animals. The drug companies say this doesn't matter because animals are different to people. On the other hand, if a drug doesn't kill an animal the drug companies say this proves the drug is safe for people. I find this illogical as well as immoral. Unfortunately, the drug companies own the medical establishment and so campaigning against animal experiments has been a struggle. I have been opposed to animal experimentation since I was a medical student (I refused to perform required experiments on animals, and persuaded one or two other students to abstain with me) and this has always made me unpopular with people who have a lot of power and money. Animal experiments enable drug companies to launch new products without testing them properly on human patients.

Your list of favourite historical figures includes quite an eclectic mix, from W.G.Grace to Che Guevera. What common thread do you see connecting these diverse personalities?

Freedom and independence. I admire people who stand up for what they believe and don't give a damn for the consequences. W.G was the best known Victorian after the Queen herself, and he didn't lead any revolutions or die in a hail of bullets but he changed his world by being himself. He could be a bit naughty but was so popular that cricket grounds put up notices saying 'Admission 6d or

1 shilling if WG plays'. Che cared and was a professional rebel. Even when he was a Minister he still worked in the docks on Saturdays.

You've been consistently critical of the relationship between the medical establishment and pharmaceutical industry since your 1975 book 'The Medicine Men'. How has this relationship evolved over the decades?

I'm not sure there is a relationship. I loathe and despise the medical establishment and the pharmaceutical industry and they hate me. Between them they've bullied, threatened, sued and tried to bribe me. They've stopped me speaking and got me fired. I don't know who it was but someone tried to kill us during the covid fraud. 'I'll rest when they bury me,' as Clarence Darrow said.

You resigned from your newspaper column over the Iraq War coverage. Could you tell us about that decision and the principles that guided it?

It was an easy decision but it was a hard decision too. I've spent most of my life writing at least one column a week (at one point I had weekly columns in four national newspapers in the UK and half a dozen other columns in newspapers and magazines) and resigning from The Sunday People was hard because I had a lot of lovely readers (and, to be blunt, they paid me a great deal of money). I wrote a column criticising the Iraq War and the editor refused to print it. That was it. I have never allowed editors to decide what I should write and I always wrote articles and columns according to what I believed in. I've always been a fan of the newspaper editor you see in cowboy films – the one who prints editorials criticising the bad guy who is tormenting the town. I miss having a column but I now try to put new material on my website every weekday (except for a two week break at Christmas). I never accept advertising or sponsors for the website (and I never allowed my videos to be monetised). My income comes from selling books which I now self-publish since, after I exposed the covid fraud at the start of 2020, most of my publishers and agents abandoned me.

Your work has often challenged conventional medical wisdom. What gives you the confidence to maintain your positions in the

face of establishment opposition?

I spent a lot of time (and money) on research. For my first book I spent more on research than I received as an advance or as royalties, even though the book did very well. My wife, Antoinette, the most compassionate and caring person I've ever met, shares my passion for truth, justice and fairness and is a brilliant and tireless researcher who can follow a complex trail with great skill and unwavering determination.

You've expressed strong views about the European Union. How has your perspective on global versus local governance been influenced by your observations in medicine?

I first became really interested in the EU in the late 1990s when I realised that national campaigns were ultimately always dependent on EU law and that there was very little point in fighting to change a law within, say, the UK unless the EU was also targeted. For example, when fighting against the use of animal experiments I found that the EU was the ultimate source of evil and legislators, administrators, drug companies, etc., would disclaim responsibility and blame the EU for every law and rule.

Your interest in Napoleon Bonaparte is well documented. What lessons do you think modern medical and political leaders could learn from his era?

It isn't widely known but when Napoleon was imprisoned on the Island of Elba and was planning to escape and return to France, the entire French army was sent to capture him. Napoleon, riding a white horse as usual, had a small faithful platoon of bodyguards with him but he rode ahead, alone and the entire French army, instead of capturing or killing him, circled round behind him as he led them to Paris. I have a copy of the leaflet his men distributed to the soldiers. It is one of the most powerful and moving documents ever published.

Your book 'The Dementia Myth' challenges common assumptions about cognitive decline. What motivated you to explore this particular topic?

When my mother fell ill with what appeared to be dementia, my wife researched her symptoms and concluded that my mother's symptoms were most likely a result of normal pressure hydrocephalus. We arranged for a total of nine neurologists to examine my mum. They were all dismissive, and even with the diagnosis handed to them on a plate they refused to accept it. When doctors finally accepted that they were wrong and that she did have normal pressure hydrocephalus, it was too late to repair the damage that had been done. The more I investigated the more I realised that many patients with alleged dementia have been misdiagnosed. There are several reasons for this. First, for some inexplicable but doubtless malign reason, doctors in the UK receive a cash bonus every time they diagnose dementia. Second, drug companies work hand in hand with charities to promote dementia in general and Alzheimer's disease in particular. I wrote 'The Dementia Myth' to draw attention to the commonest, easily cured diagnoses which are overlooked in favour of the default diagnosis of dementia.

You've been critical of medical screening programmes. Could you elaborate on why you believe they benefit doctors more than patients?

I never really saw the point of screening programmes. Having an annual medical check-up is like getting an annual bank statement. It tells you what your health is like on a particular day but it doesn't tell you what your health is going to be like in three months' time. Medical screening is a hugely profitable industry which has been shown, time and time again, to benefit no one but doctors and screening programme companies.

For readers who want to engage with your work and ideas, what's the best way to follow your current writing and activities?

Prior to February 2020 I didn't have any social media accounts. However, I was so horrified by the way the covid pandemic was promoted, that I tried to open accounts in the usual places. Even then I warned that compulsory vaccination programmes would be introduced and that, when it came, the vaccine would be dangerous. However, the censors were quickly into action. Facebook told me that I would be a danger to their community. Linkedin let me open an account and then closed it. The rest all refused to let me onto their sites. YouTube let me put up a few videos (some of which were viewed millions of times) and then expelled me for sharing too many truths. And so I am now left with the website www.vernoncoleman.com which I started in 1990. Since I am now also banned from all mainstream media, my website is the only place where my work appears. Details of new books and videos always appear on that website. Ironically, although I am banned from all social media (for the curious modern crime of telling the truth) I'm told that there are a number of fake sites using my name. When I first became aware of this I asked the platforms involved to remove the fake sites but nothing happened. So for readers who want to follow my current writing, I suggest that they visit my website which has new articles and details of campaigns posted every weekday. I am always grateful when people share the articles on my website because I am totally banned from all social media.

Appendix Four
What the papers say

(These quotes are included to balance the abuse and lies which are now littered throughout the internet.)

I've selected only quotes about me from the UK press to keep the list manageable. These were, of course, published before March 2020 when an anonymous Wikipedia editor decided, with no evidence, that I was 'discredited'.

'Marvellously succinct, refreshingly sensible.' – The Spectator

'The living terror of the British medical establishment. A doctor of science as well as a medical graduate. Dr Coleman is probably one of the most brilliant men alive today. His extensive medical knowledge renders him fearless.' – Irish Times

'His future as King of the media docs is assured.' – The Independent

'The only three things I always read before the programme are Andrew Rawnsley in the Observer, Peter Hitchens in the Mail and Dr Vernon Coleman in The People. Or, if I'm really up against it, just Vernon Coleman.' – Eddie Mair, Presenter on BBC's Radio Four

'His advice is optimistic and enthusiastic.' – British Medical Journal

'Revered guru of medicine.' – Nursing Times

'Gentle, kind and caring' – Western Daily Press

'His trademark is that he doesn't mince words. Far funnier than the usual tone of soupy piety you get from his colleagues.' – The Guardian

'Dr Coleman is one of our most enlightened, trenchant and sensitive dispensers of medical advice.' – The Observer

'Dr Coleman is more illuminating than the proverbial lady with the lamp' – Company Magazine

'Britain's leading health care campaigner.' – The Sun

'What he says is true.' – Punch

'Perhaps the best known health writer for the general public in the world today.' – The Therapist

'Vernon Coleman writes as a general practitioner who has become disquieted by the all-pervasive influence of the pharmaceutical industry in modern medicine…He describes, with a wealth of illustrations, the phenomena of modern iatrogenesis; but he is also concerned about the wider harm which can result from doctors' and patients' preoccupation with medication instead of with the prevention of disease. He demonstrates, all the more effectively because he writes in a sober, matter-of-fact style, the immense influence exercised by the drug industry on doctors' prescribing habits…He writes as a family doctor who is keenly aware of the social dimensions of medical practice. He ends his book with practical suggestions as to how medical care – in the developing countries as well as in the West – can best be freed from this unhealthy pharmaceutical predominance.' – The Times Literary Supplement

'What he says of the present is true: and it is the great merit of the book that he says it from the viewpoint of a practising general practitioner, who sees from the inside what is going on, and is appalled by the consequences to the profession, and to the public.' – Punch

'Dr Coleman writes with more sense than bias. Required reading for any Minister of Health' – Daily Express

'I hope this book becomes a bestseller among doctors, nurses and the wider public…' – Nursing Times

'Few would disagree with Dr Coleman that more should be done about prevention.' – The Lancet

'This short but very readable book has a message that is timely. Vernon Coleman's point is that much of the medical research into which money and expertise are poured is useless. At the same time, remedial conditions of mind and body which cause the most distress are largely neglected. This is true.' – Daily Telegraph

'If you believe Dr Vernon Coleman, the main beneficiaries of the hundred million pounds worth of research done in this country each year are certainly not the patients. The research benefits mostly the medical place seekers, who use their academic investigations as rungs on the promotional ladder, or drug companies with an eye for the latest market opening…The future may hold bionic superman but all a nation's physic cannot significantly change the basic mortality statistics except sometimes, to make them worse.' – The Guardian

'Dr Coleman produces mountains of evidence to justify his outrageous claims.' – Edinburgh Evening News

'Dr Coleman lays about him with an uncompromising verbal scalpel, dipped in vitriol, against all sorts of sacred medical cows.' – Exeter Express and Echo

'Vernon Coleman writes brilliant books.' – The Good Book Guide

'No thinking person can ignore him. This is why he has been for over 20 years one of the world's leading advocates on human and animal rights in relation to health. Long may it continue.' – The Ecologist

'The calmest voice of reason comes from Dr Vernon Coleman.' – The Observer

'A godsend.' – Daily Telegraph

'Dr Vernon Coleman has justifiably acquired a reputation for being controversial, iconoclastic and influential.' – General Practitioner

'Superstar.' – Independent on Sunday

'Brilliant!' – The People

'Compulsive reading.' – The Guardian

'His message is important.' – The Economist

'He's the Lone Ranger, Robin Hood and the Equalizer rolled into one.' – Glasgow Evening Times

'The man is a national treasure.' – What Doctors Don't Tell You

'Vernon Coleman is a leading medical authority.' – Woman's Own

'His book Bodypower is one of the most sensible treatises on personal survival that has ever been published.' – Yorkshire Evening Post

'One of the country's top health experts.' – Woman's Journal

'Dr Coleman is crusading for a more complete awareness of what is good and bad for our bodies. In the course of that he has made many friends and some powerful enemies.' – Western Morning News

'Brilliant.' – The People

'Dr Vernon Coleman is one of our most enlightened, trenchant and sensible dispensers of medical advice.' – The Observer

'The most influential medical writer in Britain. There can be little doubt that Vernon Coleman is the people's doctor.' – Devon Life

'The medical expert you can't ignore.' – Sunday Independent

'A literary genius.' – HSL Newsletter

'I would much rather spend an evening in his company than be trapped for five minutes in a radio commentary box with Mr Geoffrey Boycott.' – Peter Tinniswood, Punch

'Hard hitting...inimitably forthright.' – Hull Daily Mail

'Refreshingly forthright.' – Liverpool Daily Post

'Outspoken and alert.' – Sunday Express

'The man with a mission.' – Morning News

'A good read…very funny and packed with interesting and useful advice.' –The Big Issue

'Dr Coleman gains in stature with successive books' – Coventry Evening Telegraph

'Dr Coleman made me think again.' – BBC World Service

'Britain's leading medical author.' – The Star

'His advice is practical and readable.' – Northern Echo

'The layman's champion.' – Evening Herald

'All commonsense and no nonsense.' – Health Services Management

'One of Britain's leading experts.' – Slimmer Magazine

'Dr Coleman's well-coordinated book could not be more timely.' – Yorkshire Post

'Well worth reading' – Times Educational Supplement

'Dr Vernon Coleman…is not a mine of information – he is a

fountain. It pours out of him, mixed with opinions which have an attractive common sense ring about them.' – Coventry Evening Telegraph

'When the children have finished playing the games on your Sinclair or Commodore Vic 20 computer, you can turn it to more practical purposes. For what is probably Britain's first home doctor programme for computers is now available. Dr Vernon Coleman, one of the country's leading medical authors, has prepared the text for a remarkable series of six cassettes called The Home Doctor Series. Dr Coleman, author of the new book 'Bodypower'…has turned his attention to computers.' – The Times 1983

'The Medicine Men' by Dr Vernon Coleman, was the subject of a 14 minute 'commercial' on the BBC's Nationwide television programme recently. Industry doctors and general practitioners come in for a severe drubbing: two down and several more to go because the targets for Dr Coleman's pen are many, varied and, to say the least, surprising. Take the physicians who carry out clinical trials: many of those, claims the author, have sold themselves to the industry and agreed to do research for rewards of one kind or another, whether that reward be a trip abroad, a piece of equipment, a few dinners, a series of published papers or simply money.' – The Pharmaceutical Journal

'By the year 200 there will be a holocaust not caused by a plutonium plume but by greed, medical ambition and political opportunism. This is the latest vision of Vernon Coleman, an articulate and prolific medical author…this disturbing book detects diseases in the whole way we deliver health care.' – Sunday Times

'…the issues explores he explores are central to the health of the nation.' – Nursing Times

'It is not necessary to accept his conclusion to be able to savour his decidedly trenchant comments on today's medicine…a book to stimulate and to make one argue.' – British Medical Journal

'As a writer of medical bestsellers, Dr Vernon Coleman's aim is to shock us out of our complacency…it's impossible not to be impressed by some of his arguments.' – Western Daily Press

'Controversial and devastating' – Publishing News

Appendix Five
Wikipedia- the corrupt and fake encyclopaedia

There's all sorts of rubbish about me on the internet these days, some of it egregiously out of context, some of it just lies and most of it emanating from Wikipedia, Google and the other garbage distributors controlled by the conspirators. Even tradesmen look at Google and Wikipedia, recognise my name and sneer contemptuously when they see me. Bizarrely, some refuse to do essential repair work for anyone labelled 'discredited'. If governments want to remove misinformation and disinformation from the internet they should start by closing down Wikipedia which is fake and corrupt and which is used to suppress and demonise anyone daring to attempt to share the truth about left wing conspiracies.

Someone in Bangkok went through over 5,000 articles I'd written for the national press (around 10 million words altogether) to find something with which Wikipedia could berate me. All they could come up with was an article about AIDS which I wrote when I was *The Sun* doctor in the 1980s. Unfortunately for them, every word I wrote was absolutely accurate and based on medical journal papers. Everything the medical establishment said is provably wrong.

The big question is why would anyone in Bangkok bother to spend all that time reading through so many of my old newspaper cuttings?

The Wikipedia editors, some of whom are possibly linked to the CIA according to one of the site's founders, were so miffed that they couldn't find any errors that they decided to abandon facts and truth and just called me discredited and a conspiracy theorist. They added in the AIDS stuff because they wrongly thought it was a stick with which they could beat me. The really odd thing is that in the 80s I was considered an expert on AIDS. I was invited to make a keynote speech at a major conference on AIDS. And I regularly broadcast about AIDS.

But Wikipedia and Google aren't much interested in inconvenient truths.

The Wikipedia page in my name was altered after I described the coronavirus scare as a hoax in February and March 2020 and warned that compulsory vaccination would be introduced.

My books (many of them bestsellers) have sold over three million copies in the UK alone and are translated into 26 languages but the titles of my books were removed. Penguin, Pan, Corgi, Arrow and other paper-backers and dozens of major publishing houses in the UK and the USA and around the rest of the world have published my books. All were removed. All the TV programmes I'd made were removed. I was the original doctor on TV AM breakfast television but that was deleted. I was the BBC's agony uncle for two years. But that went. All the national newspaper columns I'd written were removed. The magazines I'd edited were gone. And so on and so on. The UK Government admitted it changed the law about benzodiazepine tranquillisers because of my articles. That's in Hansard but was not on Wikipedia which is truly a weapon of mass distraction and destruction.

Larry Sanger the co-founder of Wikipedia, who has since denounced the site, reckons that at least one of those involved in removing the truth from my page, and replacing facts with garbage, is linked to the CIA.

That's bad enough, but I have been approached by a Wikipedia editor offering to remove the lies and replace the truths which were removed if I hand over money. To my mind that rather suggests that Wikipedia is nothing but a protection racket. If I hand over the £500 required, another editor will simply put the garbage back. And then the protection racket will continue indefinitely.

What's the difference between this racket and the one where a restaurant owner forks over so much a week for his restaurant not to be attacked?

I regard Wikipedia as a powerful force for evil – because of its links to Google it has probably done more to suppress the truth than any other website. The site seems to specialise in demonising anyone who questions the Far Left establishment and the international drug industry. It is worth remembering that most of the people doing stuff for Wikipedia are anonymous amateurs who presumably do what they do to enjoy a sense of power and to feel important and relevant

– emotions they never enjoy in their miserable and pathetic real lives. Many entries in what is described as an encyclopaedia are written by teenagers with no qualifications, knowledge or experience.

And some editors, do what they do for 'protection' or 'bribe' money. 'Give us money and Wikipedia will say nice things about you.'

Sadly, Wikipedia is still regarded by some as a reference tool – though in my view it long ago became corrupt and entirely untrustworthy. Today the Wikipedia pages are too often written by spies and liars and read only by the naïve and simple-minded. It is worth noting that Wikipedia published a disclaimer on every page (right at the bottom in the sort of small print which tells you that your freezer warranty will expire twenty seconds after you turn on the appliance) which says (in capital letters): 'WIKIPEDIA MAKES NO GUARANTEE OF VALIDITY'.

Moreover, on the same page, Wikipedia said: 'None of the contributors, sponsors, administrators, or anyone else connected with Wikipedia in any way whatsoever can be responsible for the appearance of any inaccurate or libellous information or for your use of the information contained in or linked from these web pages.'

So, in short, Wikipedia can lie about me, destroy my life and walk away whistling. It can do the same to you too.

And Google (which has a deal with Wikipedia which means that it carries Wikipedia's garbage on its own site) can also walk away whistling.

So, there you are, dear reader. If an 18-year-old Wikipedia editor dislikes you, or picks you out at random, he can describe you as a paedophile and a serial killer and there is nothing you can do about it. Your life will be ruined but you have no recourse

If there is a more disreputable internet site than Wikipedia I have yet to find it.

(For the record, I haven't looked at 'my' Wikipedia page since 2020. I am comforted by the knowledge that everyone I respect has a terrible Wikipedia entry whereas the people I loathe seem to have wonderful entries. When I last looked, Wikipedia was so desperate to smear me that it reported that in the 1980s the Advertising Standards Authority and the old Press Council both criticised me for reporting that government agencies and medical journals had reported a link between meat and cancer. But I'd also bet good money that it doesn't mention that both are/were private, voluntary organisations without any legal authority and that I offered both a long list of scientific papers proving that I was right, but that the offer was refused. Both refused to look at the evidence. In both cases the complaints were made by the meat industry. Oh, and the ASA receives its money indirectly via advertisers. And publishers ignore the ASA's rulings and accept banned advertising. The Press Council has been defunct for well over 30 years. Wikipedia probably also reports that I received two parking tickets in the 1980s. Oh those were my wild and reckless days.)

In addition to re-editing my biography Wikipedia editors removed a Wikipedia page devoted to my bestselling series of 15 books in The Young Country Doctor series. The books, about the residents of the village of Bilbury, are set in the 1970s and have nothing to do with covid since they were mostly written a decade or two ago. Millions of people have read the books. I'm told editors also removed the Wikipedia page devoted to my series of four books about Mrs Caldicot. I think they eventually left the page devoted to the film of Mrs Caldicot's Cabbage War starring Pauline Collins, John Alderton, Peter Capaldi and company – though I understand that attempts were made to remove that. Bizarrely, a Wikipedia editor also described me as a 'conspiracy theorist' on that page.

Why would they do any of this?

None of these books had anything to do with covid-19 or covid jabs.

Was it possibly done out of spite? Or just to damage my reputation still further? Or to damage my ability to earn a living?

Who knows.

Incidentally, I'm told that my Wikipedia page was at one point edited by someone called Philip Cross.

This is what Larry Sanger (co-founder of Wikipedia) has to say about Philip Cross.

'In public discussion of Wikipedia corruption, among the topics that come up are the CIA and other government agencies editing; the 'Philip Cross' account which cannot be that of a single person; the 'Wiki-PR' company which edited Wikipedia for pay on behalf of many famous and powerful people and companies; and certain of Jimmy Wales' associates, including Tony Blair and officials in

Kazakhstan.'

And here is what Larry Sanger says in his book Essays on Free Knowledge: 'I believe Wikipedia is thoroughly corrupt – the information in it is carefully massaged through behind-the-scenes control and payoffs.'

Wikipedia has, I believe, single-handedly destroyed the credibility of the internet and degraded the word encyclopaedia.

Larry Sanger has pointed out that the search engine Google helped establish Wikipedia's 'undeserved popular perception of credibility'. Google, which Sanger reveals has 'contributed millions to Wikipedia', summarises and promotes Wikipedia material as though it were reliable and impartial. Innocent souls who give money to Wikipedia are helping to destroy the truth and sustain a dangerous sham.

Wikipedia is used to destroy the credibility of people whose work might be inconvenient for the conspirators. The brainless and undiscerning who use Wikipedia often believe they are receiving the definitive view on a subject. This is nonsense, of course. Wikipedia is inadequately researched and poorly written by amateurs, many of whom are incompetent, vindictive, ignorant, bigoted, venal and corrupt. Wikipedia is not a tool; it is, rather, a weapon for control, deceit and demonization and for spreading misinformation. Wikipedia is a danger to freedom. If Wikipedia was genuinely interested in providing honest information, the editors of every page would be publicly named and their qualifications listed. They don't do that because I suspect that the average Wikipedia editor would turn out to be 15-years-old, have an IQ of 97 and possess no qualifications whatsoever.

The anonymity offered by the internet has allowed cowardly bullies to say whatever they like, and tell whatever lies they fancy, without fear of retribution. The internet in general, and social media in particular, were designed for cowards and bullies. Many of those cowards and bullies have now become Wikipedia editors.

Here's how Wikipedia works:

After I first exposed the covid fraud in February/March 2020, I was described as 'discredited' by a solitary Wikipedia editor. There was no evidence whatsoever for this claim.

A small, local newspaper then duly described me as 'discredited' because they'd pulled the word off Wikipedia.

And a Wikipedia editor (possibly the one who had created the libel in the first place) then used the local newspaper story as evidence for the claim – putting the newspaper in its list of references.

Appendix Six

In 2024 I sent the following open letter to Dr Whitty
Open Letter to Prof Sir Chris Whitty, Chief Medical Officer,
England
From Dr Vernon Coleman

Dear Sir Chris,
So, you've admitted that you might have been wrong about covid.
How nice of you. But what a pity it took over four years for you to
reach that conclusion.

You might not have been so wrong for so long, and might not
now have to share the responsibility for so many deaths (which I'm
afraid you do), if you'd had the courage to debate the whole issue,
instead of supporting a conspiracy to suppress, censor and abuse
those of who spotted the truth way back at the beginning of 2020,
and who were struggling to share the truth with members of the
public.

As you will surely know I issued repeated challenges throughout
2020, asking you to debate the fake covid pandemic, the nonsensical
mask wearing debacle, the cruel absurdity of the lockdowns and the
wicked pseudoscience of social distancing. In February and March
2020 I warned about the semi compulsory vaccination programme
which I knew you would want to introduce. In April 2020 I sent you
a copy of my book *Coming Apocalypse* which explained in some
detail why you and governments around the world were completely
wrong. I never had an acknowledgement, of course. You will still
find the book surprisingly informative and accurate. If you and I had
debated these issues in public I could have shone a little light on
things and helped educate you and your colleagues. The errors which
were made, right from the start, were laughably inept. Your
department was guilty of scaremongering.

But you didn't want to debate, did you? Indeed, you didn't want
doctors who disagreed with you to have any voice at all. It seems to
me that you and your colleagues acted without any concern for the

truth or for freedom of speech. I wonder who was really behind the decision to forbid all debate about covid. For the record, I have given expert advice to committees in both the House of Commons and the House of Lords. But it seems that this time the decision was made not to invite truly independent, critical advice but to suppress, to ban, to censor and to demonise.

And I wonder if you know how bad the censorship and abuse was, and still is.

In March 2020 I opened a YouTube channel so that I could share my views and explain why covid wasn't anything more than the standard, annual flu. My first videos had millions of views and I made videos daily for as long as I could. I didn't monetise the videos and so they cost me much time and a little money with no financial reward. A day or so after my first video, Wikipedia altered my page on their site. They removed lists of my books, TV programmes, newspaper columns and achievements and replaced them with lies, carefully selected to do me harm. Google copied the lies and made them available to a wider audience, pretty well destroying my life. I did think about legal action but I don't think either of those internet giants take much notice of libel lawsuits and they've got rather more money than I have – especially now that my income has been cut by around 90% by their lies.

(Incidentally, you might like to know how Wikipedia works. Within hours of my first video about covid I was described by a Wikipedia editor as `discredited'. There was no reason for this. No one had described me thus. And then a small local newspaper picked up the word and ran a news story about me, describing me as `discredited'. And immediately Wikipedia used the newspaper story as the reference for their use of the word. Neat, eh? I haven't looked at Wikipedia or Google for over four years so I have no idea what new lies they've introduced.)

Then, doubtless acting under instructions, YouTube closed my channel (although everything I'd said was provably accurate) and they even told me that I couldn't look at other people's videos. In what seemed more like spite than anything else they went through their archives and removed my old television programmes from the 1980s and the 1990s. Any video which quoted me on YouTube was removed – whether it had anything to do with covid or not.

I tried to join Facebook but was told that I would be considered a `danger to their community'. I was attacked by the BBC which, promoted the vaccine and, incidentally, announced that it would not interview anyone questioning the safety and effectiveness of vaccination. (Given the evidence now confirming the toxicity of the covid-19 vaccine this was clearly a terrible error which, I believe, resulted in thousands of unnecessary deaths. Who told the BBC to do this?)

Back in 2020, I warned about the specific health problems which I knew the covid vaccine would produce. I was right. As you know the official statistics show that the death rate from covid (the rebranded flu) was no greater than the usual annual flu. (You will know that officially the flu disappeared.) Predictably, the death rate only went up after doctors started giving the toxic covid vaccine. The lockdowns, the mask wearing and the closure of many hospital departments all helped to kill people – as I predicted. The damage done to children by absurd and indefensible policies in schools and elsewhere will damage a generation.

I was banned from all social media sites though fake sites in my name were set up and no one would remove them. The abuse on social media was intense and very personal but I was never allowed to reply to any of it. Anyone who dared to interview me got into trouble; some lost their platforms, others simply lost their method of raising money.

Did you know all that was going on?

I have, by the way, been writing about this sort of thing since the early 1970s and my first book `The Medicine Men' was published in 1975.

I made videos for a platform called Brand New Tube but a brave director was told that if he didn't throw me off and silence me then his platform would be in trouble. He bravely stuck by me and shortly afterwards the platform was hacked into silence. Before that a British Army Brigade (the 77th) made life pretty miserable as part of the Government propaganda programme. I assume it was members of the 77th who were busy posting nonsense on my videos and on social media. Oh, and the Royal Society of Arts expelled me for the very modern crime of telling uncomfortable truths. Fact checkers constantly tried to find fault with what I'd said and written but although they produced a good many libellous and inaccurate reports they failed to find any inaccuracies in my reports and predictions.

Everything I've said and written about covid has been accurate (and still available via my website and in the books I've managed to publish). And my predictions and warnings have been accurate too. Nevertheless, main stream media editors refuse to print anything I've produced or to review any of my books. Quite a few of my books have been banned or suppressed and main stream media people I'd known for years won't dare talk to me. Before covid my books had been published in 26 languages by publishers around the world and serialised in hundreds of newspapers and magazines. I made numerous TV and radio series too and wrote columns for leading newspapers in a number of countries. Today, I think myself lucky when I can publish my own books. It almost seems as though editors and publishers have been told not to have anything to do with me.

In addition to the abuse online, I constantly received physical threats and deep cuts were deliberately and professionally made to the insides of the two front tyres of our car. The cuts weren't visible from outside the car and if it hadn't been for a lucky annual car service there would have been a terrible crash and my wife and I would have doubtless been killed – probably along with others.

My emails have been hacked, suppressed and edited and my website has become laughably difficult to find. I had to close down one website after it was cleverly infiltrated by an officially sponsored `bad actor' who I suspect was being paid by GCHQ though I don't expect anyone will admit that.

There's much more. But that'll do for a start. You can either assume that all of those things happened by accident, by coincidence, or you have to suspect that there has been a serious plot to suppress the truth, or anyone trying to share it.

And it's all a bit topsy turvy isn't it?

You got a knighthood for being part of a Government which even you admit may have `overstated' the risk of covid and which, more objectively, got everything wrong. And I was destroyed, both professionally and personally, for telling the truth and for trying to share the truth with as many people as possible – and for provably getting everything right. There's more than a little irony there.

If you'd like to know more about how the Government you worked for systematically silenced, suppressed, censored and abused me just please read my book *Truth Teller: The Price*.

And you might like to think about the fact that if a government silence all its critics when there is any sort of health crisis, and refuse to debate with them, then it will make mistake after mistake. And huge numbers of innocent people will continue to die unnecessarily. But then there are many who think that was the plan.

Incidentally, I have repeatedly asked to give evidence to the Government's Covid Inquiry – where you gave evidence the other day. I have, of course, been ignored though I have for decades been Britain's leading medical author (and was previously well reviewed by the media). And, as I mentioned earlier, both the House of Commons and the House of Lords have, in the past, been happy to listen to my views.

I hope you care about the fact that without debate and discussion with informed and experienced critics Governments will continue to make mistakes – even if you don't care about what happened to me.
Vernon Coleman MB ChB DSc
(www.vernoncoleman.com)

You will not be surprised to hear that I received no reply from Dr Whitty.

Appendix Seven

This is the script of a video called 'Fighting for Our Lives – We Must Unite' which was first broadcast on Brand New Tube on 22nd March 2021.

One curiosity above all others tells us for certain that covid-19 is the biggest hoax in history, a monumental fraud, a coup perpetrated by conspiracy practitioners whose aims are to win power and money over everyone, everywhere.

The curiosity is that celebrities are allowed tell us that the vaccine is safe and effective but truth-telling doctors who believe that members of the public are entitled to informed consent are suppressed, oppressed, dismissed, trivialised, lied about and demonised.

Let's be clear about one thing. The existing covid-19 vaccines do not stop people getting covid-19 and they do not stop them spreading it.

And yet politicians and government-hired hacks and the media suggest that it does. It's what scores of media doctors suggest.

But they are all lying. And they can't sue me because I'm telling the truth. Even the World Health Organisation, and top government scientists in unguarded and honest moments, have admitted that the covid injection does not stop you getting covid-19 or passing it on.

All the vaccines can do is reduce the severity of the symptoms if you do get covid-19. That's all. I repeat: anyone who says anything else is a liar. I don't care who they are. They're lying.

And all these people are either lying because they are damnably ignorant, and prepared to say whatever they are told to say, or they are lying because they've been bought.

The politicians and thousands of media doctors also insist that the vaccines are safe. That's another lie. A huge and dangerous lie. The covid-19 vaccines are safe in the way that jumping out of an aeroplane without a parachute is safe.

Right from the beginning, right from February and March 2020 when I first started writing about the coronavirus hoax, and predicted that mandatory vaccination would be introduced, discussion and debate have been silenced as the mass of people are steadily pushed into compliance by the enemies of freedom. The aim is regular, forced vaccinations – several times a year, probably one every month or two. A new vaccine for each new variant.

Meanwhile, the media won't carry interviews with doctors who insist that covid-19 isn't the plague. The TV and radio stations won't carry interviews with doctors who know that the governments and their advisors are lying. Mathematicians, singers, actors and members of the royal family can share their views. But not independent, free-thinking doctors.

There is no doubt today that covid-19 is the greatest hoax in history. I don't mean that the infection is a hoax – I believe it's as real as the flu it has replaced. The flu can kill up to 650,000 a year worldwide in a six month flu season but the flu has now disappeared – what a strange coincidence! As I've been saying for a year, I believe covid-19 is the annual seasonal flu rebranded. Again, the flu can kill up to 650,000 a year worldwide in a flu season.

The hoax lies in the deceit and lies and misrepresentations that have marked this obscene exercise in fear and that have characterised covid-19 since March 2020 when the UK Government was officially advised by its own advisors, that covid-19 was no more deadly than the flu. (The link to that is on my website if you doubt me.)

Around the world, acting like puppets, politicians and advisors built absurd predictions to terrify populations everywhere. They introduced pointless and destructive social distancing.

They introduced lockdowns and closed hospital departments knowing that this would turn cancer and heart patients into second class citizens and kill far more people than the coronavirus. Elderly people in care homes were ruthlessly, mercilessly murdered in their thousands.

Politicians corrupted the media with promises of bottomless advertising budgets. The BBC's pseudo-journalists dutifully suppressed the truth. The politicians introduced and manipulated a testing system which they knew would result in more false positives than real positives and provide an excuse for more lockdowns.

And throughout it all they lied about the science – picking and choosing the bits of evidence they found most useful. The WHO said lockdowns were bad but governments went ahead anyway. The WHO said PCR tests were potentially misleading but governments ignored that inconvenient truth. When the WHO ignored the evidence that masks do more harm than good, and recommended that they be worn, politicians decided people should wear masks at work, in shops and when travelling. The masks will result in thousands of deaths from bacterial pneumonia.

They have terrified millions with a claim that covid-19 can be spread by people who have no signs and symptoms of infection. They needed to ramp up the fear to sell their dangerous and experimental vaccine – and so they changed their minds and warned us that even people with no symptoms could spread it, though no one explained how you can spread a disease if you don't have the symptoms which spread it. Research in China, which involved just under 10 million people and was conducted by 19 scientists, found that asymptomatic spread of covid does not occur.

And throughout it all, politicians and advisors have refused to debate and they have suppressed the truth.

When I originally described the coronavirus scare as a hoax, I toyed with a different word – fraud. And that's the word I should have used because that's what this is. It's all about power and money, a huge money-making fraud which involves the destruction of economies everywhere. Political leaders and their scientific advisors are going to go to prison which is where they belong.

And the media is playing a huge part in the fraud: this has become a propaganda war. Governments everywhere have employed specialist psychologists and used sophisticated brain washing techniques. I've explained these in previous videos.

At the beginning of March 2021, a note from a Sky journalist called Sanya Burgess was passed to me. Ms Burgess told me that she was working on an article and TV package looking at the sale of books which are 'anti-vaccine and spread medical misinformation, including spreading unfounded conspiracies and the coronavirus pandemic. In my piece, I will be mentioning two of your works which I will be reporting fall under those categories.' She then mentioned my book on vaccination and my book *Coming Apocalypse* about the early days of the coronavirus in 2020.

In the old days a good journalist would start an investigation with an open mind, perhaps wanting to look at why such books are so popular, – but when you begin your research with the words 'medical misinformation' and 'unfounded conspiracies' it suggests to me that you may have already made up your mind about the way the story will go. Ms Burgess's note seemed to me to betray her purpose, her prejudice and her allegiance to government propaganda.

I'd been waiting for the authorities to target books.

They've excluded the truth from the mainstream media. They've banned public demonstrations. They've more or less taken control of most of the internet. Books were the only thing left – even though at least two of my books had been banned by more than one publishing platform, and mainstream publishers shy away from publishing anything not approved by the Government.

Ms Burgess said that she would be happy to share with me the views of the health professionals and politicians she would be talking to – though she didn't do that.

You will not be surprised to hear that I am a trifle wary of the mainstream media. Too many journalists are merely taking part in a propaganda war on the truth. I wrote columns for national newspapers for over 30 years and presented TV and radio programmes for national and regional networks and I am appalled at the way journalism has become little more than a branch of the Government's public relations programme.

But, sceptical though I was, I thought it would be worth putting a few thoughts into Ms Burgess's mind.

I pointed out that everything I have written can be backed with research and that she was starting with a misconception. I pointed out that I am not anti-vaccine but that I have merely investigated vaccines and published truths. I explained that I have never written or published any medical mis-information and told her that if she said I had then I would sue her. I pointed out that the UK Government has changed official policy because of my articles and books and that I have been right on a number of important issues – including benzodiazepine tranquillisers, mobile phones and AIDS. Indeed, I explained that since my first book in 1975, about the relationship between the drug industry and the medical establishment, my aim has always been to counter medical misinformation. I added that my work had been widely referenced and well-reviewed before the climate of truth suppression and demonization became prevalent early in 2020.

I explained to her that I have for a year been challenging government advisors to debate with me live on TV but that the offer has never been accepted. I pointed out that neither the BBC nor Sky TV would set up any such debate because they know that I am right and can defend my position successfully. I asked if she knew that covid-19 was downgraded to flu level in March 2020 (again, there's a link on my website to this), that according to the CDC in the US, the number of deaths and serious side effects with the covid-19 vaccine is between 2.5% and 3.00%. I told her that a number of important papers in eminent journals don't seem to have been reported in the press, that the NHS does not follow WHO guidelines on the PCR test, that anyone dying within 60 or 28 days of a positive PCR test – whether false or not – has been officially listed as a covid-19 death. I told her leading UK agencies have received huge sums from the Gates foundation – which has big drug company links. I told her that the UK's chief scientific officer is a former drug company executive who still had a big holding of drug company shares the last time I looked. I told her that mask wearing has been proved to cause hypoxia, bacterial pneumonia and other problems. I reminded her that the WHO says that covid-19 vaccines don't stop people getting the disease or passing it on. I pointed out that anyone who dares to question government policy is described as a conspiracy theorist and I finished by pointing out that this was not just a question of free speech but a question of informed consent.

Ms Burgess told me that my comments would be well represented in her coverage, that she would say that my work is backed by research and that I believe that the issue of informed consent is vital.

'I will also report,' she promised, 'that you feel strongly that the truth has been deliberately suppressed for political reasons.'

She did that, and I'm grateful. As far as I know that's not something anyone at the BBC has ever done.

Now let's look at the article that Sanya Burgess wrote.

She began by saying that anti-vaccination books are being sold on Amazon amid calls that there be warnings on items to combat the spread of misinformation. She didn't say who, other than perhaps SKY, had called for warnings to be placed on my book.

She then quoted a shadow health minister called Alex Norris who apparently said 'it is very sad to see these things so freely available'. He apparently went on to say 'This is anti-vax content. Much of it has been very strongly rebuffed and debunked.'

Naturally, he didn't bother to identify anything which has been rebuffed or debunked. He didn't because he couldn't.

In the past, when I was allowed to debate vaccination on TV or on the radio I always won the debates – and that, I suspect, is the reason no one wants to debate now. If Whitty or Vallance lost a debate with me – which I believe they would – then the whole charade would collapse and the Government's propaganda programme would collapse in minutes.

I didn't see the segment on SKY television but I gather that the reporter didn't ask Norris if he had bothered to read my book before criticising it.

So who is Norris and why does he feel able to pontificate on the subject? Is he now an advocate of book burning?

Well, he is a former trade union organiser who has spoken on the design of football stadia.

You might have thought that a journalist would want to speak to someone with knowledge of a subject before interviewing them. And you'd have thought that Norris might have liked to limit himself to sharing opinions on subjects about which he has some real in-depth expertise. And you might have thought that a journalist would be reluctant to allow a politician to share such nonsense.

For a real journalist, the story was 'Why are politicians and advisers determined to suppress the truth?' or 'Why are government advisors frightened to debate with critics?' or even 'What's the truth about covid-19 and the covid-19 vaccines?'

But it seems to me there aren't any real journalists in the mainstream media today. And there certainly aren't any editors with the balls to take on the establishment.

The fact is that the pro-vaxxers don't bother too much about reading the books they criticise. They're not interested in truths or science: simply in the propaganda. The trolls, some of them hired by the Government, others showing strange allegiance to some of the world's most corrupt drug companies, much prefer to suppress the truth – rather than to raise specific issues or accept a challenge to debate.

After the Sky piece appeared, ill-informed, bigoted pro-vaxxers queued up to put one star reviews on my book which told the truth about vaccines – even though they had not bought it or read it. The pro-vaxxers share this skill of being able to comment on things about which they know absolutely nothing. So many of them were doing this that one platform had to block comments which had been put on their site by people who were so prejudiced that they felt able to write a review without even looking at the book or examining the contents.

The establishment isn't interested in the truth. The policy is simple: suppress, demonise and lie. Doctors who tell the truth in our totalitarian society are shunned or attacked. It's not surprising that too few medical doctors dare to speak out.

In the old days, journalists would check, double check and then check again. In the 1970s I remember being interviewed by an American magazine called the *National Enquirer*. I received two separate phone calls from editors who wanted to make sure that their story was entirely accurate. It comes to something when there isn't a publication or broadcaster in the UK which comes anywhere near the standards of the *National Enquirer*.

Today, the media is all lies, libels and demonization. As Richie Allen said on his website richieallen.co.uk, 'a national news channel is promoting book burning and dressing it up as news. It's seeking to discredit medical experts by throwing around terms like misinformation and disputed claims, without referencing a single paragraph from the books in question. Sky is banking on its viewers being too lazy to ask for the evidence or to know the difference between news reporting and news manufacturing.'

Since mental health honesty is currently fashionable these days, I confess I am getting a trifle tired of all the abuse. Even though I feel strongly about what is happening I confess that I do regret sticking my head above the parapet over a year ago. The critics know nothing about me, what I've done, what I do, the research I do or what my motives are. They are as ruthless, as cruel, and as remorseless as they are ignorant and prejudiced. But they have cold-bloodedly destroyed my reputation just because they disagree with my sharing the truth.

I'd like to spend my days relaxing a little, writing some gentle books, growing vegetables and looking after my lady. Instead I'm still working long, long days fighting a war that most people don't seem to give a damn about. And it gets a bit wearing when the only reward is abuse, humiliation, lies, libels and demonization from blinded, largely anonymous, book burning zealots.

To be blunt I'm beginning to wonder why the hell I bother. I'm too old to give a damn about the future of the world a decade or two ahead. But I bother because I care about humanity. I guess I care too much. I have risked my reputation and finances from making these videos – none of which has earned me any money whatsoever. No monetisation, no adverts, no sponsors.

I'm sorry if I sound a little weary. But that's probably because I am a little weary; tired of being used as a punch-bag by every truth hating, cowardly, bigoted, fascist pro-vaxxer who thinks it is acceptable to ignore the science and demonise someone who is simply trying to help share the truth and oppose the enemies of freedom, democracy and humanity. And indeed tired of being abused by some who claim to be on our side but whose narrow-minded bigotry blinds them to the big picture and what we have to do to win this war. I am trying to reach the unconverted so, for example, I must occasionally use the word vaccine – if I don't then most people won't know what I am talking about. I do get offended when critics patronise me and assume they know about the science of this fraud more than I do.

I've been studying drugs and vaccines for over half a century. I'm afraid it's the trolls as much as the BBC, Sky TV and the rest of the media who will lose the war for us and who will be responsible if we lose what remains of our freedom, our democracy and our humanity.

And the major threat doesn't come from the mainstream media.

The major threat comes from the people who appear to be on our side. And this has always been the case. If we lose this war it will, I fear, be because of the back biting, the sniping and the nit picking coming from people who still don't understand how serious this war really is. This isn't an academic exercise.

During my 50 year war with drug companies I've had papers stolen from my office and I've been threatened. Editors have been urged to fire me. I've had injunctions and lawsuits. And I've learned that controlled opposition is a speciality of the drug companies.

Look at what happened recently when a Dr Bossche popped up and published a serious warning about the experimental covid-19 vaccines currently being promoted with such mis-placed enthusiasm.

I made a video in which I included a section discussing Bossche's statements. I made it clear that I knew he had worked for Bill and Melinda Gates, GAVI and GSK (the same drug company which employed Vallance, Britain's Chief Scientific Officer) but that I had, after some thought, concluded that what he had to say could be used to strengthen our position – and should, indeed, be shared as widely as possible as a weapon in the fight against vaccines.

Bossche's intervention was a God-send and could not possibly be ignored. I didn't and don't care what his motives were. His article gave us a valuable new weapon to use in our fight against lockdowns, vaccines and all the rest of the nonsense which the conspiracy practitioners are using to force us into the new normal, the Great Reset and the horrors of Agenda 21. I thought, and think, that Bossche's history gives him credibility. I don't want to have dinner with him or be his friend – his history is too vaccine orientated – but I'll use what he has to say if I can weaponise it.

And I don't think the elite realised the full danger with the experimental vaccines they are promoting. Why? Simple. They and their families will not be immune to the danger of the new deadly variants. Gates, Blair, Schwab, Prince Charles and company will all now be at risk. I don't think they saw that coming.

Critics have said that we shouldn't use anything Bossche said because of his past. That's naïve and rather stupid. Would we really not take advantage of it if Bill Gates suddenly announced that vaccines were killing people and should be stopped? Would we care what his motives might be? Mike Yeadon worked at Pfizer but his contribution, especially on the PCR test, has been invaluable.

You don't turn down a new supply of secret ammunition.

I have pointed out many times that this fight isn't an academic exercise – it's a war. Everything that is happening is heading towards genocide – the deaths of billions. Anyone who isn't for us is, by default, for Agenda 21, fascism, communitarianism and a world devoid of life, humanity, democracy, freedom and God; a world full of censorship, oppression and brutality.

As I have pointed out since the start, normal mutations or variants usually become less deadly with time. But Bossche pointed out that the vaccine induced variants will be more dangerous and will spread.

Governments and the media will use the new vaccine induced variants, and the deaths which will ensue from the pathogenic priming as well as the other problems created by the vaccines, as an excuse for more lockdowns and more vaccines. Everything that is happening is being driven by the commercial, political and ideological motives of a bunch of evil people.

Another thing I've pointed out since the start is that natural immunity is the best sort of immunity. That has always been a classic medical belief. Natural immunity provides broad protection against variants. The experimental vaccines being used make it harder for the body to deal with variants. Anyone who denies that vaccines have already killed huge numbers of people has their head stuffed firmly in the other end of their anatomy. Look at my website and see the long list of people who have been injured or killed by these experimental injections.

But today the WHO and various government agencies have turned science on its head and argue that synthetic immunity, produced by vaccines, is superior. This is nonsense, of course. But it suits the motives of the elite trying to take over the world and orchestrate the Great Reset.

Too many people still fail to realise that the masks, the lockdowns and the vaccines are merely part of the programme of death and compliance and control designed to lead the world into the Great Reset, the new normal and Agenda 21. There is no little irony in the fact that our enemies – and that's what they are – call us conspiracy theorists when they themselves are conspiracy practitioners. They have succeeded with a coup which has removed our freedom and our democracy.

The BBC and Sky and other mainstream media groups work hard to suppress the truth and oppress the truth-tellers. Trying to counter their lies wastes a good deal of time and energy – though that's probably the plan.

NOTE
This was the script of a video first broadcast on Brand New Tube on March 22nd 2021.

Appendix Eight
Just a Little Prick – The Bill Gates Story (Part One)

(This is the script of a video which first appeared (very briefly) on You Tube on July 3rd 2020. Part Two, which appears below, had to be recorded separately because our old iPad, which we were using to record all our videos, would only record videos of a limited length.)

Bill Gates is often described as a philanthropist.

Interviewers generally seem to treat him as a cross between a saint and a prophet. In a way this isn't difficult to explain. After all, the Bill and Melinda Gates Foundation is a partner with many media companies, tossing money around with remarkable generosity. In the UK the BBC and *The Guardian* are just two of the recipients of Gates largesse.

It would, of course, have been possible for Gates to have used his vast wealth to change poor countries in a very straightforward and positive way by, for example, using his billions to help with road building programmes or to help poor farmers to improve their land and their farms by digging wells. Using $10 billion to set up water supplies would have doubtless saved many lives in a simple, honest way. But you can't control the world quite as easily simply by doing practical, honest things which save lives. And Gates seems to me keen to take control of every aspect of our lives. To me he seems to be a strange hybrid of those mad fictional characters Dr Strangelove and Ernst Stavro Blofeld – the James Bond baddie.

I'm afraid I don't believe any of Gates' projects have anything much to do with philanthropy. There is too much intermixing of donations and business. What do the Gates family really want? I cannot help thinking it's more about power and unspoken plans.

Gates got rich through the Microsoft software company, allegedly because his mum knew the chairman of IBM and got Gates his big break. There are accusations that Gates stole some of the ideas for his business. Personally, I feel that Gates has made himself obscenely rich by making the world a far more stressful and annoying place than it was before Microsoft appeared. In my experience, there were other much easier to use word processing programmes but Gates steamrollered the opposition out of the way with ruthless efficiency. Gates original partner, Paul Allen, claimed that Gates tried to screw him and charged his partner, with mercenary opportunism. Before Gates arrived on the scene people who wrote software often gave it away free. Gates took over the world of personal computing, acquired a monopoly position and took full advantage of it to make himself very rich. Additionally, there have for some time been doubts in my mind about how close Microsoft is to the National Security Agency in the USA.

The Microsoft billionaire seems to have learned his hometown boy act from veteran investor Warren Buffett who didn't get to be rich by being a hometown boy but has a good line in simple charm. Gates has described himself as a health expert. He frequently offers advice and predictions about health matters though personally I'd have thought his only area of expertise with viruses involved those usually found in computers. He has stated that the world will not return to normal after the coronavirus until all or most of the world's population has been vaccinated. Because he has a lot of money, and tends to distribute it widely, politicians and bureaucrats and scientists listen to his advice and accept what he tells them – parroting his line about vaccination with great loyalty.

It would, I think, normally be unusual for a bloke with no formal medical training to give health advice to the world but Gates has managed to buy himself a seat at the table by giving huge sums of money to organisations such as the United Nations and the World Health Organisation – in my own view now two of the most evil organisations in the world. The Bill and Melinda Gates Foundation is said to be the second largest contributor to the WHO and If the United States really does stop its donations then Gates will be the biggest contributor. That sort of money buys a lot of access and, I think, an unhealthy amount of influence – especially when you also spend a good deal of money on publicity designed to show the world what a good egg you are. Gates is also linked to the World Economic Forum, which reckons that the coronavirus is a great excuse to change the world and which has a plan called The Great Reset which, like most of these plans which have emerged since the coronavirus, seems to me to have been prepared some time before the arrival of covid-19.

Gates, of course, also gives a good deal of money to Imperial College in London – the place where Neil Ferguson works. It was, of course, Ferguson whose rubbishy forecasts about the coronavirus resulted in the lockdowns, the social distancing, the ruin of the British and American economies, untold deaths in care homes and so on. Gates has also funded work done by Dr Chris Whitty, the UK's current Chief Medical Officer. And the Gates Foundation has even given money to Public Health England – a UK Government organisation, sponsored by the Department of Health, which allegedly exists to protect and improve the nation's health. Public Health England appears to be desperately keen on vaccinations which is a big surprise, of course. One of their documents carries the slogan Keep Calm and Carry on Vaccinating – which seems a little cheesy to say the least.

Before I go any further it is important to point out, and bear in mind, that Gates believes the planet is overpopulated. He thinks this is a real problem. Is it still a secret passion? Who knows? Interviewers, who often seem to come from organisations with financial links to the Bill and Melinda Gates Foundation rarely ask searching question about difficult issues.

The Bill and Melinda Gates Foundation is an odd organisation in that as well as having philanthropic aims it also invests in a good many companies designed to make a profit. Indeed, the Foundation seems to be doing very well and seems to me to operate as much like a family investment trust as a charity.

The Gates Foundation has a mass of interlinked projects and commercial holdings. And it seems to an outsider as though he is more interested in controlling the world than in helping people.

Here are just a few of the things Gates is currently doing with his money.

First, of course, there are the vaccines. I have already dealt with some of the controversies associated with the Gates's obsession with vaccines in previous videos.

Gates seems obsessed with vaccines and now seems to favour ones using very new technology. He is terrifyingly keen on giving his experimental vaccine to billions of people – ideally to the whole population of the planet. It doesn't seem to occur to him that even relatively safe vaccines have been known to cause many thousands of deaths, might enhance susceptibility to disease or indeed cause and spread infections. If it has occurred to him it doesn't seem to be something that worries him unduly.

On the surface Gates seems to see vaccination as the answer to most of the planet's health problems and sees them only doing good and incapable of doing very much harm. 'We're not going to return to normal until most people have been vaccinated,' he has said, after warning that the coronavirus would otherwise result in millions of deaths. 'You will never be free until we have a vaccine,' seems to be the mantra. Naturally, the politicians and the scientists agree with the man with the money even though experts seem to agree that a vaccine may never be found. If no vaccine is found then much of the world will remain in a state of terror and social distancing and masks and occasional lockdowns will become a normal part of life. Is that what Gates wants? The politicians and the big business people with a yearning for control will be delighted.

Moreover, Gates seems to have decided that we won't have a vaccine for 18 months – and, naturally, the world's politicians and scientists (many of whom are on the Gates payroll) agree with the world's least qualified but most powerful 'doctor'. So it seems that the artificial lockdowns and the unnecessary social distancing and masks will remain in place.

Incidentally, I usually avoid the words vaccine and vaccination because they tend to result in censorship. On this occasion, however, it seems impossible to do so.

Since Gates is convinced that the planet is overpopulated it seems odd that he would be keen on vaccinating huge swathes of Africa. You might think that vaccinating children would mean that there would be fewer deaths and that the population would go up. But Gates argues that if you vaccinate children and they don't die then mothers will have fewer babies and instead of having eight babies in the hope that two will live they will just have three, believing that the vaccines will keep them alive. I am not at all sure how this means that vaccination will result in a fall in the population but Gates says it will and the politicians and the scientists and the journalists all nod wisely, pat their wallets and agree with him. I haven't been able to find any real, solid evidence for this claim, which seems to me to be a combination of the bizarre, and the unbelievable, laced with wishful thinking, apart from the evidence from Gates himself. I don't like to point this out but religion seems to play a part in the number of children a woman has. In the UK, for example, the figures show that Muslims tend to have an average of three children per family whereas Christians usually have only two.

There are, of course, those who are concerned that Gates's mass vaccination programme is part of his plan to reduce the world's population to 500 million or so – a figure that many who are keen on population control regard as acceptable. Personally I cannot see the difference between an untested vaccine, used globally, and genocide. But then I'm perhaps a little old-fashioned in liking to see drugs and vaccines properly tested before being rolled out to large populations.

And although interviewers rarely seem to mention it there are some very worrying stories circulating about some of the vaccination programmes promoted by Gates and/or the WHO. These are not, however, worries that get aired in those parts of the media supported by grants and partnerships from the Gates Foundation. I allow absolutely no advertising or sponsorship on my videos or website. But great chunks of the media, popular and specialist, seem to enjoy close, financial links with the Bill and Melinda Gates Foundation and it is important to remember this. I have no doubt that many websites are also given money or support by the Foundation.

I will deal with Bill Gates' obsession with vaccines in the second part of this two part series entitled Just a Little Prick.

But there are many other topics which must first be mentioned.

First, the Bill and Melinda Gates Foundation has invested in a company called Monsanto.

I have always regarded Monsanto as the most evil company on the planet and I've thought of it this way for several reasons.

First, Monsanto has long been a leader in the development of genetically modified plants. These terrify me because as far as I have been able to find out they have never been properly tested to see what long term consequences there might be. What damage could there be to crops in a few years time? Could they become more susceptible to disease? And are there any risks to the people who eat genetically modified food? For some years now, Monsanto has taken to patenting its seeds and as a result small farmers who have traditionally grown their crops from their own seeds have found that they have been unable to do so. There are said to have been many thousands of suicides as a result of this – as farmers found that they weren't allowed to grow the seed they had saved from their own crops but had to buy seed they couldn't afford to buy. I have reported on this many times in the past.

And, of course, Monsanto is the manufacturer of Roundup – a doubtless effective but equally doubtless nasty weed killer. Unfortunately, there have been a number of claims that Roundup causes cancer and there were 125,000 lawsuits as a result. The German company Bayer bought Monsanto a little while ago. Bayer is alleged to have paid $63 billion for Monsanto and to have paid $10.9 billion to settle the claims relating to Roundup.

Bayer, now the new owner of Monsanto, has an interesting history which is worth a short detour while we're here. Think of this as our equivalent of a side trip to Barnard Castle.

In 1925, a group of important German companies, which included Bayer, formed a cartel called IG Farben. Their aim was to obtain control of global markets in key industrial sectors – specifically: chemicals, pharmaceuticals and petrochemicals. History shows quite clearly that it was the formation of this cartel, and the creation of IG Farben, which led directly to the Second World War (and all its associated atrocities) and ultimately the European Union. IG Farben's need for cheap labour was so great that the company built a huge factory at Auschwitz where there was a large reservoir of slave labour. Bayer, the company's pharmaceutical division tested its drugs on prisoners. IG Farben also made huge amounts of money by providing the gas for the killing of prisoners in concentration camps throughout Germany.

At the end of the Second World War IG Farben was broken up into four new companies, one of which was Bayer, and all of Farben's assets (including the profits from manufacturing the gas used in the infamous gas chambers) were transferred to the new companies – all of which were managed and run by the people who had run IG Farben.

So, the bottom line was that although IG Farben had been run by war criminals no one was really punished and things carried on much as they had done during the war. The only thing that changed was that a good deal of company notepaper had to be redesigned and freshly printed.

The new companies denied any responsibilities for the actions of IG Farben on the basis that they were new and had not existed during the war. This disgraceful self-serving legal move was accepted without a murmur of protest. Bayer, which had been a part of IG Farben, had used concentration camp victims for its experiments and for testing new drugs but the company was allowed to keep all the profits from these experiments.

By the mid-1960s Bayer had become ever richer and more powerful.

And there seemed to be no shame about the past. Bayer actually set up a foundation to honour a Nazi called Fritz ter Meer on his 80th birthday and started the foundation off with a donation of two million deutschmarks. (It was not until 20 years later that Bayer changed the name of the foundation.) It did not seem to bother anyone that Herr ter Meer had overseen the building of IG Auschwitz and had been found guilty of war crimes (including genocide) and sentenced to just seven years imprisonment in 1948. Naturally, he did not serve the full sentence. Fritz ter Meer, one of the most evil Nazis, was released in 1950 and immediately re-joined the board of Bayer.

That's the end of the detour.

Will Bayer be making a coronavirus vaccine or treatment? Who knows. Would you want it if they did?

The bottom line is that I cannot imagine why anyone who really cares for people and the planet would put any money into Monsanto or Bayer.

Many investors try to avoid what they think of as 'dirty' companies who do or have done bad things to people or the environment but this doesn't seem to bother Gates.

Oddly enough I haven't been able to find any evidence that interviewers from *The Guardian* or the BBC have asked Gates whether he is comfortable with his investment in a company widely regarded as rather worse than wicked. Have I mentioned, by the way, that both the BBC and *The Guardian* are partners with the Bill and Melinda Gates Foundation – by that I mean that they have received money from the Foundation. That is, of course, the sanctimonious *Guardian* newspaper which was founded with the aid of money from slavery.

Next, Gates has been funding scientists at Harvard who are trying to block out the sun's rays in an attempt to stop global warming.

If you haven't heard of this before just stop and think for a moment.

The scientists want to spray millions of tons of dust into the stratosphere to stop the sun's rays reaching the earth.

One plan is that every day more than 800 large aircraft would lift millions of tons of chalk dust to a height of 12 miles above the Earth and then sprinkle the dust to stop the sun's rays getting through. Another plan is to send up hot air balloons to release powder into the atmosphere.

There are, you won't be surprised to hear, a couple of problems with this.

Obviously, the first is that no one has yet proved that global warming is taking place and is anything more than a natural phenomenon. Moreover, there are a lot of scientists who believe that we are heading into a phase where the planet is actually cooling. Is it really a coincidence that the Americans and the Chinese are busy building ice breakers? Would they do that if they thought the ice was all melting because the earth was getting hotter?

And there are those who think that the Gates money and the scientists throwing powder into the sky could help create droughts, hurricanes and mass deaths. It seems fairly well agreed that altering the atmosphere to cool the planet could have unpredictable effects. In 1815 a volcanic eruption created crop shortages and disease outbreaks.

Some might say, of course, that all this could be considered a bonus by a man who wants to reduce the world population.

No one seems to have told him, by the way, that 800 large aircraft taking off every day and flying to 12 miles up, would require a good deal of aviation fuel. And what sort of dust are they planning to have sprayed? Well, some say calcium. But I have also heard talk that barium, alumina and strontium might be used. Whatever it is won't improve the quality of the air we breathe. Bottom line is that this seems to me to be a way to reduce the world's population rather than protect it – all in the guise of dealing with the climate change hoax.

Next, Gates is funding scientists at a company called Oxitec who are genetically modifying mosquitoes. This project has received authority in the US and the genetically modified mosquitoes will be released in 2022. What could go wrong? I have no idea. I don't think anyone else does either. But I can think of a number of good reasons why this is breathtakingly dangerous. There is even talk of research into mosquito delivered vaccines.

Gates is also helping to pay for researchers who are making breast milk from cultured mammary cells. This seems to me to be the ultimate in hubris. Why does Gates always wants to interfere with nature? The female body produces the perfect breast milk. There is no need for substitutes. I remember that when attempts were made to introduce powdered milk into developing countries it was a disaster. Women were told to stop natural breast feeding and to follow the example set by Western women – and to use artificial milk. One problem was that the water used to rehydrate the milk was often badly polluted. And many babies died. If Gates wants to help women and babies he would surely do better to encourage natural breast feeding.

You will by now see a pattern developing. Gates seems to me to be a mad scientist manqué. He seems to have massive faith in the idea that scientists can solve everything by interfering with nature – often using global warming as an excuse for his plans. His attitude seems to be that he knows much better than God how things should work and so he is going to use his money to pay for the improvements he thinks we need.

Next, Gates is funding the developing of fake meat. This will be very handy when his other projects such as blocking the sunshine destroys traditional farming. The Bill and Melinda Gates Foundation funds the Cornell Alliance for Science which supports the agrichemical industry. All this takes the power from small farmers and gives it to big chemical companies, in my opinion. If Gates's projects damage natural farming then his foundation's investments in laboratory food and artificial breast milk will doubtless prove to be extremely profitable.

Gates, through his Foundation, has also invested in microchipped biomedical, track and trace and payment transaction systems such as cryptocurrencies. He seems to prefer digital payment systems to old fashioned cash and appears to be enthusiastic about ID systems and health passports, which he describes as being good for keeping an eye on people, making sure that they pay their taxes and have their Gates approved vaccinations.

And I think it is fair to say that he is probably rather more enthusiastic about transhumanism than I am.

And then there is the organisation known as ID2020 which is believed by some to show more than modest enthusiasm for mandatory vaccination programmes and mandatory track and tracing programmes. Since 2016, ID 2020 has promoted digital ID. The promoters or partners are Microsoft, the company which made Gates rich and GAVI, the alliance which links drug companies and the Bill and Melinda Gates Foundation – among others. One of the Gates Foundation's aims is, of course, investing in vaccine development and surveillance.

'It's exciting,' they say, 'to imagine a world where safe and secure digital identities are possible, providing everyone with an essential building block to every right and opportunity they deserve.'

If I trusted Bill Gates I might be a trifle more enthusiastic. But I'd rather ask Donald Trump to hold my wallet than ask Bill Gates to hold my identity.

Gates and or his Foundation or Microsoft have also invested in Onfido which is preparing technology to develop a phone app to scan faces so that people can work or travel.

And I doubt if Gates would object to the suggestion that we all have medical certificates vaccinated into our bodies to prove that we have had the covid-19 vaccination.

What else is there?

Well, there is the Pirbright Institute, where they study infectious diseases affecting farm animals. The Pirbright Institute is one of those curious hybrid organisations which is government funded but also a charity and, as you have probably guessed, its major stake holders include the Bill and Melinda Gates Foundation. I was a little surprised to find Gates supporting an institute researching farm animals until I discovered that the Pirbright Institute had taken out a patent on a coronavirus with the European Patent Office. Big companies do that a lot these days and it seems institutes do, too. I wonder why anyone would want a patent on the coronavirus – though, of course, the patent might be useful for a vaccine.

And there is something called CEPI – which is the Coalition for Epidemic Preparedness Innovations. This was launched in Davos in 2017 by the governments of Norway and India, the Wellcome Trust, the World Economic Forum and the Bill and Melinda Gates Foundation. It has been given large chunks of taxpayer money from

Germany, Australia and the UK.

One of CEPI's goals is the development of platforms which can be used for rapid vaccine development against unknown pathogens. One of the board voting members is someone from the vaccine business unit at Takeda Pharmaceutical Company and the scientific advisory committee includes someone from Pfizer, of course. And CEPI and Glaxo Smith Kline have announced a collaboration, which is nice. And CEPI works in partnership with Imperial College, which is where Ferguson works and where work is being done on vaccines. You will remember Ferguson. It was his outrageously wrong prediction which led to the lockdowns and the social distancing and the desperate call for a vaccine to end all our misery. Oh and CEPI also works with GAVI which we will come to in part two of 'Just a Little Prick'. GAVI has announced its enthusiasm for identifying and registering children around the world.

Just how Gates, the world's leading expert on health, keeps up with all these organisations is beyond me. I wouldn't know whether I was at a CEPI meeting or a GAVI meeting or simply in the counting house counting out my money. But I expect our wonderful billionaire has lots of help. And there is always Mrs Gates, of course.

Gates, through his Foundation, has bought support and influence everywhere but he has, in my view, left a trail of damage and concern.

And all that brings us back to the vaccines, of course. No story about Gates would be complete without details of the vaccines – past and future.

I will deal further with Mr and Mrs Gates' obsession with vaccines in the next part of this two part series. It's an obsession which seems to me to be distinctly unhealthy though perhaps not for Bill and Melinda. I don't think it is too healthy for people in developing countries and it is probably not going to be healthy for those of us in developed countries either.

When asked when we would get back to normal after the coronavirus hoax, Gates said 'when almost every person on the planet has been vaccinated against coronavirus'. He has colourfully described the vaccine for covid-19 as the final solution. Inconveniently, many experts say that it may not be possible to make a vaccine. Some point out that making a vaccine often takes many years. And I am not the only doctor to worry that if a vaccine is made very quickly, with inadequate testing, then the global consequences could be absolutely catastrophic. Injecting 7 billion people with an experimental vaccine sounds to me like a potential recipe for a disaster previously unknown on the planet. In his less bombastic moments Gates realises this and has, therefore, insisted that there be indemnification for those making and distributing vaccines. In other words: if the vaccine kills you or destroys your brain then you're on your own. Don't expect any compensation. In the US, manufacturers and distributors have had immunity from February 2020. I'm not sure whether the immunity will cover doctors and nurses so that's something they might like to worry about. Patients should see my video entitled 'Advice for anyone not wanting to be stuffed'. Or read the transcript on this website.

Part Two of this series gets even more extraordinary. And watch it soon just in case it gets removed and mysteriously disappears.

YouTube has announced that it will remove any video deemed to be in contravention of advice being given by the WHO (that must be tricky, given the WHO's ability to change its mind but there you go).

And one of the biggest providers of money for the WHO is, of course, what's its name, oh yes, the Bill and Melinda Gates Foundation.

Still, if that happens you can always read the transcript on my website www.vernoncoleman.com – as long as that remains in place.

NOTE
This is the script of a video which first appeared (very briefly) on You Tube on July 3rd 2020.

Appendix Nine
Just a Little Prick (Part 2)

(This is the script of a video which appeared, albeit briefly, on YouTube on July 3rd 2020.)

Welcome to part two of 'Just a Little Prick', the unauthorised Bill Gates story. Obviously, the term 'little prick' refers to what happens when you have an injection and is naturally in no way meant in a pejorative way. Heaven forbid. If I were to be rude about Mr Gates his subsidised friends at *The Guardian* and the BBC would doubtless need to be revived with smelling salts.

In the first episode of 'Just a Little Prick', I dealt with a few of Mr Gates's connections, aspirations and investments. But I made it clear that he and his wife seem to have one first love: vaccines.

Some people love cats, mountain climbing or horse racing. But Bill and Melinda Gates love vaccines. They yearn to inject everyone and to them vaccines appear to be the eighth wonder of the world. I wouldn't be surprised if they spent their honeymoon watching vaccines being made or watching vaccinations being given to tiny African children. I bet they spend their evenings drooling over vials of vaccines. And at Christmas they probably give each other unusual vaccines they've found.

Unravelling the Bill and Melinda Gates Foundation and its links with the world of vaccines and vaccinations has taken weeks and given me a headache. Thank heavens there isn't yet a vaccine for headaches.

Among the many partnerships and so on which the Bill and Melinda Gates Foundation has developed in recent years there is one with an organisation called GAVI.

Now GAVI is rather odd in that it is a partnership between the Bill and Melinda Gates Foundation, the World Health Organisation (which itself is very well financed by the Bill and Melinda Gates Foundation) and the World Bank and a variety of other bodies.

So, for example, GAVI also has close and loving partnerships with what I think are some of the world's biggest, dirtiest, most disreputable multinational drug companies including GlaxoSmithKline and Pfizer.

Perhaps not surprisingly, the organisation 'Doctors Without Borders' has I think criticised GAVI, alleging that large multinational drug companies working with the Bill and Melinda Gates Foundation put high mark ups on their prices and that GAVI spends oodles of money subsidising large companies. One of GAVI's stated aims seems to be to create a healthy market for vaccines.

You will probably not be surprised to hear that Gates has close links with a number of multinational drug companies but you may, or may not, be surprised to hear that he doesn't seem to me to be terribly fussy about the company he keeps. On the other hand it would I suppose be quite difficult to find a drug company partner that didn't have a reputation that would make Al Capone blush with shame. If you get into bed with a drug company you have to be prepared to wake up in the morning with a bit of scratching and itching and so on.

In a previous video entitled 'Would You Trust These People with Your Life?' I detailed some of the bad things that GSK has done over recent years and I pointed out that if it were a human being GSK would be described as a recidivist. It would probably have regular appointments with a parole officer.

GSK is one of the world's biggest pharmaceutical companies and in my view if it made teaspoons you'd need to be a special sort of person to buy a teaspoon from them.

In 2014, for example, GSK was fined $490 million dollars by China after a Chinese court found it guilty of bribery. The court gave GSK's former head of Chinese operations a suspended prison sentence and they gave suspended prison sentences to other executives too.

Sadly, that misadventure in China wasn't GSK's only little 'Oh dear, whoops, how did that happen?' mistake. Here are some others.

In 2009 in Canada, a five-year-old girl died five days after an H1N1 flu shot and her parents sued GSK for $4.2 million. The parents' lawyer alleged that the drug was brought out quickly and without proper testing as the federal government exerted intense pressure on Canadians to get immunised.

In 2010, GSK paid out $1.14 billion because of claims over a drug called Paxil. And they settled lawsuits over a drug called Avandia for $500 million.

In 2011, GSK paid $250 million to settle 5,500 death and injury claims and set aside $6.4 billion for future lawsuits and settlements in respect of the drug Avandia.

And then there are the accusations of fraud, misbranding and failure to report safety data.

In 2012, GSK pleaded guilty to federal criminal offences including misbranding of two antidepressants and failure to report safety data about a drug for diabetes to the FDA in America. The company admitted to illegally promoting Paxil for the treatment of depression in children and agreed to pay a fine of $3 billion. GSK also reached a related civil settlement with the US Justice Department. The $3 billion fine also included the civil penalties for improper marketing of half a dozen other drugs.

There's more interesting stuff about GSK on my video entitled 'Would you trust these people with your life?'

Oh, and there are a couple of other things you should know about GSK.

First, GSK is one of the top earning vaccine companies in the world. And in 2010, there were reports of narcolepsy occurring in Sweden and Finland among children who had the H1N1 swine flu vaccine. It is reported that not all the safety problems were made public.

In Ireland, the Irish Government kept inviting people to get vaccinated even when it was clear that the pandemic was on the wane and it was nowhere near the catastrophe portrayed by influenza researchers, governments, industry and the media. One member of the Irish parliament, told the Irish Prime Minister. 'The Health Service Executive decided to purchase Pandemrix and continued to distribute it even after they knew it was dangerous and untested.'

It is perhaps worth noting that Professor Neil Ferguson, the Eddie the Eagle of mathematical modelling though perhaps without the innocent and patriotic charm, had predicted that the swine flu could lead to 65,000 deaths in the UK alone. In the end, the swine flu killed 457 people and had a death rate of just 0.026 per cent of those infected. Just another of Ferguson's cock-ups. Cock-ups seem to be a speciality of his in more ways than one.

Second, Sir Patrick Vallance, is the Chief Scientific Adviser in the United Kingdom and, I suspect, a key figure in dealing with the coronavirus in the UK and the plans for a vaccine. Vallance worked for GSK between 2006 and 2018. By the time he left GSK he was a member of the board and the corporate executive team. Fines and so on which I have listed took place while Vallance was working as a senior figure at GSK.

As I say, you can find out lots more exciting stuff about GSK and about Astra Zeneca in my video entitled 'Would You Trust These People With Your Life?' If the video disappears, you can, as always find the transcript on my website www.vernoncoleman.com

Oh, and there's one more thing I nearly forgot to mention. Glaxo Smith Kline was fined £37.6 million for cheating the National Health Service. I wonder what Vallance thought about that.

The Bill and Melinda Gates Foundation also has a relationship with Pfizer and to be honest with you, Pfizer's record isn't anything you would want to boast about. If you worked there you'd keep quiet about it I think and say you worked for the tax people or robbed banks for living.

So, for example, in the UK, Pfizer was fined £84.2 million for overcharging the NHS by 2,600% and in the US Pfizer was hit with a $2.3 billion fine for mis-promoting medicines and paying kickbacks to doctors.

You might think that a foundation wanting to have a clean reputation might avoid relationships with companies like those.

But Bill Gates doesn't seem to mind about all these little peccadillos; the cheating and the deceiving and so on. And in a way why should he? He has a team of PR people willing and able to make sure that his halo is constantly being repaired and polished and I doubt if any of his many press and broadcasting partners will want to damage their financially advantageous relationship by mentioning anything which might caught embarrassment. After all, we must not forget that the Foundation he shares with Melinda, Mrs Gates, seems to me to have investments with bought much of the world's media; doling out fairly huge chunks of cash to no doubt grateful partners. Did I remember to mention that those two sanctimonious organisations the BBC and *The Guardian* are partners with the Gates Foundation?

It cannot be that Gates isn't aware of the problems associated with vaccination because his own foundation has allegedly had its own little peccadilloes to think about. I've described some of those controversies in other videos.

In India there was trouble over a Gates funded vaccine programme. A government investigation claimed the programme, an observational study, violated the human rights of those being injected and failed to report properly adverse effects. That, as we have seen, is not entirely unusual drug company practice. A parliamentary investigation concluded that the Gates funded Program for Appropriate Technology in Health had been engaged in a scheme to help ensure 'healthy markets' for GlaxoSmithKline and Merck (another drug company).

An eminent Indian editor said 'it is shocking to see how an American organisation used surreptitious methods to establish itself in India. Another complaint was that Indians were used as guinea pigs.

In Africa a meningitis vaccine project, funded by Gates, led to reports of up to 500 children allegedly suffering seizures and convulsions and becoming paralysed.

And back in India it was reported that over 490,000 people developed paralysis as a result of the polio vaccine that was given. Remarkably and horrifyingly it was claimed that 80% of polio cases were derived from the vaccine.

There are complaints that the Gates Foundation has taken over public health for the benefit of big drug companies. The links between the Gates Foundation and other organisations and the pharmaceutical giants seem never ending.

Gates has long argued that the world is overpopulated and to help further this end the Gates Foundation is said to have funded Marie Stopes, an organisation, which performs over three million abortions a year and has also worked with a charity called Gynuity which is experimenting with a second trimester abortion trial in Africa.

But it is vaccines which seem to interest Gates most and despite all the known hazards the enthusiastic Gates remains gungho about vaccines. He must know that there are very real dangers with vaccines but curiously it doesn't seem to worry him. I wonder if he really has any idea what he is talking about when he discusses vaccines. There seems to me to be little awareness of the risk-benefit ratio.

For example, I have seen an interview in which he agrees that if 7 billion people are vaccinated against the coronavirus there could be 700,000 people damaged by the virus. There could of course be many deaths but I don't think Mr Gates likes to talk about that scenario.

He says that there could be 700,000 people with side effects and he dismisses this as though he is talking a bit of soreness or a slight rash.

Not necessarily so, Mr Gates. I've been studying and writing about vaccines for 50 years and the side effects from vaccination are often life changing. It is perfectly possible, for example, that there could be 700,000 people with severe brain damage after the first tranche of the vaccination programme has been completed.

I wonder if Gates has any idea what a brain damaged person looks like; how devastating it is not just for them but for their relatives.

And of course the covid-19 disease, the subject of the Gates determination for a global vaccine, has, as I keep reminding everyone, killed far, far less than the ordinary flu can kill in the same sort of time period.

What is all this about? Who is doing what for why and who is profiting and how?

Well, the drug companies are making money. Loads of it. The Bill and Melinda Gates Foundation is getting more control over global healthcare. And Bill and Melinda are becoming ever more powerful and ever more able to pursue whatever other goals and agendas may be dear to them. And wherever they go they are treated like royalty. And Bill Gates himself is said to be richer now than he was a decade ago. Indeed, during the decade of vaccines promoted by Gates, his personal worth is said to have doubled to over $100 billion.

The bottom line, however, is that I can't help suspecting that if Gates hadn't made so much money and hadn't doled so much of it out to buy influence, everyone would laugh at him, ignore him or dismiss him as a nutter. Is there a hidden agenda? How much does Gates' fear about overpopulation influence what he does? And how much does that family interest in eugenics affect the aims of the Gates Foundation. Many rich people do wonderful things with their money – but they do it without trying to change the world and without wanting to alter the way people live.

Although Gates is a university drop out with no more medical degrees than your fridge, he is regarded as a saviour and his views on vaccination are treated as though they had been carved in stone and handed down from on high. What Gates wants is what we get. It seems to me that Gates is ignorant, deluded, arrogant and enormously dangerous. In my view, he is doing, and will do, infinitely more harm than good.

And the other half of this strange joke is that whereas although I am medically trained and have studied vaccines and vaccination for half a century my questioning, cautious view, asking only for more medical or scientific evidence to be produced in support of the claims which are made, is regarded as unacceptable and I am the one libelled, demonised and dismissed as a nutter, targeted by trolls, demonised as too questioning and regarded as too dangerous to be allowed onto Facebook lest I terrify the 'community' with too many truths.

Putting aside my scepticism and doubts about vaccination (and my conviction, after much research, that vaccines are neither as safe nor as effective, as we are assured by their ignorant supporters) I am deeply concerned about the safety of any coronavirus vaccine. I feel that anyone who accepts a coronavirus vaccine as proposed or supported by Bill Gates or his Foundation should perhaps be placed in protective care for their own protection. I pray that no parents will allow their children to be given a vaccine that has been hastily produced. Those who believe in vaccination should demand that any vaccines are thoroughly tested for safety and efficacy – and that all test results be made public.

Still, there is a bright side to all this.

When the inevitable biopic of Gates' life is made I hope they will use my title 'Just a little prick'. It seems so suitable for a man who appears to be dedicated to vaccinating the world.

NOTE
This video was broadcast on July 3rd 2020, though it was taken down so quickly that if you blinked you would have missed it.

Appendix Ten
Free Blood Clots with Every Covid Jab

(This is the script of a video which first appeared on Brand New Tube in June 2021)

In America you can get a free doughnut if you live in the right place and agree to have yourself jabbed with the toxic, experimental brew known as the covid-19 jab.

But there are no free doughnuts available in the UK.

Here all you get if you have a covid-19 jab is a free blood clot.

Free clots with every jab.

They should make honest adverts promoting the blood clots.

A clot for a clot. My kingdom for a clot. They could hire some of those media doctors to explain how wonderful clots can be. A clot in your leg. A clot in your lungs. A clot in your brain. Kill you quick, kill you slow.

Let's bring some honesty into government propaganda.

Could those queues be really full of people wanting to be jabbed? Or maybe they're all out of work actors who've been offered £10 to stand in a queue for three hours. For another fiver they'd hold up signs saying 'jab me, jab me'. For £20 they'd say Fauci and Whitty were human. I don't believe the number jabbed is anywhere near as many as they claim. I don't believe anything the Government, its advisors, the BMA, the BBC or anyone working for the mainstream media has to say.

The problem is that we're living in a world asylum controlled by psychopaths and I hardly know where to start. I don't know about you but I feel quite pleased with myself when I manage to struggle through another day.

I have become very cautious. I tip toe round the garden to avoid falling over and breaking something because I don't want to go to hospital. I back away from barky dogs because I don't want one to bite me requiring a hospital visit. I'm going to buy a second-hand tank so that I can drive around without worrying about being rammed by some idiot whose mask has made him drowsy. Incidentally, I realised the other day that the only time I will ever wear a mask is when the authorities tell me I must not – then we'll know they're necessary.

I'm terrified of needing to go to hospital. A nine hour wait in the casualty department and then, if you're lucky, you get to see a nurse. The doctors have all disappeared and are hiding in Aberystwyth or the Colorado mountains. I don't want to be tested. I'm terrified I'll fall asleep and someone will creep up and jab me behind the arras with the evil poison in a syringe. You probably won't believe this but I've even bought a surgical suture kit so I can sew myself up if I slice myself with the hedge-trimmer or a chain saw. Honest. I've got sutures and thread and lancets for tidying things up. And a nice bottle of antiseptic to splash on the wound. Do it yourself invisible mending. I've got a very nice bottle of malt whisky to use as an anaesthetic and a good bottle of brandy to get me through the post-op hours. You think I'm kidding but I promise you I'm not. Colin Barron's got Lulu and a Whitty wig and I've got a boxful of operating theatre supplies.

The empty headed cretins who believe that we're living through a pandemic are enjoying their days in cloud cuckoo land.

I can't believe how many stupid, gullible people there are around. And how readily they believe the nonsense they are told. They must all have at least one foot firmly planted in the loony bin. There are battalions of bed wetting numpties around who dutifully wear their grubby masks, which they are told to wear to try to hide the Bell's Palsy they'll get from taking a toxic experimental jab. If the rules ever do soften for a while millions will be so terrified they will wear their masks and do the distancing sidestep for eternity because they believe they will live forever if they do. They might as well be immortalised in formalin like one of those hapless animals preserved in the name of what Hirst calls art and the rest of us call pointless.

There are people in the UK who still believe things they're told by government ministers such as Johnson and Hancock when in truth the world's politicians are about as much use a hundredweight of crisp dingle berries. I wouldn't trust Macron to clean my car and I wouldn't trust Biden to blow his own nose even if someone put a hanky in his hand and told him what to do. The people manipulating these sorry quarter wits, the Global Economic Forum, the Gates Foundation and so on are laughing at everyone; they're taking the piss and no one seems to give a damn.

The only people quoted in the media these days are invertebrates such as Dr Dolly Parton and Dr Mrs Queen who, despite knowing nothing at all about anything other than wigs and corgis, are happy to assure us that the covid jabs will do us even more good than spinach. They haven't bothered to consult the information collected by their own governments which show that the jabs have killed thousands and injured hundreds of thousands. I've been writing about iatrogenesis for many decades and there is no drug in history which has been promoted as hard as the covid-19 jab and no drug in history – and vaccines count as drugs – that has killed and injured as many people. I doubt if napalm has killed as many people as the covid jabs.

And then there are complete cretins who want children to be given a deadly, experimental, inadequately tested, vaccine that only has a temporary licence and that doesn't do what the cretins think it does to protect them against a disease they probably won't get and that almost certainly won't kill them if they do get it. I wonder how many know what the word 'experimental' means. For the record it means that no one knows what will happen to the people who take it. That's an experiment. If I throw Matt Hancock off the top of Big Ben I don't know precisely what will happen. Will he die of a brain injury or blood loss? That's the same as the covid-19 jab. The jabs have been given emergency authorisation despite the fact that the covid-19 responsible was officially downgraded and declared no deadlier than the flu.

Establishment figures are falling over themselves and each other to insist that mandatory vaccinations must be brought in. One columnist says that care workers must be jabbed because the ones who won't accept it, don't care enough. 'More than 30% of carers in her borough of Hackney have refused a vaccination that would she says protect them and others from a virus that she claims has laid waste to the planet.' That sentence would win her applause from the BBC. The virus hasn't laid waste to the planet. The figures show it killed no more people than the flu. And the NHS admits that the vaccine won't necessarily stop people getting the virus or spreading it.

Do journalists know the truth, I wonder. Are they too naïve to realise that governments and their advisors know that if you tell a big enough lie no one will recognise it as a lie because no one believes anyone could lie that much and keep a straight face.

Hancock the moron says we should aim for the double jabbed cretins to be able to avoid quarantine. Wonderful. Do journalists not know that Israel says it is facing a new covid-19 outbreak despite having the world's most vaccinated population.

Patrick Henningsen's magnificent '21st Century Wire' website contains an article from the *Wall Street Journal* reporting that 450 US colleges and universities have announced policies mandating that all students be fully vaccinated before the autumn term. The snag, reports the journal is that the mandated vaccinations aren't legal or morally acceptable and violate the basic principles of medical ethics. Go to 21s Century Wire to read the report headed *WSJ: American University Vaccine Mandates Violate Medical Ethics.*

Worse still there are double, double cretins and ignorant psychopaths around who insist that 12-year-old children should be allowed to decide for themselves whether they want to be jabbed. They want children to be jabbed without parental consent. Children who aren't considered old enough to smoke, go into pubs, vote, have sex or watch dirty movies are told they're old enough to decide whether they want to be jabbed with stuff that is entirely experimental and so complex that not one in 100,000 adults understands it and which has, according to government figures, already killed thousands of people around the world and maimed hundreds of thousands more. How long before they start offering kids a new game console if they agree to roll up their sleeves and risk death and disablement? Alternatively, the kids will probably be told they can remain unvaccinated and be ostracised, lonely and laughed at, and will have to live in a damp, dark cellar for six months.

Adults don't have the foggiest what they're being jabbed with but 12-year-olds are mostly illiterate and don't know whether to put their socks on before or after their shoes. And now we want them to decide whether or not to be jabbed.

There is no such thing as informed consent these days. And it is illegal to give this stuff to a human being without their full and informed consent. The vast majority of doctors and nurses who have been jabbing people are criminals who will, when justice is served, find themselves sitting in cells alongside world famous war criminal Tony Blair. It's a crime to give treatment without informed consent. It's a double crime to give treatment which is experimental without obtaining full informed consent. And it's a triple crime to do it to children.

It was, of course, the evil Blair who gave the Brexiteers victory in the UK because every time he opened his mouth everyone knew he was lying about the Common Market. And now he's our greatest champion. The pro-vaxxers ought to lock him up but they're stupid and they think it helps when he opens his mouth and lets his brains dribble out. Every time he says anything promoting vaccines and death rays and mustard gas, another million people decide to say no thank you very much to whatever it is the malignant bastard is selling. Blair has the eyes of the devil, the soul of a psychopath and the principles of a politician. A man who, like Bush and Powell took deceit to new depths.

Excuse my language, by the way but it is acknowledged to be impossible to mention Blair without using at least one expletive. Indeed, most people outside the UK think his first name is 'Thatfuckingtwat' because they're so used to hearing people describe him as 'Thatfuckingtwat Blair'. The odd thing is that if Blair says anything about covid-19, such as that the unvaccinated should stay in lockdown, presumably as a punishment for having working brains, the BBC clears everything to give him airtime. But if 100 independent doctors stand up and have something to say then the BBC ignores them.

Blair provides the mark for evil, of course, but the rest aren't much better.

I hate this damned covid jab.

It is everything that is wrong with medicine. It's deadly, not properly tested and there is a risk that the vaccinated will kill us all. The idiots who've let themselves be jabbed should have a big V tattooed on their foreheads so that we can identify them and keep well away. Or maybe a big I standing for Idiot.

Let me explain how much I hate it.

There is a small fish found in the river Amazon called the candiru, aka the toothpick fish. It's a tiny fish which lives as a parasite in the gills of bigger fish. If you go swimming in the

Amazon and feel the need to urinate and decide to relieve yourself in the river, something bad, really bad can happen. The little candiru will be attracted by the smell and will travel up the stream of urine into your urethra and there it will stick out its little spines and makes its home. The pain is apparently horrific. The flow of urine from the bladder will cease and serious surgery will be required if you are to be saved. This is not a fun thing to happen. It's not something you laugh about later.

Well, I'd rather bathe in a pool full of candiru than have one of the deadly, experimental covid-19 jabs because at least with a tiny fish living inside my urethra I'll get to keep my soul and I'll have a better chance of staying alive.

We have to stop all this and you're the only people who can do it. It's no good me preaching to the converted, and you're the only people I can reach since I'm banned from anything resembling mainstream media.

Send videos and articles off my websites to everyone you know and everyone you don't know. Everyone. It's how we'll win this war. Share the truth with people and they'll be astonished at the extent of the lies they've been told. My websites contain up-to-date figures of the numbers who have been killed or injured by these jabs.

Encourage those who are brave enough to tell the story of how they've been harmed by the vaccine. Encourage them to admit they made a mistake. If you see such videos offer sympathy and support. Their courage will help us enormously.

And remember, people who rely on the mainstream media will have been lied to consistently – especially by the UK's state broadcaster, the Government's propaganda arm, the utterly unscrupulous, ruthless and deadly BBC. There are, remember, no proper journalists working for the BBC – just pseudo-journalists.

Remember too just how confusing everything is.

You can't go to Spain, Guatemala or Texas or the Isle of Wight unless you've been to Cornwall. You can't have you hair cut while getting married unless you've washed behind your ears three times and own a bicycle. If you live north of the equator you can't hug more than three people at once and you must stay indoors between the hours of 9 am and 3 pm on Saturdays unless you're at Ascot and there is an R in the month. You must wear a mask, socks and galoshes while eating and drinking but you can remove your mask to eructate or answer questions at the police station.

It's hardly surprising that people get confused and frightened.

The rules about working from home are just as bad. Office workers and doctors are all working from home, and surgeons will probably soon tell patients to be prepared to perform surgery on their own kitchen table. You download a video on YouTube and a surgeon guides you through the whole procedure. The first cut isn't necessarily the deepest by the way. Matt Hancock, who is allegedly in charge of fibbing in the UK, will probably tell us that firemen can also work from home if they wish. You ring 999 and ask for the fire brigade and one of the firemen asks you to take your fire round to his place. Alternatively, you can download an App and take pictures of the fire and the firemen will watch your home burn to the ground and make comments on what they are seeing.

The world has gone stark raving mad.

My videos on BNT are controlled and suppressed by governments, with increasingly ruthless efficiency. So spread the word far and wide. Be daring and put videos on your Twitter or Facebook. Take a chance.

And if someone you know is being threatened with a vaccination they don't want remember there are four ways to stop this happening.

First, tell the doctor or nurse or busy body involved that you will make an official complaint (something everyone in any bureaucracy is terrified of these days).

Second, tell them that you will send details of their perfidy to the press and all over social media – naming them personally.

Third, tell them that you will sue them personally.

And, fourth, if it's a doctor or a nurse tell them that you will make a formal complaint to their licensing body.

And after all that hand them a loo roll because they'll need it.

NOTE
The text above is the script of a video which appeared on Brand New Tube in June 2021.

Appendix Eleven
Proof the Covid-19 'Vaccine' Programme
Should be Stopped Now

(The text below is the script of a video which appeared on BrandNewTube on 1st June 2021. The entire platform, with all the videos I'd recorded after my channel on YouTube was taken down, disappeared after one of the owners was 'warned' to take down my videos 'or else'.)

I've been warning about the covid-19 jabs for many, many months. My first videos detailing the very real dangers were published last year. In this video I'm going to prove, beyond any question, that the whole experimental jabbing programme should be halted immediately. The lunatics have truly taken over the asylum and they could kill billions with these jabs alone.

But instead of halting the roll out of a vaccine that hasn't been properly tested, doesn't work and isn't needed, the authorities in some countries are already jabbing children and in others are pushing for children to be jabbed. This is total lunacy. Jabbing adults with this toxic brew is madness but at least most adults have a choice. Children are being jabbed with dangerous poison straight out of the witches' cauldron in Macbeth and they don't have the faintest idea what is happening to them. There is absolutely no informed consent and they are being given an experimental vaccine that doesn't do what people believe it does, to protect them from a disease which I have proved, in a previous video, is nothing more than the rebranded flu.

Wicked lies are being spread about giving the experimental jab to children. Attempts are being made to put children under peer pressure to accept, ask for or even demand the covid-19 jab.

Those who are putting children under pressure should know that it is against international law to coerce someone to accept medical treatment. It isn't just unethical and irresponsible – it is illegal.

Young adults are already having jabs they don't need because their mates are having them. Peer pressure.

Michael Caine says the jab doesn't hurt – in my view surely the most patronising remark ever used in a health campaign. The young are being jabbed because it's free and they're told that if they have it they can go to discos and pubs and big events. The brave thing to do is surely to say 'No!'

The evidence – and I'll produce all the evidence that is needed in this video – the evidence proves that any parent who allows their child to be vaccinated against covid-19 should be arrested for child abuse. Any doctor or nurse who jabs a child with one of the experimental covid jabs should be arrested for assault and child abuse and imprisoned for a very long time.

Every teacher pushing the jabs for children, and every doctor or nurse prepared to give them should be asked these simple questions:

Ask if they know that this is what the NHS in the UK says about the covid-19 vaccine: 'We do not yet know whether it will stop you from catching and passing on the virus.' That's in the official booklet they send out. So everyone who says the so-called vaccine will stop you getting covid or stop you passing it on is ignorant or stupid or both.

Ask if they know that the CDC in the US reported early on that the covid-19 vaccines (and I'll use the word vaccines so that those who aren't properly awake will know what I'm talking about – though you should know that the definition of vaccine has had to be changed to accommodate these new toxic substances) caused a huge variety of dangerous side effects. I listed these back in 2020. Indeed, the incidence of death and serious side effects was reported to be over 2.5%. Logically, that means that if you vaccinate 100 people then two and a half of them will die or have notable side effects. Huge numbers stand a real risk of being seriously injured or killed. That puts these jabs into the same sort of category as napalm. If Dr Crippen had been alive he'd have been offering these jabs.

Ask if they know that although the injection is usually given into a shoulder muscle it can, and invariably will, enter the blood stream. If you have a bruise after a jab then that's proof of bleeding. Rubbing the site after this vaccine could, in my view, speed up the rate at which the toxin enters the blood and causes massive problems. Many of those giving the jabs know little or nothing about the substance they're injecting. Some vaccinators undoubtedly put the tip of the needle into a small blood vessel thereby squirting the material directly into the circulatory system. Is it possible that the people suffering the most immediate, dramatic consequences are those in whom this has happened? How many vaccinators check that the needle tip isn't in a blood vessel? How many vaccinators realise that these jabs are like no other they have ever given? I say that as a medical doctor who has been writing about vaccines and vaccination for over half a century.

Ask if they know that Professor Byram Bridle, a professor of viral immunology and most assuredly not an anti-vaxxer, has said that the spike protein from these jabs is a toxin which can spread throughout the body, entering the spleen, liver, bone marrow and ovaries. It is the fact that the spike protein affects the platelets which can cause clotting, bleeding, heart problems and neurological problems.

Ask if they know that breast milk is affected by this toxic jab – and that the antibodies in breast milk can cause bleeding in infants.

Ask if they know that the BBC deliberately refuses to tell its viewers and listeners anything which questions the value of vaccination.

Ask if they know that up until the end of May 2021 these vaccines had been responsible for 4,406 deaths in the US and 1,213 deaths in the UK. Those are official government figures and they are low because less than 1 in 100 adverse events in the US is reported. Many deaths have been ignored or dismissed as coincidental. In the US there had been 1,214 cases of anaphylaxis. Horrifyingly, 14,986 had needed hospitalisation and there had been 34,474 urgent health problems. In the UK there had been 1,213 deaths caused by the vaccines and 859,481 total adverse reactions. With the Astra Zeneca vaccine alone, 192 people had gone blind. Those are all official government figures so the fake fact checkers, bought and paid for in their thousands, can huff and puff all day but the figures won't disappear. The idiot journalists who claim the deaths and serious injuries are coincidental might like to apply that nonsensical judgement to the alleged deaths from covid-19. The truth is that the total killed and injured by these damned jabs will turn out to be far higher than the figures I've given. The figures for Europe and places such as Israel are just as scary. Weekly deaths all around the world have soared as more and more people are injected with this toxic junk. Women everywhere are noticing changes to their monthly cycle. And that's crucial.

Ask if they know that over half of GPs said they would not have the vaccine. In the UK, the Government has admitted that despite putting NHS staff – hospital doctors, nurses, porters and bureaucrats – under pressure at least 20% have refused to be jabbed. I bet the 20% of wise people mainly consists of clinical staff rather than administrators. The GPs who said they wouldn't be jabbed were probably the honest ones. How many pretended they had been jabbed but weren't? The UK Government is now talking about making jabs mandatory for NHS staff but the jabs are experimental and it seems unlikely they'll be able to force that through. More bullying and lying.

Ask if they know that perfectly healthy children are probably no more at risk of dying of covid-19 than they are of being killed by lightning? No previously healthy child under the age of 15 has died of covid-19 in the UK. Most children have hardly any symptoms if they do catch it. Why would you vaccinate – or whatever – against something so irrelevant? It's like giving a toxic potentially lethal jab to stop kids getting ink on their clothes.

Ask if they know that the claims for long covid have been wildly exaggerated? There is little or no evidence showing that it is a real risk – or indeed any more of a risk than the usual post viral fatigue syndrome which commonly follows the flu. Oddly enough the symptoms of so-called long covid are exactly the same as the problems caused by the jabs. But we're not allowed to mention that.

Ask if they know that the UK acquired herd immunity in April 2021.

Ask if they know that even if they get it, children don't transmit covid-19 as readily as adults.

Ask if they know that teachers are less at risk of covid-19 than other working age adults.

Ask if they know that the latest figures from the MHRA in the UK show that in the UK the side effects involved include serious neurological problems, heart attacks, strokes, blindness and many other serious disorders. I think it is an insult to the patients who have been damaged to describe their side effects as mild. All this is particularly relevant when you remember that covid-19 has a mortality rate which is much the same as that for the ordinary flu.

Ask if they know that the WHO has said early on that the

vaccines don't stop people getting covid-19 or passing it on.

Ask if they know that in my view at least no one who has been jabbed should be allowed to give blood for transfusion. In my professional view, the blood transfusion stock has already been contaminated.

Ask if they know that no one knows whether the covid-19 jab will interact dangerously with the many other vaccinations given to children.

Ask if they know that there has been no testing to find out if the covid-19 might interact dangerously with other prescription drugs such as Ritalin or anti-asthma medications. Or, indeed, the other hundreds of prescription and over the counter drug.

Ask if they know that at least 66 fully tested and approved vaccines have been withdrawn and discontinued in the US for safety reasons. And those were ordinary vaccines – not experimental jabs.

Ask if they know that governments around the world have paid out billions of dollars in compensation to patients who have been severely injured by vaccines – or to the relatives of patients who have been killed by them. You don't do that if vaccines are safe.

Ask if they know that a vaccine recommended during the alleged swine flu pandemic, – given to us by Ferguson who gave us the fake covid pandemic – resulted in over 1,000 cases of narcolepsy before being withdrawn.

Ask if they know that another drug given to children before full trial results were available was associated with the deaths of 19 children because of possible antibody dependent enhancement. The vaccine was withdrawn. Could this happen with the covid-19 jabs? Your guess is as good as anyone else's. Your goldfish's guess is as good as Hancock's in the UK.

Ask if they know that many people are catching covid-19 after being jabbed.

Ask if they know that in October 2020, Kate Bingham, the head of the UK Government Vaccine Task force was reported as saying: 'There is going to be no vaccination of people under 18'. And that was before all the evidence became available showing the potential dangers of the vaccines.

Ask if they know that the Pfizer vaccine has been linked to altered menstrual cycles and abnormal bleeding in women and to myocarditis in males – both in Israel where the jabs have been given to young people. I see, by the way, that according to the BBC a new Pfizer research centre for vaccines has opened in Bristol. The disgraceful Hancock opened it and the BBC refers to it as a centre of excellence for studying vaccine preventable disease. They should have called it a death camp. Pfizer is one of the most evil companies in the entire universe and paid out one of the biggest fines in history. They were fined $2.3 billion for mis-promoting a medicine and paying kickbacks to doctors. What rancid, rabid people they are. Pfizer was also fined £84.2 million for overcharging the NHS by 2,600%. Easy to do if you're a lying, cheating, thieving crook I suppose.

No informed consent, no long-term testing. Just huge profits and massive salaries for the bosses.

Why would anyone have anything made by Pfizer injected into their body?

Ask if they know that former health secretary Jeremy Hunt is alleged to have said that the Government should look into offering covid vaccines to children because children can spread the disease to older people. The jabs don't stop people spreading covid.

Ask if they know that the BBC claims that if children are jabbed then adults with whom they come into contact will be protected. But, again, that's utter rubbish because even the NHS admits that the jabs don't stop anyone getting covid-19 or passing it on. The BBC is the most disreputable media organisation in history – desperate to keep their licence fee they will do and say anything to keep the Government happy. Like other journalists guilty of sharing an undiluted diet of lies deceits and blatant misinformation the people working for the BBC already have blood on their hands. Are journalists stupid or ignorant or are they just lying? Either way it's unforgiveable.

Ask if they know that the technology used in some of these vaccines, mRNA technology, has never been properly approved for humans. And as I have said many times it is still experimental. That means that anyone who has the jab is taking part in a dangerous experiment.

Ask if they know that children still have developing immunological and neurological systems and are even more vulnerable than adults. Could fertility be damaged? Could auto immune disease develop? One scientific paper has suggested that the vaccines might trigger neurodegenerative disease.

Ask if they know that the Government is analysing waste water to find the coronavirus as a way of tracking the infection. They say that genetic fragments of the virus can be detected in sewage. So it's a safe bet that the damned experimental vaccine will be in the sewage too and if it's in the sewage it will be in the drinking water. Take a look at my video about vaccines in drinking water.

Ask if they know that the warning about shedding which came from Dr Bossche, and which I shared in my video entitled 'Covid-19 Vaccines are Weapons of Mass Destruction and Could Wipe Out the Human Race', is now very likely to be accurate – those who sneered were wrong.

Ask if they know that the drug companies making these vaccines, including Pfizer, Astra Zeneca and so on, have been fined billions of dollars for fraudulent activities. Why would anyone trust anything these companies say? Companies making bombs and land mines have probably killed fewer people than these monsters. Every drug company employee should have a warning sign tattooed on his or her forehead. And yet seemingly sane people are putting their lives and their children's lives into the hands of these inhuman monsters. It's like hiring the McCanns to babysit your toddler. Why don't people think for themselves? At least half the population would chain their ankles together if someone in a suit told them to do so.

Ask if they know that GPs who are enthusiastically promoting the jabs could make £50,000 a year each from jabbing their patients – or telling their staff to do it.

Ask if they know that media organisations promoting the jabs are receiving huge amounts of money from the Government and that many, such as the BBC and *The Guardian* have financial links with the Bill and Melinda Gates Foundation which is making millions out of vaccines. The BBC actually boasts that it deliberately hides information from viewers and listeners and, as a matter of some insane and indefensible policy, deliberately suppresses the truth about vaccines. The BBC really must go.

Ask if they know that it is an offence to give a drug – including a vaccine –without the patient giving their informed consent. But in my view 99.999% of the individuals who have been jabbed were not given the information required to give informed consent. So all those giving the jabs are criminals.

Ask if they know that in December 2020, a petition filed with the European Medicines Agency suggested that there is plausible evidence to suggest that the spike proteins in the MRNA vaccines could trigger an immune reaction against syncytin-1, a protein which is responsible for the development of a placenta in mammals and humans. How will this affect young girls? Your local grocery store clerk can give you as good an answer to that as your doctor. No one knows.

Ask if they know that according to the journal *Nature*, for every 1,000 people under the age of 50 who are infected with the coronavirus, almost none will die. Indeed, the risk of a young person dying of covid-19 is not very different to the risk of their being struck by lightning. I assume that doctors and nurses do not recommend that children carry lighting rods around with them.

Ask if they know that the covid-19 jabs were only given emergency licences because there was thought to be a global pandemic. But the Government in the UK knew in March 2020 that the coronavirus was no more of a threat than the flu. The proof is on my websites. These jabs are experimental and the experiment does not conclude until 2023. Actually, it won't even stop then because these jabs are entirely new and no one knows what will happen in ten, twenty or more years' time. The development of type 1 diabetes after vaccination can take three or four years.

Ask if they know that there are plans to give everyone jabs several times a year. That will include children.

Ask if they know that there are side effects with all vaccines. At least one media doctor claims that the side effects of vaccines present themselves early rather than later. That's not true. Side effects can develop long after a vaccination was given and this is why when vaccines are first introduced it is usual to test them for several years.

Ask if they know that there are serious medium and long term dangers with these jabs. Despite the reassurance being given by celebrities and media doctors it is possible that many, many patients will die or fall seriously ill when they come into contact with what is called the 'wild' coronavirus.

All that relates to the covid-19 jabs but the attention given to the covid-19 jab has highlighted the lack of evidence showing that vaccines given to children are safe and effective.

In June 2020 the BMJ published a paper headed *Routine Vaccination during covid-19 pandemic response.* The authors reported that 'During the 11 week period following the emergency declaration there were fewer deaths in US children compared to 2019. The difference is 'statistically highly significant.' The most pronounced mortality decline occurred in infants under one year of age. The authors suggest that the question of vaccination (as a link to infant death) needs investigation and conclude: 'More study is required and, in time, perhaps changes in the immunization schedule.'

That won't happen, of course. The maniacal pro-vaxxers and truth deniers hate science, facts and truth and will happily see thousands of children slaughtered so that their beloved drug companies can make oodles of money.

Meanwhile, the *British Medical Journal*, having published a paper questioning the value of vaccination will now, presumably, be placed on the anti-vaxxer list of proscribed organisations and individuals.

In 2017, the Danish government and a Danish vaccine maker, funded a study of the DTP vaccine. Gates and his pet WHO claim that the DTP vaccine saves millions of lives but the truth seems to be very different. After looking at 30 years of data the scientists concluded that the DTP vaccine was probably killing more children than died from diphtheria, pertussis and tetanus prior to the vaccines introduction. The vaccine had ruined the immune systems of children rendering them susceptible to death from pneumonia, leukaemia, bilharzia, malaria and dysentery. None of those diseases is officially recognised as vaccine injuries.

So, the Danish government should also be included on the Anti-vaxxer list – and banned by fascist organisations such as the BBC, Facebook, YouTube, Twitter and so on.

We all have to share this information.

You have to share this video or the transcript with teachers, doctors, nurses, journalists and parents.

Print out copies of the transcript and hand them to everyone you see. Everything I've told you is absolutely true. Any anonymous critic who says it isn't, or who presses the thumbs down button is a liar or a shill or a drug company hack or all three.

Please help share this vital information before it's too late.

NOTE
The text above is the script of a video which appeared on
BrandNewTube on 1st June 2021. Many of my videos appeared on
BrandNewTube which was, sadly, taken down and removed entirely.

Appendix Twelve
Looking After Yourself

In order to survive in the New World (which won't have much in the way of doctors or hospitals) you need a well-equipped medical cabinet box in your home. Don't keep it in the bathroom, by the way. Bathrooms tend to be damp and the worst place in the world to keep medicines. If you have a medicine cabinet or box then I suggest you keep it in a bedroom. If there are small children around it might be wise to arrange to keep your medicines in a lockable box.

Please note that I consider that acquiring a supply of antibiotics and an Epipen are the two most important things you can do to save your life or the life of a loved one.

Everyone in the world should have an Epipen – it's the effective way to deal with a huge allergy reaction or anaphylactic shock. It's the easiest way to save a life. (I don't get any kickbacks, by the way. I have no idea who makes the Epipen and I don't care. It works.)

It's especially important to have an Epipen if you travel, if you live more than five minutes away from medical help or if you live in a country with inadequate health care (such as the UK). If you have an anaphylactic shock reaction an Epipen can save your life.

Our GP refused to prescribe an Epipen (even though I've had an anaphylactic shock before – and I can promise you it isn't fun) so I bought one online. It cost a biscuit short of £90 – nearly half of one week's old aged pension in the UK but worthwhile.

The Epipen contains adrenaline and is quite easy to use. You must read the instructions carefully but, basically, if you see someone having an anaphylactic shock reaction you take the top off the pen and jab the needle part of the pen (which isn't a pen at all) into the patient's thigh. You just follow the instructions printed on the side of the pen. You can do this to yourself, of course. You can tell by looking at the pen if it has deteriorated and needs replacing. I am so convinced that the Epipen is the one piece of equipment that can most easily be used to save a life that I am rarely more than a few feet away from mine. I keep it in my study and if I leave the house I have one in my shoulder bag (which contains a plentiful supply of notebooks, a collection of pens and pencils and half a dozen books to read if it looks remotely possible that while out of the house I might have to spend two minutes standing in a queue).

Antibiotics are also essential. Sepsis is an increasingly common cause of death and governments recommend that anyone exhibiting signs or symptoms of sepsis should be given antibiotics within one hour. In countries where there is no reliable health care (such as isolated desert islands and the UK) this is unlikely to happen. (GPs are reluctant to prescribe antibiotics for the reasons explained in this book, and patients attending hospital in an emergency may have to wait days to be seen by anyone more qualified than an admissions clerk.)

Serious infections need to be treated quickly – usually within an hour or two of symptoms developing. It is the failure to treat infections speedily which may be one of the reasons why the incidence of sepsis has reached epidemic proportions. Sadly, many infections which could be treated effectively are not treated quickly enough and patients die unnecessary. GPs (whose working hours are similar to those of part time librarians) now refuse to see patients at home either at night, at weekends or even during the working day. Many doctors refuse to see patients face to face insisting on providing half-hearted and totally inadequate advice after a telephone or internet consultation. (It has been shown that patients who are 'treated' this way are more likely to die.) Patients who are lucky enough to obtain a face to face appointment with a GP often have to wait several weeks to be seen – even in an emergency. (I wish I was joking but I am not).

Of course, the real reason for not prescribing life-saving antibiotics is that restricting drug availability is part of the depopulation plan. The bottom line is that we all need to have access to antibiotics without needing a prescription. Unfortunately, in most countries antibiotics are only available on prescription and doctors refuse to prescribe them appropriately. However, there are solutions. A bloke I met in a pub told me that he had obtained a supply of antibiotics for possible emergency use for himself or a member of his family by visiting a reputable online medical service which provided antibiotics for travellers. He told me, seemingly without shame, that he had filled in an online form saying that he would be travelling abroad and would need a supply of medicines to help deal with any emergency health problems. The medicines supplied included a well-known broad spectrum antibiotic. Another man I met in a pub told me that he had obtained antibiotics for emergency use by telling an online doctor that he had a serious tooth infection when this was not true. These methods of obtaining antibiotics do involve some mild deceit, of course, and I would not dream of using either of these tricks. I'd rather die of septicaemia than obtain antibiotics in an improper manner. I feel sure that you too, dear reader, will feel the same way. But I mention these techniques merely as theoretical examples of what is happening in the world. (It is important, of course, to be careful when obtaining antibiotics or any other drugs online. There are many unscrupulous people around who will sell you fake drugs. Buy only from a registered and properly licensed source.)

In olden days travellers used to consider it wise to take a supply of essential medicines with them when travelling abroad to what were known as Third World Countries. These days, people travelling to places such as Britain need to take a supply of essential medicines with them. In the distant past a number of charities collected up unwanted drugs and sent them off to less fortunate countries where the local citizenry were deprived of decent health care. We can only hope that before long an enterprising charity collects up antibiotics in Africa and sends them to the deprived citizens of the United Kingdom, the United States, Canada or the European Union.

And remember: keep well clear of any health care workers who are wearing their work clothing outside their place of employment. There is clear evidence that antibiotic resistant organisms are being carried out of hospitals on the clothing of staff members. It would make sense for the authorities to arrest (for attempted murder) any hospital or clinic staff who go shopping or catch public transport while wearing the clothes they wear at work.

If you need a good first aid book (which you do) then I recommend *The Ship Captain's Medical Guide* which is published by the Maritime and Coastguard Agency in the UK and made available through The Stationery Office in the UK. It is the only really useful publication any government has ever produced and is intended primary for use on vessels where there is no medical professional on board. It provides assistance and directions for crew members if it becomes necessary for them to assess and treat an illness or accident. Despite the fact that it carries the name of a drug company I also recommend *the Merck Manual of Home Health Handbook* which is probably the most comprehensive medical textbook available to the public. (It has well over 2,000 pages and if you drop it on a foot you'll need to look up foot trauma in one or both books.)

I cannot stress too firmly that there will soon be no health care. The medical establishment has already decided that people must be left to die because of the (mythical) threat posed by global warming. It is, therefore, necessary for you to know how to look after yourself and those close to you.

Put together a collection of the medicines you think you might need. And a supply of bandages and dressings is essential too.

Printed in Great Britain
by Amazon

62579350R00191